NEGOTIATING PARENT-ADOLESCENT CONFLICT

THE GUILFORD FAMILY THERAPY SERIES
Alan S. Gurman, *Editor*

Negotiating Parent-Adolescent Conflict
A Behavioral-Family Systems Approach

Arthur L. Robin, PhD
Children's Hospital of Michigan and
Wayne State University School of Medicine

Sharon L. Foster, PhD
West Virginia University

Foreword by K. Daniel O'Leary

The Guilford Press
New York   London

© 1989 The Guilford Press
A Division of Guilford Publications, Inc.
72 Spring Street, New York, NY 10012

All rights reserved

No part of this book may be reproduced, stored in a retrieval system,
or transmitted, in any form or by any means, electronic, mechanical,
photocopying, microfilming, recording, or otherwise, without written
permission from the Publisher.

Printed in the United States of America

Last digit is print number: 9 8 7 6 5 4 3

Library of Congress Cataloging-in-Publication Data

Robin, Arthur L.
    Negotiating parent–adolescent conflict: a behavioral family systems approach /
Arthur L. Robin and Sharon L. Foster.
    p. cm. — (The Guilford family therapy series)
Bibliography: p.
Includes index.
ISBN 0-89862-072-4
1. Adolescent psychotherapy. 2. Family psychotherapy.
I. Foster, Sharon L. II. Title. III. Series.
[DNLM: 1. Adolescent Psychology. 2. Behavior Therapy—in
adolescence. 3. Family Therapy—in adolescence.   WS 463 R655n]
RJ503.R63 1989
616.89'022—dc19
DNLM/DLC
for Library of Congress   87-31502
CIP

To Ruth—A. R.

To Tom—S. F.

And to the families who have helped us—A. R. and S. F.

Foreword

Conflicts between adolescents and their parents are natural and expected. We have not been prepared for the extent of this conflict, however, as judged by the increase in the number of "run aways." Robin and Foster have been working with adolescents since they have been in graduate school, a decade or more ago. They combine a wealth of information in both research and clinical areas. Much of this information is conveyed in this book, *Negotiating Parent–Adolescent Conflict: A Behavioral–Family Systems Approach*. Robin and Foster have adopted an integration of cognitive–behavioral and family systems approaches. Central to their model are concepts such as family structure, belief systems, problem solving abilities, and communication patterns. These concepts are of special interest to me for as the former advisor of both Robin and Foster, I have seen a change in two individuals who had a full appreciation for an operant behavioral approach before they came to Stony Brook, and they received further training therein at Stony Brook from Professor Howard Rachlin. Their inclusion of concepts such as enmeshment, disengagement, and power along with the traditional cognitive-behavioral concepts is welcome. True to their backgrounds, they have an empirical focus that is used to evaluate the heuristic value of the concepts in their model and the effects of therapeutic approaches with adolescents. The authors provide sufficient detail that a practitioner can learn how to conduct interviews, decide what assessment measure to use, and learn how to integrate the objective and subjective components of the assessment. The tour de force of the book is contained in the chapters on problem solving training and functional interventions. Finally, the authors provide suggestions on dealing with resistance.

This book is a gem! It is loaded with useful information both for clinicians and researchers. Adolescents are a tough lot. They certainly have the capability of refusing to do things their parents request, and the carrot-and-stick methods only go so far with adolescents—and they often backfire. There is a fine line between producing change because all parties involved see the change as beneficial and producing change that only the parent or the adolescent sees as desirable. This book goes a long way in helping professionals help parents *and* adolescents negotiate adolescence and make changes that are seen as desirable by all.

K. Daniel O'Leary, PhD
State University of New York at Stony Brook

Acknowledgments

Many individuals over the years contributed to the work that underlies this volume. Dan O'Leary supported our initial investigations in this area when we were graduate students, nurturing our interest and sharing his farsighted vision of the need for new assessment and treatment procedures for parents and teenagers in distress. Ron Prinz participated in these early endeavors, both in conducting therapy and in developing the assessment battery on which we still rely. He also graciously allowed us to reproduce many of his measures in this volume. Ron Kent lent his methodological expertise to the design of our early studies. And in the years that followed, our graduate students and colleagues continued to stimulate our interest and contribute to further methodological and theoretical refinements of our work.

Numerous others assisted in seeing this volume to fruition. Seymour Weingarten offered his encouragement throughout the writing process, prompting us when writing bogged down. The Department of Pediatrics at Wayne State University School of Medicine and the Department of Psychology at West Virginia University provided secretarial and technical support in preparing numerous drafts of the manuscript. Alan Gurman, Seymour Weingarten, and Russ Barkley read and provided comments and suggestions on earlier drafts of our work. Pearl Weisinger supplied valuable editorial feedback, and she and the rest of the Guilford production staff turned the volume from our original manuscript to the bound book you hold in your hands.

Finally, no endeavor of this sort would be possible without the unflagging support of our spouses, Ruth Robin (A. R.) and Tom Barton (S. F.). Despite busy careers of their own, both were patient and flexible over the many hours, days, evenings, and weekends it took to transform this volume from dream into reality.

Contents

NEGOTIATING PARENT-ADOLESCENT CONFLICT

CHAPTER ONE

Introduction

Relations were deteriorating between Mr. and Mrs. Smith and their 14-year-old daughter Sally. Sally had begun to talk back, disobey rules, spend time with undesirable friends, act moody, and display an inordinate amount of interest in boys. The family was embroiled in a seemingly endless series of arguments, mostly about petty issues but with a cumulative negative effect on members' perceptions of their relationships with each other. Mr. Smith reacted with impulsive flashes of anger to Sally's rebellious behavior, while Mrs. Smith counseled reason and calm. Two spouses who previously thought they had a good marriage were often finding themselves at odds over how much freedom to give Sally and how to discipline her. When Mrs. Smith eavesdropped on Sally's telephone conversation with her friend Barbara, she heard Barbara telling Sally about how the girls smoked marijuana, went to all-night parties, and shoplifted cosmetics from a local store. A bitter argument ensued when Mr. and Mrs. Smith confronted their daughter concerning her choice of friends. At the suggestion of a neighbor, the Smiths contacted the parent–adolescent communication clinic, which offered free treatment to families willing to participate in clinical research. During the Smiths' initial visit to the clinic, the clinician requested that they discuss and attempt to resolve for 10 minutes the issue of who should be Sally's friends. The following is an excerpt from their conversation:

MR. SMITH: Well, I guess I'll begin. I think, Sally, that I'd like you to stop seeing friends that I think are bad kids.

(10 seconds of silence)

MRS. SMITH: Do you have anything to say about that?

SALLY: Yes, they're not bad kids. And I ain't stopping being friends with them because you want me to. They're trying to straighten out and they want me to help.

MRS. SMITH: Well, the only time you see them is at school. . . .

SALLY: *(Interrupting)* They still want me to help.

MRS. SMITH: Well, Sally, I'd like you to have them come over to our house so I could see what they're like before you go out with them after school.

SALLY: Well, he's the one that thinks they're bad kids. He's the one. . . .

MRS. SMITH: *(Interrupting)* Well, I'm not particularly happy with them either. . . .

MR. SMITH: *(Interrupting)* I think Mom might think they're bad kids too.

MRS. SMITH: No, you're wrong. I don't think they're bad. I think that they have serious problems—didn't they tell you they smoke pot and shoplift?

SALLY: That was rotten, listening to me on the phone. I was going to tell you anyway.

MR. SMITH: I think Mom was doing what was best for you, Sally. We only want what's best for you.

SALLY: Mom, they think that you're real good-looking and all that stuff. They think good things about you and you think bad things about them.

MRS. SMITH: That's because we've heard bad things about them. What bad things have they heard about Dad?

SALLY: No bad things except he is going through his second childhood.

MR. SMITH: Well, Mom thinks I'm going through my second childhood too.

SALLY: You are.

MRS. SMITH: *(Jokingly to Sally)* He's growing out of it.

SALLY: Thank God.

MRS. SMITH: But from the things you've told us about your friends. . . .

SALLY: *(Interrupting)* But I told you they are trying to straighten out.

MR. SMITH: Sally, I think helping friends is great, but I think these girls may help you in bad ways. You just have to get new friends. . . .

SALLY: *(Interrupting)* No way. Forget it. . . .

MR. SMITH: *(Interrupting)* I'd like to finish. . . .

SALLY: *(Interrupting)* No way. No. You can't. I've been friends with them for 4 years. You think they would be able to get me into that stuff?

MR. SMITH: That's a good point. But they are changing and so are you. I just want you to grow up right. This is a critical time in your life. You just can't risk these things.

MRS. SMITH: Your Dad is right. . . .

SALLY: *(Interrupting)* You don't understand what I'm saying. Barbara's parents don't stop her from seeing her friends. It's not fair.

MRS. SMITH: *(Interrupting)* We do understand. Barbara's parents don't care about her. We care. . . .

SALLY: *(Interrupting)* If you understand, then why do you want me to stop seeing my friends? You really don't care. You just don't want to be embarrassed.

Such family situations pose a serious challenge for the behaviorally oriented clinician. How are we to understand, assess, and treat conflict between young adolescents and their parents? Should we view Sally's behavior as a response to her parents' poor child-management skills and invoke the paradigm of parent training in contingency management? Should we see Sally's behavior as a reflection of unresolved marital conflict between her parents and proceed to intervene with a family systems approach? Or should we conceptualize Sally's behavior in terms of deficits in self-control, assertiveness, and/or social skills and intervene with an individual cognitive–behavioral approach designed to remediate these deficiencies? Conceptualization of family problems will clearly influence our choice of assessment and treatment strategies.

This volume outlines a behavioral–family systems model of parent–adolescent conflict, an assessment methodology, and a treatment program. It is an integrationist approach that blends cognitive–behavioral and family systems theories with developmental considerations concerning adolescence. An analysis of the interchange between Sally and her parents highlights some of the critical components of this theory, assessment, and treatment program.

Sally and her parents argued over a specific issue—her friends. She wants to spend more time with her friends, but her parents fear the friends' negative influence over their daughter. Choice of friends is one of many issues, often petty, about which the family squabbles. These issues reflect the general theme of Sally's growing independence from the family. A previously harmonious family is now undergoing a transition as their daughter becomes more independent. Previously stable interaction patterns no longer produce mutually satisfactory relationship outcomes for the Smiths; normal family functioning has been disrupted. The therapist therefore needs tools to assess and treat specific disputes as examples of more general independence-related conflicts.

The Smiths' difficulties illustrate the underlying concept of the family as a homeostatic system undergoing stress and change because of the normal maturation of children into adolescents and young adults. From an organizational framework, Sally's role within the family is changing. She is no longer a little girl, yet she is not a responsible adult. Her parents need to grant her more rights and responsibilities, but it is difficult to know how to sequence and structure this process. As Sally approaches adulthood, she will assume more control and decision-making power within the family hierarchy. Treatment will help smooth out this transition, which is particularly problematic for the Smiths.

Let's look more closely at how the Smiths have chosen to deal with the disruption produced by their daughter's independence-seeking behavior. To do this, we examine their communication around the "friends" issue. Mr. Smith began the discussion with an authoritarian command for Sally to stop seeing her friends, calling her friends "bad kids." Sally rebutted. The accusatory, commanding tone of the parents' remarks continued throughout the interchange, evoking complementary defensive remarks from Sally. The family was unable to specify the problem in clear-cut, nonaccusatory terms and point the discussion in a productive, solution-oriented direction. Because of this difficulty, issues such as friends remain unresolved, periodically reemerging to provoke bursts of anger and hostility. In short, Sally and her parents exhibited deficits in positive problem-solving communication skills. Until their skills improve or some external event changes their situation drastically, their conflicts will continue.

During their conversation, the Smiths gave some indication of what they think about each other and the process of adolescent independence seeking. Mr.

and Mrs. Smith appear to believe that their daughter is incapable of making wise decisions concerning her friends, that the consequences of permitting her to continue to spend time with marijuana-smoking, partying, shoplifting friends would be ruinous, and that their close supervision of her behavior reflects their basic love for her. Sally appears to think that her parents' restrictive rules are a sign they don't care about her, that they should permit her to do whatever she pleases with her friends, and that she is capable of making wise, responsible decisions without her parents' guidance. Each member's position is characterized by absolutes and by unreasonable assumptions and attributions. Statements reflecting their distorted cognitions impede their discussion and elicit negative emotional responses.

There is another subtle dimension to the interaction. Sally's independence seeking also sets the stage for heightened tension between Mr. and Mrs. Smith. During the discussion, Mr. Smith voiced strict prohibitions regarding Sally's friends. When Sally disagreed with her father, her mother cautiously mediated the dispute ("Well, Sally, I'd like you to have them come over to our house"). Sally sided with her mother against her father ("Well, he's the one that thinks they're bad kids"), a coalition that Mrs. Smith accepted ("No, you're wrong. I don't think they're bad"). With her comments about how her friends complimented her mother, Sally tried to elicit a more sympathetic reaction from her mother, cementing the coalition. Together, mother and daughter discussed Mr. Smith's "second childhood" in a denigrating manner. Mother and daughter were consistently taking sides against father in what we call a "cross-generational coalition." Mr. Smith accepted their put-down but tried to reestablish a coalition with his wife ("Well, Mom thinks I'm going through my second childhood too"). When Mrs. Smith signaled that a limit had been reached ("He's growing out of it"), the negative remarks directed at her husband ceased. Then, Mr. Smith again stepped in as the "heavy" ("Sally, I think helping friends is great, but . . ."), eliciting a hostile, defiant response from Sally. Mrs. Smith backed her husband up ("Your Dad is right") but soon began to soften his assault ("We do understand. . . ."). Mr. and Mrs. Smith were now working as a team, taking sides against Sally, in what we call a "within-generational coalition."

This illustrates a repetitive sequence of triadic interaction where Sally's independence seeking involves her in a parental dispute: (1) father attempts to exercise control over Sally; (2) Sally defies her dad, and his tactic fails; (3) mother mediates the dispute; (4) mother and daughter align, putting father in his place; (5) mother sets the limits on putting father in his place; (6) father recovers and again attempts to exercise authority over Sally, restarting the cycle. Each person plays a crucial role in the cycle, and their behavior is interdependent.

What is the payoff for each person's behavior in this cycle? What functions do their behaviors serve? Without further information we cannot answer these questions definitively. However, we postulate that behavior in such cycles always serves potentially specifiable functions. Speculating here, Sally may be trying to see which of her parents will be more sympathetic to her position.

Gaining her mother's sympathy and attempting to denigrate her father may increase the probability that she will ultimately be able to spend time with her friends. Mr. and Mrs. Smith also disagree about effective and appropriate parenting strategies. Mrs. Smith may use the failure of her husband's authoritarian tactics to build a coalition with her daughter, thus demonstrating the superiority of her calm, rational approach. Backing off when authority is required may serve to maintain a close relationship with her daughter.

Viewing the Smiths' conflict purely in terms of skill deficits and cognitive distortions, we would miss this sequence of interactive behavior (Barton & Alexander, 1981). An understanding of family structure and the functional characteristics of family interaction sequences is crucial to effective use of skill-training interventions. Blending selected strategic–structural family therapy concepts (such as triangulation, coalitions, and cohesion) with behavioral constructs not only supplements our model of parent–adolescent conflict but also broadens the descriptive and analytic skills needed for in-depth treatment planning.

Thus, we see the Smiths' conflict as resulting from poor communication and problem-solving skills, augmented by unreasonable beliefs and problems in family structure. Each family member's behavior serves a function for him/her; interlocking functions perpetuate the family's nonproductive cycles. How can a therapist help to break these patterns and establish more productive processes in their place?

The form of treatment outlined in this volume has its foundations in behavioral and cognitive–behavioral approaches developed for a variety of specific problems over the past two decades. What might a "typical" treatment program for the Smith family look like? The therapist might begin by teaching Sally and her parents steps of verbal problem-solving to resolve specific disputes. Over successive sessions the family might apply these steps to a variety of conflictual issues. As they emit put-downs, accusations, interruptions, or any other negative communication habits, the therapist might stop the discussion, give feedback concerning the negative response, and help the family emit more positive communication behaviors. To change the absolutistic, unreasonable beliefs of the family, the therapist might introduce cognitive restructuring, which combines rational–emotive (Ellis & Grieger, 1977) and cognitive therapy techniques (Beck, Rush, Shaw, & Emery, 1979) for challenging the logical premises of unreasonable beliefs or conducting experiments designed to disconfirm them.

During this process, the therapist also gauges the family's reactions to the introduction of skill training and cognitive change techniques. Taking a behavioral–family systems integrationist stance, the therapist looks for reciprocal parent–adolescent influence processes such as the sequence of interaction outlined earlier. When such a sequence becomes clear-cut, the therapist can plan goals and strategies to change it. For example, if the therapist decided to change the triadic interaction in the Smith family so that mother and father reached agreement on discipline before approaching Sally, the parents might be required to conduct their own problem-solving discussion before discussing a problem with their daughter. Occasionally, a behavioral–family systems analysis may lead the therapist to conduct marital therapy concurrently with, prior to, or following family therapy.

This is a book about helping families such as the Smiths. It represents our attempt to provide a comprehensive framework for conceptualizing, assessing, and treating parent–adolescent conflict based upon a social-learning, behavioral–family systems integration. It is the product of almost a decade of research and clinical practice with parents and adolescents in conflict. It represents a continually evolving attempt to refine our theories, assessment methods, and treatment procedures to be specific and flexible enough to be useful with individual families, yet broad enough to be generalizable across many families.

This book is about clinical work with families. It also deals with research strategies and empirical evaluation of the tenets we propose. In the development of our work, research and practice nurtured each other. By integrating research data with clinical procedure, we hope to emphasize our strong adherence to empiricism, which grew from our roots in behavior therapy.

Thus, this book is designed for the practitioner and the researcher, as well as the advanced graduate student or resident in psychology, psychiatry, or social work. Most of all, it is geared toward the scientist–practitioner, regardless of his/her academic discipline.

The chapters focus on three general topics related to parent–adolescent conflict: theory, assessment, and treatment. Within each area, some chapters and chapter sections are more practical and clinical in focus, while others examine existing research in more detail, highlighting conceptual and methodological issues. Readers interested in studying clinical aspects of the theoretical framework and assessment and treatment packages should read Chapters 2, 4, and 6, the first half of Chapter 5, and Chapters 7–13 most carefully. Readers who wish to evaluate carefully the research underlying the approach will probably find Chapter 3, the second half of Chapter 5, and Chapters 14 and 15 most useful.

CHAPTER TWO

Theoretical Orientation

The discussion of the Smith family in the introduction highlighted several key factors in a comprehensive behavioral–family systems analysis of parent–adolescent conflict. These include (1) the family as a homeostatic system, disrupted by the developmental phenomenon of adolescent independence seeking; (2) the role of family structure and hierarchy in understanding changes brought about as children become adolescents; (3) deficits in problem-solving communication skills; (4) cognitive distortions; and (5) the function of each member's behavior within the total system, particularly the function of the adolescent's rebellious behavior within the parents' marriage. This chapter outlines in greater detail the principles of normal family functioning and the development of parent–adolescent conflict. (Chapter Three reviews research relevant to behavioral–family systems hypotheses.)

BEHAVIORAL–FAMILY SYSTEMS MODEL

Two predominant models of family functioning have received increasing attention in recent years—the behavioral and the systems models. Behaviorally oriented theorists have explained family processes in terms of molecular contingency arrangements, social-learning principles, and behavior exchange theory (S. B. Gordon & Davidson, 1981; Jacobson & Margolin, 1979; Patterson, 1982; Robinson & Jacobson, 1987). Family systems theorists have explained these same processes in terms of circular, cybernetic systems with an emphasis on molar-level structural analysis (Aponte & VanDeusen, 1981; Bodin, 1981; Minuchin, 1974; Stanton, 1981; Steinglass, 1987). While there are definite differences between these two theoretical approaches, they both share a common emphasis on observable regularities in interpersonal processes and may be viewed as having potential areas of rapprochement (Foster & Hoier, 1982). The detailed molecular analysis of contingency arrangements inherent in the behavioral tradition provides an excellent basis for a functional analysis of families' interactive behavior. However, this tradition has often failed to address the circular nature of interaction patterns and the hierarchical structure of families, which overlay contingency arrangements. By contrast, the cybernetic, molar and analysis of hierarchy inherent in the systems tradition provides a rich conceptual basis for a structural analysis of families. Unfortunately, the molar concepts of a systems approach are often difficult to relate to an operational analysis of specific sequences of interactions within families. We have therefore found it useful to integrate concepts from both schools in building a comprehensive behavioral–family systems theory of family functioning, adding notions of contingency arrangements, social-learning principles, and cognitive–behavioral theory to the analysis of the family as a circular system with a definite structural configuration.

Families can be seen as social systems of members, held together by strong bonds of affection, who exercise mutual control over each other's contingency arrangements. A family has a definite structure or organization that permits it to accomplish definite goals within a developmental time frame. Individual members of a family have repertoires of problem-solving communication skills and cognitive sets (belief systems), which both determine and are in part determined by their interactions with other members. The family takes as its implicit goals the preservation, growth, development, and nurturance of its members. From an evolutionary viewpoint there may be broader goals related to the preservation of the species, but these transcend our level of analysis. Preservation, growth, development, and nurturance translate into providing age-appropriate primary and secondary reinforcers to individual members of the family and into arranging the environment to encourage the acquisition of age-appropriate repertoires of social, motoric, academic, and emotional behaviors and attitudes.

Adolescence is a period of exponential physiological, cognitive, emotional, and behavioral change. A complex constellation of biological changes within the maturing child set in motion a reverberating series of psychosocial changes within the family. These psychosocial changes can be examined in terms of the adolescent's developmental tasks, the major one of which involves becoming independent from parents. Prior to the adolescence of its young members, a family has established self-maintained and self-maintaining patterns of mutual influence over each other's behavior. The independence-seeking behavior of young teenagers interrupts these previously established homeostatic patterns of family relations. The system reacts to these changes by attempting to reestablish control and balance. Some conflict is normal during this time of adjustment. The manner in which families react to the challenges of teenage individuation determines whether the normal perturbation of early adolescence is resolved or whether it escalates to clinically significant proportions.

Three factors are hypothesized to influence a familiy's reaction to developmental challenges: problem-solving communication skills, belief systems and cognitive distortions, and family structure. Difficulties in any of these dimensions propel a family towards clinically significant conflict. The model pictured in Figure 2–1 integrates behavioral and family systems constructs within a developmental context. Biological maturation provides the impetus for changes in the family system, which creates a "developmental crisis." Periodic conflict, characterized by verbal disputes over independence-related issues, is the manifestation of the "crisis." The skills, cognitions, and structure of the family constitute the independent variables that explain how a normal developmental

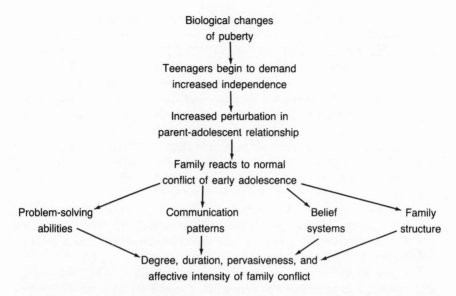

Biological changes
of puberty

Teenagers begin to demand
increased independence

Increased perturbation in
parent-adolescent relationship

Family reacts to normal
conflict of early adolescence

Problem-solving   Communication   Belief   Family
abilities   patterns   systems   structure

Degree, duration, pervasiveness, and
affective intensity of family conflict

FIGURE 2-1 Behavioral–family systems model of parent–adolescent conflict. From Foster and Robin (1988). Reprinted by permission.

crisis can become a clinical problem. In the pages that follow, we elaborate on elements of this model and describe specific hypotheses derived from it.

Developmental Factors

In addition to individuation from parents, the adolescent must master several other critical developmental tasks to become a competent, healthy adult (Conger, 1977, p. 220).

1. Adjustment to the physical changes of puberty and growth and the psychological changes of sexual maturity
2. Development of a system of values and a sense of identity
3. Establishment of effective social and working relationships with same- and opposite-sex peers
4. Preparations for a vocation or career

The adolescent faces these challenges in the context of important biological changes. Simultaneously, the adolescent is developing cognitively. Early adolescence marks the emergence for most youths of formal operational thought (Inhelder & Piaget, 1958)—the ability to think and reason logically in ways that younger children do not display. This mode of thinking characterizes adult cognitive processes.

In light of these developmental changes and challenges, it is not surprising that families are confronted with transitions during this period. Previously quiescent children now have the abilities to present logical arguments to their parents. Peer-delivered reinforcers may conflict with parental consequences. Access to new situations may require the acquisition of new skills for the teenager; peers rather than parents may assume primary status as role models. Thus parents will be confronted by a teenager's new ways of thinking, new physical appearance, new behaviors, new requests for increased autonomy and independence, and new availability of important peer-related activities.

Just as each family goes through individual developmental stages, the family as a whole has certain developmental stages. Carter and McGoldrick (1980) differentiated six phases of family development, each with its own tasks and crises.

1. *Between families: the unattached young adult.* During this phase, the unattached young adult must assert independence from his/her family of origin, formulate personal and life goals, and develop a personal identity before joining with another to form a new family.

2. *The newly married couple: the joining of families.* When two young adults marry, they become a new family. They must establish a marital system and realign their relationships with extended families and friends to include both spouses.

3. *The family with young children.* During this phase, the spouses must accommodate to accept new members. The marriage adjusts to make space for children, the spouses assume parental roles, and their relationships with their extended family are redefined to include parenting and grandparenting roles.

4. *The family with adolescents.* As children reach the adolescent years, the family's boundaries are challenged, necessitating increased flexibility to permit age-appropriate independence. Parent–child relationships must shift to permit adolescents to move easily in and out of the system. At one moment, adolescents boldly wish to make autonomous decisions concerning rules and regulations governing their conduct; however, when hurt or upset, they may just as quickly return to seek their parents' support, consolation, and advice. These boundary shifts may refocus the parents' attention on midlife marital and career issues as well as foreshadow a shift toward concerns for approaching old age.

5. *Launching children and moving on.* When young adults exit from the nuclear family, a great deal of flexibility is required. The routines of the marriage must be renegotiated, the parents and grown offspring must develop adult–adult ways of relating, relationships must be changed to include in-laws and grandchildren, and the entire family is typically faced with disabilities and deaths of parents, grandparents, and so forth.

6. *The family in later life.* As the parents age, generational roles within the family continue to shift. The parents must accommodate their marriage to physiological declines, deal with the possible loss of spouses, siblings, and friends, and review their own lives. The family must adapt to this aging process and accept the experience of the elderly, without either relying too heavily upon them for support and assistance or relegating them to a trivial role.

Looking at the family as a developing unit provides a context for understanding the ramifications of an adolescent's individual development (Grotevant & Cooper, 1983). These transitional processes set the stage for the etiology of conflict. It may be relatively simple or very difficult for the adolescent to complete developmental tasks successfully, depending upon cultural and familial contexts. Adolescents growing up in modern American society, faced with multiple, often conflicting, social, economic, and moral pressures, may have more difficulty completing these tasks than adolescents growing up in tribal African society, but the tasks remain constant across cultural settings. Considerable empirical evidence has converged to suggest that the pivotal factor influencing completion of the other tasks is the adolescent's ability to become independent from his/her parents, the first and primary task (Conger, 1977).

The adolescent's growth and development presents challenges to the family. As noted, the family's boundaries are challenged; adolescents wish to move in and out of family relationships flexibly. Adolescent independence is a key theme around which parent–teen conflict occurs. Disagreements about specific issues such as curfew, dating, and chores, frequently reflect adolescents' growing desire for increased independence. Conflict is heightened when adolescents wish to obtain autonomy in decision making at a faster rate than their parents feel they are capable of handling responsibly. Problems also occur when parents fail to become involved in the process, allowing adolescents as much autonomy as they wish. Under these conditions, teens may become involved in peer cultures that encourage antisocial behavior, resulting again in increased family conflict. Readers interested in further discussion of the reciprocal influences of adolescent development and family development might consult Grotevant and Cooper (1983) or Youniss and Smollar (1985).

Skills

The competencies and cognitions of family members underlie their social interactions. They are the "atoms" or "molecules" of a behavioral–family systems theory, the stuff of which interactions are made. When combined in certain proportions and quantities, they may react explosively to create a full-blown family conflict or fuse harmoniously to produce mutually satisfactory relationship outcomes.

Problem-solving and communication skills are particularly salient to the study of parent–adolescent relations because many conflicts between parents and teenagers take the form of a series of specific disputes that require resolution to restore a new pattern of family functioning. Rational problem solving is a cognitive–behavioral process whereby an individual follows a logical sequence of steps to reach a solution to a given problem (D'Zurilla, 1988; D'Zurilla & Goldfried, 1971). While investigators have described the steps of problem solving in a variety of ways, they generally concur that certain basic skills are necessary (Spivack, Platt, & Shure, 1976).

1. *Problem finding:* recognizing the presence of an interpersonal problem
2. *Problem definition:* formulating the problem in clear-cut terms, collecting information relevant to the formulation of the problem, and communicating the formulation to others
3. *Generation of solutions:* generating a variety of creative alternatives for resolving the problem through the use of brainstorming or related techniques
4. *Evaluation:* projecting the benefits and costs of implementing the solutions, viewing them from a variety of perspectives
5. *Decision making:* choosing and negotiating a solution that maximizes the benefits and minimizes the costs for everyone involved in the problem
6. *Implementation planning:* specifying the details required to implement a chosen solution effectively
7. *Verification:* evaluating the effectiveness of the solution in resolving the problem and recycling through the earlier steps if the solution fails to solve the original problem

While family members may not always cycle through these steps in a formal manner, they need to be reasonably proficient at each skill in order to resolve disputes. The more intense the dispute, the greater family members' problem-solving skills must be to resolve their difficulty effectively.

Applying problem solving within an interactional context also requires skills in expressive and receptive communication. Family members need to express their feelings and opinions assertively yet unoffensively, to listen to each other's statements attentively, and to decode messages accurately. Accusations, denials, threats, commands, poor eye contact, and so forth, impede effective communication by provoking anger and reciprocated negative statements. Reflections, paraphrases, brief acknowledgments, empathetic remarks, and appropriate eye contact and posture facilitate effective communication.

Deficits in any problem-solving and communication skills may result in increased conflict and argument. For instance, not defining a problem in clear-cut terms may lead different family members to address different problems and be confused as to what topic is indeed being considered. Families who cannot brainstorm a variety of solutions may become bogged down in their original positions, unable to perceive alternatives for overcoming their conflict, while families who prematurely evaluate the first new ideas they suggest are likely to inhibit novel ideas. Inability to project the consequences of solutions can result in impulsive adoption of an impractical, implausible course of action doomed to failure. Difficulty in negotiating compromises can result in the breakdown of an entire discussion.

How parents and teenagers structure the use of problem-solving communication skills in decision making is also important. Decision-making power can be exercised on a continuum ranging from authoritarian–autocratic through permissive–laissez faire (Elder, 1962). With an authoritarian–autocratic structure, parents impose their decisions upon the adolescent. With a permissive–laissez faire structure, parents abdicate decision-making authority completely. Intermediate on the continuum is a democratic structure, where the parents encourage the adolescent to participate meaningfully in decision making about issues pertaining to the teenager. Research in child development suggests that in contemporary Western civilizations, using democratic problem-solving skills to resolve independence-related disputes promotes less conflict and greater achievement of the developmental tasks of adolescence than using either authoritarian–autocratic or permissive–laissez faire problem-solving skills (Conger, 1977; Grotevant & Cooper, 1983).[1] We postulate that when parents attempt to restore disrupted homeostatic functioning by resorting to excessive imposition or abdication of authority, clinically significant conflict is likely to result.

There are several reasons why democratic problem-solving and positive communication skills promote more effective resolution of parent–adolescent conflict than either authoritarian or permissive approaches:

1. Democratic approaches complement the natural developmental thrust of adolescence, which is towards gradually increasing independence from the nuclear family. Authoritarian approaches oppose this developmental thrust, while permissive approaches provide too much independence too soon without appropriate parental shaping of independence-related behaviors.

2. Democratic decision-making structures imply easy, flexible adaptation to rapid changes, while authoritarian or permissive structures indicate rigidity and resistance to change. Rigid systems are slower to restore homeostatic functioning than flexible systems, and adolescent development mandates frequent, significant shifts in homeostatic functioning.

3. Positive problem-solving and communication skills permit orderly, rational discussion of relevant issues, while excesses in negative communication skills sidetrack constructive problem-solving exchanges into reciprocal bursts of accusatory–defensive comments (Alexander, 1973). Problems remain unresolved, lingering to elicit further conflict and negative affectual reactions whenever the situations recur. Family members come to expect biting, sarcastic responses from each other and may anticipate such responses by expressing even mundane matters in a defensive manner.

Cognitions

Within a social-learning theory cognitions are conceptualized as private events subject to the same principles of behavior that govern overt behavior (Dobson, 1988; Kendall & Hollon, 1981). Family members' beliefs, expectations, and

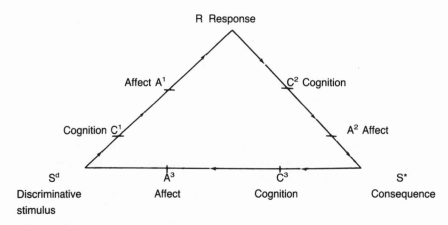

FIGURE 2-2 Cognitive–behavioral three-term contingency analysis.

attributions concerning parenting, child rearing, and family life are habitual responses learned from life experiences and are subject to control by environmental and internal antecedents and consequences. Figure 2–2 presents a model that integrates cognitive events into a three-term contingency analysis. This model begins with a basic three-term contingency of discriminative stimulus, response, and consequence. Cognitions and affect are interposed as mediators of motoric responses. The model also differentiates between cognitions and affect that precede and that follow responses. By convention, thoughts that precede the occurrence of a response (or consequence) and relate to the likelihood particular responses will occur have been labeled "expectations," while thoughts that are subsequent to the response (or consequences) and involve interpretation of the outcome have been labeled "attributions."

To illustrate the role of cognitive factors in parents–teen relations, consider the case of a 13-year-old who repeatedly fails to clean up her room. Her mother reacts to this failure by withdrawing the daughter's allowance. The girl complains bitterly. From the mother's perspective, the dirty room is a discriminative stimulus in whose presence she might think, "If she doesn't learn to clean up her room now, she will grow up to be a slob; this would be a major catastrophe." Such an expectation, representative of a "ruination" theme, might elicit a great deal of anger, which then might prompt parental punishment. From the daughter's perspective, the loss of her allowance serves as a discriminative stimulus for the attribution, "Mom is just not fair; my room isn't that bad that I deserve to lose my allowance." This thought, representative of an "unfairness" theme, might elicit anger, mediating her bitter complaints.

Three aspects of cognitions in family interaction deserve special attention: (1) the relationship between thoughts and feelings; (2) cognition as information processing; and (3) basic assumptions and themes underlying dysfunctional cognitions.

Positive cognitions elicit positive affect while negative cognitions elicit negative affect. Over time, multiple negative interactions will occasion repeated negative cognitions, and if family members consistently perceive their relationships in negative terms, they will experience prolonged negative feelings towards each other. An interactant's expression of negative affect may then become a discriminative stimulus for reciprocal expression of negative affect by the others. Eventually, interlocking cycles of punishment and avoidance may no longer be under control of the original antecedents that elicited the negative cognition and affect, creating a "snowball" effect, as in families who report that they argue all the time at the slightest provocation.

To think is to process information and interpret events. Information may be processed accurately or inaccurately, depending upon the capabilities and learning histories of the individual, affective states, and a host of other variables of which we only have a rudimentary understanding at the present time. Beck and his colleagues (Beck, 1967, 1976) have described a number of common distortions in information processing, including arbitrary inference, selective abstraction, overgeneralization, magnification and minimization, and absolutistic thinking. The extent to which family members distort information in particular interactions will influence the ways in which behavior is influenced by cognitions. Definitions and examples of these logical errors applied to family conflict follow:

Arbitrary Inference

This refers to drawing a specific conclusion in the absence of supporting evidence or when the evidence is contrary to the conclusion.

Example.   A teenager lets his hair grow long and listens to rock music; his father concludes that because his son wears long hair and listens to loud music, the boy is in danger of becoming involved in taking drugs.

Selective Abstraction

This consists of focusing on a detail taken out of context, ignoring other more salient features of the situation and conceptualizing the whole experience based on this fragment.

Example.   A 16-year-old girl comes home by her curfew of 12 a.m. for seven weekends, but on the eighth weekend is 1 hour late without telephoning. Her parents conclude that she is irresponsible and ground her for a month.

Overgeneralization

This refers to drawing a general conclusion on the basis of one or more isolated incidents, then generalizing the conclusion to related and unrelated situations.

Example.   A 14-year-old asks his parents for permission to go to a local shopping mall to meet his friends; his parents refuse because they feel that the teenagers who loiter there are "a bad crowd." The 14-year-old concludes that parents are unreasonable people who always say "no," and he decides that he'll have to lie to them from now on to obtain privileges.

Magnification and Minimization

These refer to gross errors in evaluating the significance of events.

Example of Magnification.   A couple who rarely disagree have a single argument. Their teenage daughter concludes that her parents are going to divorce and becomes extremely upset, acting out in school to distract her parents from their problem.

Example of Minimization.   An adolescent who has received numerous failing grades in school brings home a report card with two B's, three C's, and one D. His overly critical father concludes that his son's average still is not very high, and fails to acknowledge the boy's improvement.

Absolutistic, Dichotomous Reasoning

This refers to the tendency to polarize all experiences in extremely negative or positive categories. Usually others' actions are classified as negative.

Example.   A mother suspects that her 16-year-old daughter is kissing, petting, and possibly experimenting with sexual intercourse with boys. She views any premarital sexual activity as sinful, preferring to follow the old adage, "Nice girls don't do it."

Distorted information processing is a situational response to particular environmental antecedents. At another level of analysis are an individual's basic assumptions about family relationships. Basic assumptions refer to cross-situational expectations and attributions about how parents and teenagers should interact. They are consequences of a lifetime learning history. Ellis, Beck, and their colleagues (Beck, 1967, 1976; Dryden & Ellis, 1988; Ellis & Grieger, 1977) have found that certain assumptions are consistently associated with particular types of psychopathology. Ellis, for example, has coined 10 "irrational ideas," which he believes mediate anxiety and fear (e.g., "If everyone does not always approve of everything I do, it is a catastrophe"). Parents and teenagers also adhere to certain absolute assumptions concerning their relationships. While a detailed taxonomy of assumptions must await empirical investigation, we offer here a tentative list of dysfunctional cognitive themes.

Perfectionism

Parents expect their offspring to behave in a flawless manner. For example:

- "Teenagers should always respect their parents."
- "Teenagers should always behave responsibly."
- "My son is intelligent and should get all As in school."

Ruination

Parents believe that if their adolescents engage in some proscribed behavior, catastrophic consequences will ensue: Youths will ruin their lives and/or greatly damage their families. Teenagers believe that their parents' restrictions will ruin their lives. For example:

- "If we permit him to smoke marijuana, he will become a drug addict."
- "If she dates before 16, she will become promiscuous, pregnant, and ruin her reputation."
- "If my father doesn't permit me to stay out all night, my friends will think I'm too straight, reject me, and leave me very lonely."
- "If we permit him to stay out late, he will become an irresponsible adult."

Fairness

Adolescents believe that their parents should always treat them fairly and that it is a terrible injustice if their parents propose unfair rules and regulations. For example:

- "My parents should always treat my brother and me equally."
- "My parents should be at least as lenient as my friends' parents."
- "My father was permitted to date when he was 14; it's not fair to make me wait until I'm 16."

Love/Approval

Family members believe that they should confide secrets in each other and always approve of each other's behavior. Disapproval or failure to confide are interpreted as signs of the absence of love. For example:

- "My son should tell me what's bothering him, and if he doesn't, it must mean he doesn't really love me."
- "If my mother really loved me, she wouldn't question what I do."
- "My parents really don't care about me; they are just afraid that if I mess up they will be embarrassed."

Obedience

Parents believe that their teenagers should always comply with their requests willingly and without question. For example:

- "My daughter should always do what I say because I know what's best from my experience."
- "Young people have no right to challenge their parents' decisions."

Self-Blame

Parents believe that their adolescent's mistakes signify their basic inadequacies as parents. For example:

- "If he fails at school, I'm a bad mother."
- "If she turns to drugs, it must be because I haven't given her enough love."

Malicious Intent

Parents believe that their adolescents misbehave or rebel on purpose to hurt them. Teens abscribe hurtful motives to parental criticism and/or rules. For example:

- "My daughter is trying to drive me crazy."
- "My son is rebelling to punish me for not doing what he wants."
- "My mom makes me come in early because she doesn't want me to have any friends."

Autonomy

Teenagers expect that they should have as much freedom from parental restrictions as they desire, and become indignant if their freedom is curtailed. For example:

- "I'm all grown up at 16 and should be able to go out with anyone I like."
- "You don't have the right to set my curfew because I'm not a baby anymore."

Cognitive distortions influence parent–adolescent conflict in at least two ways. First, the inflexible nature of family members' belief system translate into rigid positions on specific issues. Parents may mistakenly think that they can never permit a teenager to go on dates because terrible consequences will result; adolescents may mistakenly think that their parents can never be trusted with important personal information. Individuals' inflexible stances rapidly polarize the family during problem solving, interfering with resolution of disputes. Second, the anger and hostility elicited by exaggerated negative interpretations of relationship events or illogical reasoning make it difficult to approach specific disputes calmly and to communicate positively, even when appropriate skills are within family members' repertoires. The teenager who believes her parents were extremely unfair to restrict her curfew is prone to lose control and express her hostility in an accusatory manner. The father who believes his son is ruining his entire future by smoking marijuana will have difficulty remaining rational in a discussion of this issue. The result will be overly negative exchanges of dis- satisfactions, inducing reciprocally negative affect. The more rigid and distorted the cognitive processes are, the greater the degree of expected conflict.

Why do family members continue to adhere to unreasonable expectations and to make overly negative attributions of each other's behavior, if these distortions promote anger, hostility, and conflict? Faulty information processing appears to be an overlearned, cross-situational cognitive style resistant to change. Further, cognitive distortions may function to help certain families regain homeostatic functioning through avoidance and positive reinforcement in the face of adolescent independence-seeking behavior. Under the avoidance hypothesis, parents' cognitive distortions serve as excuses for them to restrict their teenagers' autonomy in the hope of avoiding the occurrence of perceived catastrophic outcomes. The mother who distorts her daughter's sexual ex- perimentation in absolutistic, negative terms feels justified restricting the girl's contacts with boys to "protect" the girl from pregnancy and eventual ruination. The father who minimizes his son's improved academic achievement may hope to spur his son to study harder, in order to avoid future academic and career failure.

For some families, events that occurred in the parents' families of origin may have provided the impetus for the avoidance function. A mother who gave birth to children as a teenager is likely to restrict her daughter's sexual ex- perimentation out of fear that the daughter will repeat the mother's pattern. Parents who were treated poorly by their parents when they were children may believe they must be "superparents" to avoid ruining the children; they take any sign of adolescent rebellion as evidence that they have failed to be superparents.

Under the positive reinforcement hypothesis, family members' cognitive distortions may lead to behavior that restores previously disrupted schedules of interaction and reinforcement in the system. By restricting her daughter's con- tacts with boys, the mother may intermittently coerce her daughter into spending more time at home, restoring the higher level of mother–daughter contact that had been disrupted by the girl's increased interest in boys. The effects of this contact might be even stronger if the girl's father were providing insufficient interpersonal reinforcement to his wife. The teenager who reacts to her parents' argument by acting rebelliously in school may restore positive contacts between her parents by uniting them in the cause of disciplining her. Even if an individual does not consciously plan a relationship outcome based upon the action that follows from a cognitive distortion, the action may produce that outcome, strengthening the sequence of interactions and the mediating cognitions. The interlocking nature of the functions served by cognitive distortions is complex and idiosyncratic to particular families. At the present time we do not know enough about these functions to place them within an empirically based taxonomy; however, clinical experiences do suggest their importance.

Structure

Organization is necessary to accomplish family goals. Families are structured in a hierarchical manner punctuated by the differential distribution of power (Haley, 1976; Minuchin, 1974; Steinglass, 1987). Power is the relative social influence of each member on the outcome of a particular interaction. An individual's influence or power may be founded on rules, on patterns based on generational differences or external systems (e.g., society), on the history of that particular family system (e.g., a matriarchical tradition), on the control of reinforcers, and/or on coalitions (e.g., two family members support each other to achieve a particular outcome) (Haley, 1976; Stanton, 1981). Terms capturing types of hierarchical organization provide shorthand descriptions of general patterns of influence across a variety of situations, although situation-specific patterns may sometimes deviate from the general description.

In contemporary American families, for example, power is ordinarily founded on generational boundaries and on control of reinforcers. Parents are higher in the dominance hierarchy and control more of decision-making processes than do children, who may themselves establish a dominance hierarchy within the sibling subsystem. Parents control their children's access to important reinforcers and punishers and impose significant contingency arrangements on their children. Grandparents often serve as "consultants" or advisors to the parents, although in some families they may be the primary decision makers and care givers. Cultural contexts and societal expectations serve to define the basic repertoires of behavior that constitute the roles of "parents," "spouse," "child," and "breadwinner" in a family.

The structure of family relationships is drastically altered as the family responds to adolescent individuation. Adolescents seek to upgrade their positions of power within the dominance hierarchy from a subordinate to a more egalitarian status. Parents' positions as the executives or leaders of the family are challenged by the teenagers' demands for increased decision-making power over rules governing their behavior.

To understand the implications of family structure for a behavioral–family systems theory, two concepts derived from structural family therapy bear further discussion: alignment and cohesion. *Alignment* refers to joining or opposing one member of a system who is carrying out some function (Aponte & VanDeusen, 1981). Within each family, members have patterns of working together or in opposition on certain activities or goals. Alignments may take various forms, most commonly coalitions or triangulation. A *coalition* consists of a joint set of actions of two family members against a third. In the Chapter 1 case, Mrs. Smith and her daughter united to criticize Mr. Smith's authoritarian behavior. Although Sally and her mother may have had different reasons for punishing Mr. Smith, they united to obtain a common outcome. Coalitions are likely to form when two members who seek common relationship outcomes from a third conclude that the advantages of cooperative action outweigh the advantages of individual action.

Coalitions occur to some extent in all families but create problems when they cross generational boundaries and thereby run counter to the natural parent-controlled dominance hierarchies common to Western societies (Haley, 1976, 1980; Minuchin, 1974). Problem coalitions may include (1) parents who fail to work together (a weak parental coalition); (2) an alliance between a teen and a laissez faire parent, characterized by interactions where the teen involves the allied parent in decision making and overrules regulations promoted by the more authoritarian parent; (3) teen coalitions with nonparental adults to weaken parent decision-making influence (e.g., grandparents, teachers); and (4) overly rigid parental coalitions in which the teen's attempts to state his/her wishes are consistently punished, thus stymieing the natural development of increased autonomy.

In *triangulation* each of two opposing parties seeks to join with the same third person against the other; they compete for the allegiance of the third person, who alternately aligns with one and then the other of the two opposing parties (Aponte & VanDeusen, 1981). For example, a couple may argue about a variety of relationship issues, and each spouse may attempt to persuade an adolescent daughter to align with him/her against the other. The daughter may vacillate between supporting her mother and backing her father.

Triangulation occurs in all families, but can become a problem under either of two circumstances: (1) the adolescent and one parent each consistently attempt to garner the support of the second parent during a conflict; (2) each parent consistently seeks the adolescent's support to mediate marital conflict. Stepfamilies often provide the most blatant examples of the first circumstance: When an adolescent boy argues with his stepfather and the stepfather attempts to discipline the boy, the adolescent may appeal to his natural mother to intervene on his behalf, "triangulating" her by forcing her to side with either her natural offspring or her new husband. The second instance is illustrated by the couple engaged in a mutually accusatory marital dispute, with each spouse turning to the teenager for support ("Didn't Dad to this?" or "Did you ever hear Mom say that?")

Cohesion refers to a continuum describing the amount of closeness and contact among family members (Aponte & VanDeusen, 1981). This continuum ranges from *enmeshment* at one end to *disengagement* at the other. In the enmeshed family there is close involvement in the affairs of other members, lack of privacy, and emphasis on conforming to family norms. Everyone minds everyone else's business. Privacy is minimal; mind reading runs rampant. Family members are fine-tuned to discriminate minute changes in each other's behavior and affect. In verbal interchanges they often interrupt each other, completing each other's thought. Behaviorally speaking, members exercise very tight stimulus and consequence control over each other's responses on a molecular level. They provide social reinforcement and punishment on continuous or high frequency schedules, and there is a great deal of contingent, moment-to-moment reciprocity of behavior and affect.

At the other end of the continuum, members of a disengaged family have infrequent interaction with each other, are distant and uninvolved in each other's affairs (Aponte & VanDeusen, 1981). Members are often unaware of others' behavior and affect. Reserve, privacy, and interpersonal distance characterize family interactions. Members exercise loose stimulus and consequence control over each other's behavior, and provide reinforcement on infrequent, intermittent schedules. There is a low degree of contingent reciprocity of behavior and affect.

The extremes of enmeshment and disengagement are hypothesized to exacerbate conflict as the family attempts to react to adolescent individuation, while the central balanced range of cohesion is considered more adaptive (Olson, McCubbin, Barnes, Larsen, Muxen, and Wilson, 1983; Olson, Sprenkle, & Russell, 1979). In highly enmeshed families or dyads within families, parents are likely to experience difficulty permitting adolescents to make independent decisions, go places with peers, and have age-appropriate privacy. In these families, increased adolescent autonomy results in a significant loss of reinforcers for the parents, a loss the adolescent may also experience if peer contact is insufficient to replace familial involvement. Adolescents may experience a great deal of difficulty assertively requesting increased privileges; the sensitive adolescent may fear loss of parental approval and contact. If autonomous behavior has been punished in the past, the adolescent may feel anxiety and guilt about making new requests. Parents who derive major interpersonal benefits from the confiding, dependent behavior of their children may respond with bitter conflict when the adolescent attempts to gain a new kind of autonomy. Adolescents may have to rebel in extreme ways in order to establish some degree of independence. The transition from a parent-dominant to a more egalitarian hierarchy can provoke a serious crisis within a highly enmeshed family as a result of the emotional reactions elicited by the "stretching" of reinforcement schedules and "loosening" of stimulus control.

By contrast, in the disengaged family, independent functioning has been a long-established norm, and the adolescent's increased requests for decision-making freedom do not pose a direct threat to existing mutual control contingencies. However, too little parental control over a teenager's decision making can lead to poor decisions if the teen lacks sufficient judgmental skills to make mature, self-enhancing choices. The teenager may, through poor decision making, become involved in realistically dangerous situations with drugs, delinquency, alcohol, academic failure, sexuality, and so forth, without the parents' awareness or concern. When an external community agency such as the school or police complains to the parents about the adolescent's misbehavior, the parents are likely to react in a powerful, negative manner to reestablish control. Severe parent–teen conflict may continue until the system again gradually drifts toward disengagement.

Those teenagers from disengaged families who value parental attention but have not received it because the parents are preoccupied with their own lives may learn that their parents will pay increased attention to them only when the adolescent's antisocial behavior causes extrafamilial agencies to complain to the parents. These adolescents may repeat their antisocial behavior in order to coerce the community into contacting their parents, who then are coerced to apply increased, albeit negative, attention to the teenagers. When antisocial adolescent behavior ceases, parents are rewarded for their attention via negative reinforcement. Thus disengagement can indirectly encourage the kinds of maladaptive but functional interlocking contingency arrangements that are described in the next section.

FUNCTIONAL ANALYSIS

To this point, we have discussed individually the elements of conflict—problem solving, communication, cognitions, and family structure. The clinician faced with a conflictual family must paint an overall picture of the problems, integrating the particular shapes, colors, and textures with broad strokes of the brush which produce a finished work of art. Within our model, this integration is based on an examination of the functions that cement together recurring sequences that represent the kind of operationalization of the concept of homeostasis. These sequences describe how each member's behavior influences and is influenced by the others' responses, within the constraints of the family's organizational structure, skill deficits, and cognitive sets.

What maintains such recurring sequences of interaction or homeostatic patterns? How do we answer the question, "What is the function of the sequence for each member?" While there are no completely acceptable, empirically sound answers to this question at the present time, we find it useful to apply constructs from social-learning theory and applied behavior analysis in attempting to deal with the issue of function. These constructs vary considerably in their degree of complexity and detail.

At the most molecular, complex level are the constructs of positive reinforcement, negative reinforcement, punishment, and avoidance. These constructs are applied to family interactions by looking for *interlocking, interdependent* sequences of behavioral operations.

Positive Reinforcement

Positive reinforcement is defined as the presentation of a stimulus contingent upon the emission of a response, leading to an increased probability that the response will recur. If family member A's behavior serves a positive reinforcement function in a dyadic interaction with B, A's behavior results in a consequence from B that increases the probability that A's behavior will recur in the future in similar situations.

Example 1.   A teenager completes a chore and receives praise from a parent. The teenager is more likely to complete chores in the future. Completion of chores serves to obtain positive reinforcement in the dyadic relationship between the teen and the parent.

Example 2.   A son's disobedience towards his mother eventually results in increased attention from his otherwise distant dad. If the son's disobedient behavior is maintained in part by eventual paternal attention, the father can be viewed as positively reinforcing the son's disobedient behavior.

Negative Reinforcement

Negative reinforcement is defined as removal of stimulus contingent upon emitting a response, which increases the probability that the response will recur. The stimulus removed is typically aversive. If A's behavior is negatively reinforced by B's behavior, the cessation of a response by B increases the chances that the behavior of A that changed B's response will recur.

Example 1.   A teenage girl suddenly loses a lot of weight and refuses to eat properly. Her parents have been having severe marital arguments for several months. They stop arguing over marital issues and unite to help their daughter resume eating. Marital fights were aversive to the daughter; eliminating the marital fighting negatively reinforced the teenager's anorectic behavior, and she continued to refuse to eat. Cessation of eating served a negative reinforcement function for the daughter in the mother–father–daughter triadic interaction.

Example 2.   A mother and father lecture their son about a rule violation. He tells them he will do as they ask but later breaks his promise. In this example, the son's promise terminated parental lectures, thus negatively reinforcing his untruths.

Punishment

Punishment is defined as the presentation of a stimulus contingent upon the emission of a response, leading to a decreased probability that the response will recur. The stimulus that suppresses behavior is typically called a punisher or aversive stimulus.

Example. Bill took the family car out on Friday night to go driving with his friends without parental permission. His father forbade him to use the car for 1 month and cut off his allowance for 3 weeks. Bill never again took the car without permission. The loss of the use of the car and allowance served to punish Bill's behavior of taking the car without permission.

Avoidance

Avoidance is defined as any response that prevents the occurrence of a previously established aversive stimulus.

Example 1. John refuses to do his homework; his father threatens to ground him for 1 week. John then does his homework to avoid the grounding. Homework compliance serves an avoidance function in the father–son dyad.

Example 2. A husband and wife do not enjoy time spent together in recreational activities. They have few common interests and rarely communicate positive feelings to each other. When their two teenage sons begin to fight with each other, the parents decide that they should stay home on weekend evenings for their sons' safety. By staying home with the children, they avoid unpleasant recreational time together. Dealing with sibling fighting serves an avoidance function in the parents' marriage.

At a slightly more molar level, social-learning theorists have formulated the constructs of reciprocity and coercion, which depict sequences of mutual reinforcement, punishment, and avoidance (Gottman, 1979; Patterson, 1982; Patterson & Bank, 1986; Patterson & Reid, 1970).

Reciprocity

Reciprocity refers to an exchange of behavior between two family members. The concept of reciprocity has been defined in two ways: as a contingency arrangement and as rate matching. Contingent reciprocity implies changes in the probability of one person's behavior based on another's behavior. In other words, if person A directs behavior X at person B, there is a greater probability that B will, at some later time, direct behavior X back to A than if the prior event had not occurred (Gottman, 1979, p. 63). The time frame of contingent reciprocity may be moment-to-moment, hour-to-hour, day-to-day, or longer, and the behavior to be reciprocated may be positive or negative.

Example 1 (Contingent Reciprocity). A father accuses his son of being irresponsible by smoking marijuana; the son accuses the father of being old-fashioned; the father accuses the son of being disrespectful; and the son counters that the father doesn't deserve respect. This dyad is reciprocating negative, accusatory behavior on a moment-to-moment contingent basis.

Example 2 (Contingent Reciprocity). On Monday Jill asks her parents for permission to go to a concert with Bob the next Saturday evening. They hesitate but reluctantly agree. She is pleased that they trusted her. For the next few days she behaves in an overly friendly, helpful manner towards her parents. They praise her for her "positive attitude." She continues to talk nicely to them and help with housework. Jill and her parents are reciprocating positive behavior over a relatively long time frame.

The rate-matching concept of reciprocity describes an interaction in which persons A and B exchange behavior at equitable rates (Gottman, 1979). Over many interactional episodes, their exchange of behavior will be proportional (Patterson & Reid, 1970). If A positively reinforces B's behavior 50% of the time, in the long run B will positively reinforce A's behavior 50% of the time. If B punishes A's behavior 90% of the time, A will punish B's behavior 90% of the time. If A expresses hostility to B 25% of the time, B will express hostility to A 25% of the time. A tight contingency is not implied, although a loose contingency exists; rate-matching reciprocity implies a general quid pro quo in dyadic relationships.

Example 3 (Rate-Matching Reciprocity). Mrs. Barker relates to her son Tom in a sarcastic, accusatory manner, often criticizing his behavior. He "repays" her with argumentative, noncompliant behavior. In contrast, Mr. Barker rarely disciplines his son, leaving that role to his wife. He tends to converse with Tom about positive subjects such as athletics and current events. Tom confides in his dad and treats him respectfully. Mrs. and Mr. Barker disagree often; Mrs. Barker accuses her husband of undermining her attempts to discipline Tom. Mr Barker passively listens to his wife to appease her and avoid conflict, then promptly ignores what she suggests. Reciprocity of negative behavior occurs in the father–mother and mother–son dyads, but reciprocity of positive behavior predominates in the father–son dyad.

Coercion

Coercion refers to interlocking contingencies cemented together by negative reinforcement. For example, imagine a dyadic interaction where person A makes an aversive demand of person B, and B complies with the demand. A's aversive, demanding behavior is positively reinforced, and B's compliance is negatively reinforced. The positive reinforcement for A is B's compliance with the request.

The negative reinforcement for B is the removal of A's aversive demand contingent upon B's compliance. Over time, A learns to escalate aversive demands, and B learns to escape these demands by complying with them. B usually also experiences strong negative emotional reactions to coercive interchanges. If B talked back to A, and A withdrew the request, A's withdrawal of the request would be negatively reinforced by the cessation of backtalk. Backtalk would be negatively reinforced by the withdrawal of the demand. Both examples represent coercive processes. (See Patterson, 1982, for an elegant, data-based model of coercive processes to account for the aggressive behavior of pre-adolescents and their parents.)

Example 1. A mother repeatedly demands that her recalcitrant husband discipline her son when he disobeys her, and eventually threatens to get a divorce. Then the father talks to the boy. She stops threatening him after he talks to his son.

Example 2. A father pays very little attention to his teenage son, and when he does talk with the boy, it is usually to make a request or a criticism. The boy first tries to engage his father's interest through positive approaches (i.e., relating daily events, developing joint activities, etc.). The father, overinvolved in his career, ignores the boy's positive overtures. Eventually, the boy tries to engage his father's interest through aversive means. He begins to fail in school, smoke marijuana, and shoplift small articles. Faced with demands from the school and police, the father finally begins to pay attention to his son. The boy stops his antisocial activities. The boy's escalating antisocial behavior was coercive; it was designed to force his father to pay attention to him. The father's paying attention to his son was negatively reinforced when the boy ceased his antisocial activities, removing an aversive stimulus for the father. This example also illustrates how coercive repertoires may develop through a successive approximation process. When the father failed to reinforce earlier more positive adolescent attention-seeking responses, the son resorted to coercive responses that created an aversive situation that could not be ignored.

ADOLESCENT INVOLVEMENT IN MARITAL AFFAIRS

Adolescent involvement in marital affairs is one sequence of interaction that has drawn particular attention. Some families regularly involve children in parental disputes; others do not. Patterns of child involvement in marital affairs develop gradually over a family's developmental life cycle and assume characteristic modes of functioning. Systems-oriented theorists believe that when children become accomplices in marital fights, problems inevitably result, often taking the form of a specific child symptom (Haley, 1976, 1980; Madanes, 1981). They postulate that parents draw children into disagreements over discipline, form cross-generational coalitions, or develop triangulated relationships. The child's symptom becomes a metaphorical representation of the parents' underlying marital pathology, a "protective" mechanism to prevent divorce, avoid overt marital tension, and maintain homeostatic functioning.

Social-learning theorists recognize the role marital discord can play in childhood behavior problems but dispute the inevitability of this relationship (Blechman, 1981; Emery, 1982; Porter & O'Leary, 1980). Only under certain conditions does marital conflict cause or maintain parent–adolescent conflict. These conditions have to do with the functions served by the adolescent's rebellious independence-seeking behavior within the marital system.

All parents face a myriad of decisions regarding child-rearing practices. During the course of family development, disagreements between parents naturally arise over discipline, schooling, recreational activities, mealtime habits, medical care, and other problems of daily living. The frequency and anger intensity of such disagreements may increase when adolescent independence seeking disrupts homeostatic functioning, particularly if parents have a history of disagreement over granting the child's requests, setting rules, and responding to misbehavior. Typically, one parent favors a certain activity, choice, or behavior for an adolescent or the family while the other proscribes it. Each parent may turn to the adolescent offspring for advice, support, or counsel in making a decision, forming temporary cross-generational coalitions and/or patterns of triangulation. Adolescents become adroit at exploiting their parents' differences of opinion, as when a daughter whose father opposes dating asks her mother for permission to go to the movies with her boyfriend, before her father comes home from work. While most spouses are able to resolve their disagreements, occasionally parents find themselves repeatedly embroiled in arguments revolving around how to handle their adolescent's behavior.

Children's behavior serves important functions in all marriages. Three common functions are positive reinforcement, negative reinforcement, and avoidance. The functions are usually benign and nonpathological. For example, couples derive a great deal of positive reinforcement from sharing and discussing their children's successes in scholastic, athletic, social, or recreational pursuits. Children's behavior can also serve a negative reinforcement function in the marriage: a couple may stop an argument (an aversive situation for the child) when a school-age child asks for help with homework, or a teenager acts sullen and depressed. Alternatively, parents may avoid unpleasant responsibilities by using their children as an excuse. A child's illness provides a common excuse for parents to cancel an obligation. Managing the children's illness behavior then serves an avoidance function for the parents.

We suggest that all of the structural and functional patterns of childhood involvement in marital affairs, which system theorists postulate lead to pathology, in fact occur regularly in nondistressed families. Nondistressed parents, however, generally recover from disagreements, work as a team, maintain their authority as family executives, and display a fair amount of consistency in their child-rearing functions. Pathology develops because of the manner in which children's behavior accomplishes certain marital functions, not because of the mere existence of these functional links. Long-standing histories of marital strife, consistent cross-generational coalitions, severe triangulated relationships, and reliance on punishment and avoidance to influence others predispose families toward problematic involvement of adolescents in marital functions. For example, spouses who disagree often over child-rearing issues, with each attempting to impose his/her will on the other by instructing the children to follow his/her rules without regard for the other parent's position, are likely to develop significant conflict. The children's misbehavior comes to serve a punishment function within the marriage: Each spouse punishes the other's noncompliant behavior by encouraging the children to behave in a manner unacceptable to the other. Alternatively, if spouses fight repeatedly and bitterly over sexual, activity-related, or household issues, with the recurrent threat of separation or divorce, children are likely to react strongly to the potential loss of the reinforcers that accompany a stable family environment. Adolescents may emit behaviors designed to avoid parental separation and subsequent reinforcer deprivation. Depending upon the adolescent's personal history, characteristics, and exposure to models of antisocial or illness behavior, these avoidance repertoires might involve externalizing behaviors such as delinquency, substance abuse, excessive disobedience at home, academic failure, or internalizing behaviors such as anxiety, depression, or psychophysiological reactions. The teenager's behavior comes to serve inappropriate avoidance and negative reinforcement functions within the system, by leading to temporary decreases in parental hostilities and avoidance of threatened separation.

Thus it would appear that parental deficiencies in resolving child-rearing and marital issues predispose families toward inappropriate involvement of teenagers in marital affairs. This expands the earlier hypothesis concerning deficits in parent–teen problem-solving communication skills and cognitive distortions to include the marital dyad. Poor problem solving, negative communication, and distorted thinking beget conflict. When the deficits encompass both the marital and the parent–teen dyads, cross-generational coalitions, triangulation, and problematic teen involvement in marital interactions can result. When the deficits are limited to the parent–teen dyads, teenagers are unlikely to become inappropriately involved in their parents' affairs. In multiproblem families there is usually a history of marital disord prior to the disruption of homeostatic functioning by adolescent independence seeking; the adolescent striving for independence adds a new twist to the already existing strife, complicating the clinical picture considerably.

CONCLUSIONS

In this chapter we have presented a model that defines parent–adolescent conflict as predominantly verbal disputes concerning specific issues; these conflicts are regarded as a natural developmental phenomenon that results when young adolescents begin to individuate from the nuclear family. The manner in which the family reacts to this biologically driven, culturally mediated developmental transition of its younger members determines whether a period of "normative crisis" subsides or escalates to clinical proportions. Escalation is hypothesized to occur when family members display deficits in problem-solving communication skills, distorted cognitive processes, or problems in family structure. We have outlined how skills, cognitions, and structure are the building blocks for interlocking sequences of interaction that repeat themselves over time and constitute the "functions" or mechanisms by which problem behaviors are maintained. In the next chapter we turn to the evidence in support of this model.

NOTE

1. Most of the commentary in this book applies broadly to mainstream Western cultures, but whether it is equally applicable to subcultures (such as blacks and Hispanics) in Western society, or to non-Western cultures, is an empirical question. It is quite possible that distinct culturally specific routes exist for managing the transition from childhood to adult life, and that the adaptiveness of these different routes varies depending upon cultural norms and practices.

CHAPTER THREE

Empirical Evaluation of Behavioral–Family Systems Theory

The hallmark of a behavioral approach to clinical phenomena is empiricism. Theories, assessment devices, and therapies are derived from principles of scientific psychology and are expected either to withstand the scrutiny of scientific research or to be modified or discarded. The behavioral–family systems theory of parent–adolescent conflict is no exception. A number of studies test our theory. In this chapter we summarize existing research and suggest future directions for theory-testing studies.

Specific testable hypotheses are essential to evaluate a multifaceted theory. Experimental and/or correlational tests of these hypotheses provide evidence for or against them. In the case of parent–adolescent conflict, the ideal experiment is both unethical and impractical: randomly assign a large group of families to conditions where skills as well as cognitive, structural, and functional variables are manipulated to induce maximum versus minimum conflict. Longitudinal and cross-sectional studies of naturally occurring groups of families differing on relevant variables represent reasonable alternative strategies.

In longitudinal research, an investigator might select a representative sample of families with preadolescents and assess relevant aspects of family functioning periodically throughout their growth and development from age 9 or 10 until age 19 or 20. To date, few longitudinal studies have been conducted. In cross-sectional research, an investigator compares the amount of parent–adolescent conflict in intact groups known to differ on relevant independent variables. While differences among groups do not logically imply that the independent variables caused the conflict, they are at least consistent with causal hypotheses. Through careful selection of variables in a programmatic research effort, competing hypotheses can be eliminated and quasi-causal inferences made. Most of the research to be reviewed here falls in this category.

Investigators often test theories of psychopathology by providing intervention consistent with a particular theoretical framework. If the intervention proves successful, they interpret the results as supporting the underlying theoretical premises. However, such inferences represent a serious error in logic. The effectiveness of a particular intervention does not necessarily support the underlying theoretical model of the development of the clinical problem, although it is certainly consistent with the theory. Aspirin ameliorates headache pain, but we would not conclude that headache pain is caused by a lack of aspirin. We do not therefore consider our reasonably successful treatment outcome research (see Chapter 14) as confirmatory of the behavioral–family systems theory of parent–adolescent conflict.

BEHAVIORAL–FAMILY SYSTEMS HYPOTHESES

Many specific testable hypotheses can be derived from the theory presented in this volume. Here we restrict our review to five general assertions that have been or are in the process of being researched.

1. Families are homeostatic systems. The biological changes of puberty lead to adolescent independence seeking, which disrupts homeostatic functioning, and parent–adolescent conflict erupts as families attempt to restore homeostatic functioning.

2. Deficits in positive problem-solving and communication skills lead to unresolved disagreements and heated verbal arguments.

3. Strong adherence to unreasonable beliefs or misattributions about family life promotes conflict. This link occurs because unrealistic expectations or malevolent misattributions induce angry reactions to parent–adolescent disagreements, impeding effective communication or problem solving and promoting reciprocity of negative affect and behavior.

4. Distressed families exhibit greater reciprocity of negative and less reciprocity of positive behavior and affect than nondistressed families.

5. There is not always a relationship between parent–teen and marital conflict. However, marital discord is occasionally a causal and/or maintaining variable in parent–teen conflict. This relationship is most likely either when marital conflict is severe and long-standing or when adolescents' conflictual behavior comes to serve inappropriate homeostatic functions in parents' affairs.

Families as Homeostatic Systems

That families are homeostatic systems is a basic concept. As discussed earlier, from a behavioral–family systems perspective, homeostatic functioning is a convenient construct that represents circular sequences of interactive, three-term contingencies where each member's behavior influences and is influenced by the others' behavior. Over time these mutual control contingencies are self-maintaining. Principles of reinforcement, punishment, discrimination, extinction, and other learning phenomena have been widely explored with both animals and humans since the publication of the book *Schedules of Reinforcement* (Ferster & Skinner, 1957). The applicability of these concepts to the understanding and modification of human behavior is reflected by the proliferation of journals such as the *Journal of Applied Behavior Analysis, Behavior Modification, Behavior Therapy,* and others. Reciprocity and coercion, representing interlocking patterns of behavior, have also been empirically explored, and will be summarized later.

The second portion of the homeostasis hypothesis (that the biological changes of puberty spur adolescent independence seeking, which disrupts family homeostasis and increases conflict), has received indirect support from developmental research. Steinberg (Steinberg, 1981; Steinberg & Hill, 1978) studied the relationship between physical maturation and family interaction in cross-sectional and longitudinal investigations with adolescent boys and their parents. His results suggested that the pattern of mother–son and father–son relations throughout puberty were quite different. From the onset of puberty until the pubertal apex, mother–son conflict increased, as evidenced by increased adolescent interruptions and decreased mother–son explanations; overall family rigidity also increased. In addition, adolescents deferred less to their mothers. During the later part of puberty, mother–adolescent conflict subsided, with the mother (not the adolescent) backing off, suggesting increased adolescent dominance over mothers. Although fathers also interrupted sons more and gave explanations less from the onset to the apex of puberty, the adolescents became less assertive and more deferential toward the fathers. This pattern of paternal dominance and adolescent deference continued into late puberty.

The hypothesis that adolescent independence seeking disrupts family homeostasis could also be evaluated by assessing homeostatic functioning across the family life cycle and demonstrating significant disruption during adolescence. Although no longitudinal studies directly address this question, cross-sectional investigations of marital satisfaction in separate groups of families at various stages of the family life cycle provide an indirect test. If marital satisfaction can be assumed to represent one measure of homeostatic functioning, we would predict less satisfaction in couples with adolescent children than in couples with younger or older children. Data supporting this prediction were reported by Snyder (1981) and Margolin (1981).

Alternatively, disruptions of homeostasis might be evaluated by asking families to participate in analogue (as opposed to naturalistic) tasks designed to induce stressful deviation from normal family patterns, then assessing the reaction of the system. Minuchin, Rosman, and Baker (1978) reported a study testing the structural family theory of psychosomatic illness using a laboratory task to assess the effects of disruptions of family homeostasis. In one part of the study, families with diabetic children participated in a three-phase interview: (1) parents discussed a family problem while the children watched behind a one-way mirror; (2) the interviewer took sides with one spouse against the other to exacerbate conflict while the children continued to watch behind the mirror; and (3) the children entered the room to participate in the parental dispute. The family transactions throughout the three phases of the interview were then assessed.

Three groups of families were included: (1) nine families with psychosomatic diabetic children; (2) seven families with nonpsychosomatic diabetic children; and (3) eight families with diabetics whose illness was under good medical control but who had been referred for behavioral problems. "Psychosomatic diabetes" was diagnosed by physicians as a condition where a child had recurrent bouts of ketoacidosis triggered by emotional stress and not controlled by massive doses of insulin. Diabetic acidosis is preceded by a rise in the concentration of free fatty acid found in the blood; free fatty acid is also a marker for emotional arousal. The free fatty acid levels of the family members were monitored throughout the interview to document the relationship between family stress and psychosomatic crises.

Compared to the other two groups, the psychosomatic diabetics displayed elevated free fatty acid levels throughout all phases of the interview. When the psychosomatic diabetic children were present in the room with their parents, their free fatty acid levels continued to rise; afterwards, the levels did not return to baseline. The free fatty acid level of the parents of the psychosomatic diabetics was also elevated during phases one and two of the interview; however, the parents' free fatty acid levels decreased when their children were brought into the conflictual discussion; no such effect was noted for the other two groups. Presence of the children decreased the parents' physiological indices of emotional arousal, at the cost of the continued rise in the children's arousal, propelling them toward disease.

Thus, disruption in family patterns can, at least in some families, produce physiological arousal. Assuming that this arousal is experienced as negative, family members should attempt to reduce this aversiveness. Behaviors that serve to decrease unpleasant autonomic arousal should be negatively reinforced. In this case, the presence of the child in the psychosomatic families served just such a function for the parents. This investigation thus supports the assumptions that changes in homeostatic family interaction patterns may elicit stress responses in individual family members and that family members contribute to complex interlocking contingency mechanisms that can support particular interaction patterns.

Problem-Solving Communication Skill Deficits

The hypothesis that deficits in problem-solving communication skills lead to verbal disagreements and arguments over independence-related issues has been tested by comparing the skills of families referred for treatment of relational problems and families satisfied with their relationships. In early studies, investigators frequently explored observational categories they assumed represented higher order constructs in family interaction, but with low face validity as communication skills, such as duration of talk time and number of successful interruptions. Nonetheless, several of these studies showed that, when given a task requiring the family to arrive at a consensual solution to a problem, distressed families took longer to reach agreements (Ferreira, Winter, & Poindexter, 1966) and were less likely to reach consensus (Hetherington, Stouwie, & Ridberg, 1971; Riskin & Faunce, 1970b).

Other studies have examined more specific behavior assumed to represent "skilled" and "nonskilled" communication. These investigations have found that those parents and adolescents referred for relationship distress report more negative communication, more intense specific disputes, and more negative interaction time and display more negative problem-solving communication behavior and less positive supportive behavior in analogue observations than families satisfied with their relationships (Alexander, 1973; Prinz, Foster, Kent, & O'Leary, 1979; Robin & Weiss, 1980; Vincent-Roehling & Robin, 1986). When the specific components of negative communication and problem solving have been examined, distressed families were found to emit fewer problem-specification, problem-solution, evaluation, agreement, praise, humor, and accept-responsibility statements and to emit more commands and put-downs than nondistressed families (Robin & Weiss, 1980).

Furthermore, families referred to a clinic for parent–child relational problems have been found to display more negative communication than families referred for other adolescent psychological problems. Finally, direct correlations between the levels of independence-related conflict and problem-solving communication behavior have been significant and moderate (−.43, −.39, and −.34 for mothers, fathers, and adolescents, respectively; Adams, 1987; Nayar, 1982).

Taken together, the results of these correlational and cross-sectional studies support the behavioral–family systems hypothesis concerning deficits in problem-solving communication skills, but are less than definitive because of their correlational nature, the failure to distinguish carefully between "skill" and "performance" deficits, and the laboratory-analogue nature of the observational studies, limiting generalizability to real-life problem solving.

Cognitive Distortions

Recent evidence supports the link between unreasonable beliefs, misattributions, and family conflict. Investigators comparing the degree of adherence to unreasonable beliefs of clinic-referred and nonclinic families with 12- to 17-year-old adolescents find that clinic-referred parents adhere more strongly to beliefs concerning ruination, perfectionism, and malicious intent than nonclinic fathers, and that clinic-referred teenagers adhere more strongly to beliefs concerning ruination, unfairness, and autonomy than nonclinic referred teenagers (Robin, Koepke, & Moye, 1986; Vincent-Roehling & Robin, 1986). Research with parents of younger abused and neglected children has also established a link between unrealistic expectations, malicious attributions, and abusive behavior (Azar, Robinson, Hekimian, & Twentyman, 1984; Bauer & Twentyman, 1985; Twentyman, Rorhbeck, & Amish, 1984).

While these investigations indicate that families in conflict endorse unreasonable beliefs and misattributions, they do not establish the process through which such distorted cognitive processes contribute to conflict. For example, do such beliefs in fact induce anger, which then interferes with positive communication and effective problem solving, or is there some other mechanism? Laboratory-analogue studies that experimentally manipulate cognitive content and affective states and assess the resulting influences on family interaction are needed to establish this link. Barton and Alexander (1979) reported on such a study. In this investigation, families with delinquent and nondelinquent teenagers played a game after competitive versus cooperative instructions were given. Competitive instructions (i.e., that only one member could win) produced more defensive behavior for delinquent than for nondelinquent families, supporting the hypothesis that adversarial thoughts lead to negative behavior in troubled families.

Additional studies that assess cognitions more directly during ongoing interaction are needed to address the role of cognition in family communication. In addition, a broad-based approach should be used to establish the range, diversity, and prevalence of cognitive distortions in clinic versus nonclinic families. Finally, in some cases of extreme adolescent misbehavior, so-called "unrealistic beliefs" are more accurately described as "realistic appraisals" of severe problem behavior. For example, ruinous concerns about sexuality would be realistic for a sexually active teenager who has been pregnant in the past and currently refuses to employ birth control. Researchers need to develop methods to assess when unrealistic beliefs are truly unrealistic.

Reciprocity

Patterson, Reid, and their colleagues' pioneering work illustrated patterns of reciprocity in families of younger children, exploring both reciprocity and coercion through sophisticated conditional probability and correlational analyses (Patterson, 1976, 1979, 1982). Rate-matching and contingent reciprocity have also been explored using observations of married couples as well (Gottman, 1979; Wills, Weiss, & Patterson, 1974).

Several studies examined reciprocity with parents and adolescents. Correlational analyses provide strong evidence for rate-matching reciprocity between parents and adolescents for defensive and supportive communication (Alexander, 1973), ratings of mutual appreciation, compliments, personal attack, anger and hostility, and complaints about unfairness (Prinz, Rosenblum, & O'Leary, 1978), quantity of positive and negative interaction time at home assessed via family members' daily records (Robin, Nayar, & Rayha, 1984), positive and negative problem-solving communication behavior displayed during audiotaped discussions, and anger-intensity levels reported for specific disputes (Nayar, 1982; Rayha, 1982). Examinations of whether distressed and nondistressed families differ in reciprocity of positive and negative behavior have produced mixed results. Alexander (1973) found modest evidence for greater reciprocity of defensive behavior in families with delinquent adolescents and greater reciprocity of supportive behavior in families with nondelinquent adolescents.

We reanalyzed data from a previous investigation of parent–teen communication, by collapsing observational categories into "positive," "negative," and "neutral" (Robin & Weiss, 1980). Analysis yielded no clear-cut differences between distressed and nondistressed mother–son dyads for rate-matching reciprocity and for contingent reciprocity of positive behavior. The likelihood that distressed mothers and sons, however, would respond to a negative remark with another negative behavior was significantly greater than the base rate of negative behavior, indicating contingent reciprocity of negative behavior. Nondistressed dyads did not display this pattern. Clearly, much remains to be done in this area, particularly with respect to the selection of the appropriate degree of molarity or molecularity in the unit of interaction to be examined for reciprocity.

Marital and Parent–Adolescent Conflict

One way of testing the hypothesis that marital discord will determine and/or maintain parent–teen conflict under certain (but not all) circumstances is to assess the correlations between marital and parent–adolescent conflict in families. If there is an occasional but not inevitable relationship between the two variables, we would predict moderate overall correlations in large-sample research. Investigators then need to examine subsamples of families with severe and mild marital conflict to search for different patterns of parent–adolescent conflict. Laboratory-analogue studies could also experimentally manipulate specific variables in the marital relationship and examine the effects on parent–adolescent interactions as a way of determining the functions of adolescent behavior in the marital system.

At the present time, only correlational studies have been conducted. Most showed a relationship between related marital communication or discord and childhood behavior problems. A few others explored patterns of parent–parent interaction during parent–adolescent discussions, finding that observed patterns of parent comments differ in clinic-referred and nonreferred families, including voicing more disagreements and aggressive statements to each other (Hetherington et al., 1971) and agreeing less often on solutions to hypothetical problems assessed by questionnaires (Hetherington et al., 1971). Unfortunately, these studies fail to indicate whether these communication patterns were related to general dissatisfaction with each other or were limited to discussions when parents were trying to reach agreements with their child. Nor did these studies provide functional analyses of behavior or comparisons of families with different severity levels of marital discord. The research of Minuchin et al. (1978) with psychosomatic families, reviewed earlier in this chapter, comes closest to capturing functional relationships between children's behavior and parents' marital discord.

Emery (1982) reviewed the correlational research relating marital distress and childhood behavior problems. These studies typically employed broad clinic- and/or non-clinic-referred samples of families with boys and girls of all ages, making it difficult to draw specific conclusions about adolescents. Many of the studies also suffered from a variety of methodological flaws, including biased sampling, same judges rating both marital and child problems, use of psychometrically unsound measures, and failure to operationalize sufficiently the basic constructs under study.

Nonetheless, Emery summarized a number of general findings of the research:

1. Prolonged, openly hostile marital conflict is associated with greater child behavior problems than less prolonged, more general, and less openly hostile marital conflict.
2. Marital discord is more closely related to externalizing, undercontrolled childhood behavior disturbances than to internalizing, overcontrolled disturbances.
3. Marital turmoil has a greater effect on boys than on girls, but failure to consider adequately the possible differences between girls' and boys' reactions to marital conflict limits this conclusion.
4. A particularly warm relationship with at least one parent can mitigate, to some extent, the detrimental effects of marital conflict.
5. Age does not appear to relate to the severity of child behavior problems associated with marital conflict.
6. Marital conflict may be a third variable mediating many previously found correlations between individual parental pathology and childhood behavior problems.

Two of our investigations specifically examined the relationship of parent–adolescent and marital conflict. Foster and Steinfeld (1980) found little relationship between global marital distress (assessed using the Locke–Wallace Marital Adjustment Test) and parent–adolescent conflict (assessed using a comprehensive battery of observational and self-report measures of parent–teen relations) in distressed families referred for behavioral family treatment of parent–adolescent relational problems. Using the Marital Satisfaction Inventory, a multidimensional measure of marital discord, Rayha (1982) found that the Conflict over Child Rearing and Dissatisfaction with Children scales correlated moderately with families' reported anger intensity of parent–teen disputes and with observations of negative communication–problem solving. Scores on these scales also discriminated between families with and without parent–teen conflict. However, none of the more specific marital satisfaction scales produced either significant correlations or significant between-group differences.

Because of differences in populations, measurement techniques, and procedures, caution is warranted in generalizing from these studies. Nonetheless, the weak-to-moderate correlations support the behavioral–family systems position that there is not an inevitable relationship between parent–adolescent and marital conflict. The two studies we conducted specifically with adolescents suggest that, at least in families presenting for our clinical research programs, marital conflict does not necessarily covary with parent–adolescent conflict, although there are families where such patterns exist. Studies of this sort, however, cannot discriminate families in which marital conflict is avoided successfully via parent–teen interaction patterns, since these parents presumably would report general satisfaction with their marriages because conflict is detoured. Future investigations need to examine more closely the conditions under which adolescents' conflicts with their parents serve important functions in the parents' marriages.

Summary of Evaluations of Theoretical Hypotheses

The evidence reviewed here provides partial confirmation for each of the five hypotheses derived from the behavioral–family systems theory of parent–adolescent conflict. Hypotheses concerning deficits in problem-solving communication skills and the relationship of parent–teen and marital conflict have received the greatest degree of research attention, with considerably less emphasis on cognitive distortions, homeostasis, and reciprocity. Research reviewed here has distinct strengths and weaknesses. Its greatest strengths include developing psychometrically sound tools for assessing theoretical constructs and attacking extremely complicated questions creatively. The greatest weaknesses include reliance upon cross-sectional rather than longitudinal designs, inclusion of small numbers of families relative to the number of variables assessed, and failure to address directly the functional relationships among family members' behaviors. These weaknesses need to be corrected to produce more definitive conclusions from future research.

IMPLICATIONS FOR ASSESSMENT AND TREATMENT

The behavioral–family systems theory of parent–adolescent conflict grew inductively out of our experiences assessing and treating families, shaped by our basic commitment to integrating a behavioristic, empirical tradition with family systems concepts (Foster & Hoier, 1982). Since the theory is intended to guide practitioners, it has many more specific implications for intervention than can be enumerated here. Several of the most salient implications are summarized:

1. A multidimensional model of conflict mandates a multidimensional assessment battery and a multidimensional treatment program. If skills, cognitions, structure, and function are all critical dimensions of family interactions, tools are needed for assessing and treating each dimension of the problem. Assessment tools should not only meet psychometric and behavioral assessment measurement standards but should also tap multiple vantage points with multiple

measurement methods. Interventions should be available to teach skills, restructure cognitions, change family structure, and address the functions of adolescent misbehavior within the entire family system.

2. All families in conflict are not equivalent. Some will display the greatest problems in skills, others in cognitions, and others in structure and function. The therapist must be able to combine diverse intervention components flexibly to meet the needs of idiosyncratic presenting problems of particular families. Treatment components need to be clearly specified and relatively independent of each other in order to permit such synthesis.

3. Since parent–adolescent conflict represents a family's attempt to regain homeostatic functioning during the period of a teenager's increased independence seeking, the therapist should be prepared to encounter resistance during intervention. Conflictual interactions represent a self-maintaining homeostatic state which the therapist interrupts. In addition, change involves response cost to family members in the form of homework, attending to and altering their interaction patterns, and possibly experiencing anxiety associated with developing new relationship routines. Faced with possible chaos, families may fail to comply with therapeutic interventions privately, despite their public protestations that they wish to change.

CHAPTER FOUR

Assessment—
Overview and Interviewing

Thorough assessment is an integral part of the behavioral–family systems approach to parent–adolescent conflict. The information collected during this initial phase of therapy provides the foundation for treatment geared to the family's specific problems and interaction patterns. In addition, during assessment the therapist begins the therapy process by establishing appropriate expectations for treatment, providing the family with a constructive experience of discussing their difficulties, and relabeling or reframing family members' attributions and beliefs about the nature of their problems in ways that will be conducive to later interventions.

The assessment phase generally lasts between $1\frac{1}{2}$ and 3 hours, depending upon the family, and has several specific goals. The first of these to collect information regarding the presenting problems, the issues of dispute, problem-solving communication skills, cognitive and affective experiences, family structure, and the recurring interactive sequences that comprise the functions of behavior within the family system. These are the primary content areas derived from the behavioral–family systems model of parent–adolescent relations reviewed in Chapters 2 and 3. A second goal is to determine which strategies employed in the treatment program are appropriate for the family at that time. Third, the therapist explains the treatment approach and its rationale to the family to enable the members to understand the relevance of a behavioral–family systems intevention for their particular difficulties.

In addition to specific assessment goals, the therapist has more general goals related to the process of engaging the family in therapy. These goals revolve around setting the stage for later treatment by establishing the basis for a productive working relationship with all family members. This aspect of assessment is frequently quite difficult and entails maintaining an impartial style and avoiding the appearance of alliances with particular family members while simultaneously remaining involved and attentive to all parties' concerns.

The approach taken to achieving these goals is based upon the paradigm of behavioral assessment (Ciminero, Calhoun, & Adams, 1986; Haynes, 1978; Mash & Terdal, 1988; Nelson & Hayes, 1979). In order to understand the rationale underlying the development and evaluation of instruments considered in the next three chapters, it is important to develop an appreciation of this paradigm.

Behavioral assessment differs from traditional assessment in several important respects (Goldfried & Kent, 1972; Nelson & Hayes, 1979). Traditional assessment generally adheres to either a dynamic or trait conception of personality. Unobservable, intraorganismic variables are hypothesized to account for behavior. By contrast, behavioral assessment espouses a situational or interactionalist conception of personality. Behavior is seen to be a function of environmental contingencies, interacting at times with organismic variables, not a function of traits, intrapsychic phenomena, or psychodynamic processes. The therapist is interested in assessing problematic behaviors (overt and covert), current and historical antecedents for these behaviors, and consequences of these behaviors.

Under a traditional approach, the target events of interest are assumed to occur cross-situationally, since they are the products of processes or traits carried around within the person. Responses to assessment measures are consequently viewed as signs of the underlying constructs that determine behavior. As long as the assessment measures appear to tap the relevant constructs, the assessor need not attend to situational variables. Within behavioral assessment the cross-situational consistency of behavior is an empirical issue; no a priori assumptions are made, although early behavioral assessors tended to discount the possibility of cross-situational consistency (Mischel, 1968). Situational factors related to the content and use of assessment tools are consequently of paramount concern to the behavioral clinician. Responses to assessment instruments are viewed as samples of criterion events, not signs of underlying constructs. Thus, issues pertaining to the representativeness, directness, and methods of sampling these criterion events, as well as psychometric considerations of reliability and validity, are germane to behavioral assessment and predominate the discussions that follow.

We have employed three primary methods of assessment: the clinical interview, standardized self-report questionnaires, and direct observation. From this chapter through Chapter 6, we will describe how we use these three methods to assess the content areas derived from a behavioral–family systems model of parent–adolescent conflict. This chapter focuses on the clinical interview, a primary assessment method, while Chapter 5 focuses on self-report and observational methods. Chapter 6 provides guidelines for integrating assessment information derived from all three methods to form a comprehensive picture of the family.

THE BEHAVIORAL INTERVIEW

The behavioral interview provides one of the most useful and efficient methods of collecting relevant information for intervention. Rather than seeing verbal reports as reflections of underlying personality dynamics or unconscious processes, the behaviorally oriented interviewer is concerned with the relationship of client reports and therapist observations in the session to behavior in situations and settings outside therapy. Consequently, behavioral assessment interviewing often focuses on pinpointing the occurrence, dimensions, and interrelatedness of specific events, thoughts, and affective reactions, rather than on discussing global, inferential constructs.

The versatility of the behavioral interview makes it particularly useful for family assessment. Through the interview, the therapist can begin to accomplish several goals important to setting the stage for therapy: gathering information, screening the family to determine whether problem-solving communication treatment is appropriate, explaining the treatment and its rationale, and establishing a good working relationship with all family members. These goals are generally addressed during four stages of assessment interviews: (1) greeting and overview of the session, (2) information gathering, (3) providing feedback to the family and describing a relevant treatment approach, and (4) setting goals and establishing a treatment contract.

While the interview ordinarily follows this sequence, occasional deviations are necessary. In some cases, for example, information gathering may be sacrificed in order to build rapport with a reluctant adolescent or to intervene in a crisis situation. This underscores the idea that, despite the structured, didactic approach of the treatment program, intervention is an interactive process in which the therapist must guide the progress of therapy while simultaneously assessing the family's ability at each given moment to follow this guidance. Common problems that are encountered in assessment interviews and that influence this interactive process are described throughout the chapter.

Greeting and Overview

Members of a family entering treatment are often not uniformly committed to therapy. Frequently one or both parents have decided that their adolescent must be "fixed" and bring him/her to the therapist, implicitly or explicitly requesting a cure. Teenagers may be ill-informed about where they are going and why. "Psychiatrist," "psychologist," and "mental health center" are often synonymous with "crazy," particularly for a young teenager. The adolescent may feel tricked or forced into seeing the therapist and/or may have argued unsuccessfully about attending the session prior to the family's arrival. Parents, too, may wonder why they should attend the session if they feel that their offspring is solely to blame for the presenting problem, may question whether therapy is appropriate, and may feel nervous about confiding in a stranger with their adolescent present. The goals of the initial greeting phase of the first session are to (1) reduce the anxiety any family members may feel, (2) correct misinformation, (3) describe briefly the format of the assessment phase, and (4) permit the therapist to interact positively with each family member.

In our experience, the adolescent is the family member most likely to be reticent and misinformed. As in the clinical process of systematic desensitization, anxiety can be reduced by beginning the session with neutral or positive topics and working into more conflict-laden issues as the family appears to relax. With the adolescent, this process can begin in the waiting room. A supply of teen-oriented magazines and comic books can give the therapist a lead-in for informal chat with the adolescent en route to the interview room. Noticing the adolescent's clothing (e.g., running shoes, a ski jacket with lift tickets) or an item s/he may have brought to the session can also be used to begin a conversation. Therapist comments that are brief, informal, and use simple, colloquial language are most likely to elicit friendly responses from a teenager. For example, "I see you were reading 'Doonesbury.' I really like that cartoon. Do you read it at home?" is preferable to a more adult-oriented comment like " 'Doonesbury' is very witty, particularly the politically oriented cartoons." Informal conversation with the parents can revolve around parking, locating the building, and so forth. This initial phase, usually lasting no more than 5 minutes, introduces the parents and the adolescent to the therapist's style and allows the therapist to communicate interest in the family in a nonthreatening fashion.

Once the casual greeting is finished, the therapist can give an overview of the session. It is often useful to assess any misconceptions and concerns that family members have about participating in the assessment. In our experience, one parent initially contacts the therapist to set up an appointment. The therapist then asks this individual to communicate information about the initial session to the other parent and to the adolescent. Asking relevant family members what they had been told or understood about the session often elicits misconceptions about both assessment and treatment in general. The therapist can introduce the topic by saying something like

THERAPIST: I spoke with you, Mrs. Johnston, and explained a little bit about how I work and what to expect from this session. But I didn't get a chance to speak to you, Mr. Johnston, or to you, Bill. So that I don't repeat any information, perhaps you could tell me what your mother [wife] told you about today's meeting.

If family members respond with an accurate thumbnail sketch, the therapist can then give an overview of the session.

THERAPIST: That's pretty close. What I would like to do now is to give you an idea of how we'll spend our time together today. One of the things I do is to teach families how to get along better. To see if what I do might be helpful to you, I'll need to find out more about how all of you see your family—what you like about how you get along and how you would like this to improve. Today we'll talk for about an hour. During this, I hope you will ask questions or bring up anything that concerns you about what I say. Do you have any questions before we get started?

The session overview will vary depending on how the family has been referred to the therapist and how the therapist structures the assessment phase. In our outcome research, families most often respond to newspaper notices advertising a specific program. By their presence, the family is indicating their evaluation that the program may be beneficial for them. In these cases, the therapist should provide a basic description about the program during the course of the session. In research settings, assessment is generally conducted in a long single session, sometimes lasting $1\frac{1}{2}$ to 3 hours, and in this case, the therapist should also explain that the family will complete questionnaires and hold a sample discussion during this time.

Such lengthy sessions may not be feasible in clinical settings, and the therapist may need two or three interviews to collect sufficient information to plan a treatment strategy. In addition, the therapist may wish to obtain and score questionnaire information and an interaction sample before outlining the treatment approach. Inexperienced family therapists may require additional time to complete a family assessment. In these cases, the therapist should be sure to inform the family, either during the overview or at the end of the session, that the first two or three meetings will be devoted to getting a clearer idea of the problem and that the therapist will at the end of this time propose an intervention (see Jacobson & Margolin, 1979, for an example of how this is presented in marital therapy).

An alternate approach for structuring the initial session is to interview the adolescent and parents alone during portions of the session. This allows the parents and therapist to discuss topics that the parents prefer not to raise with the teenager present, such as marital problems or interpretations of the adolescent's difficulties. In addition, teens who contribute only monosyllables during the family interview may become more verbal when interviewed alone and voice concerns they are afraid to talk about with both parents present. In some circumstances, the therapist may even begin the assessment session by seeing the adolescent alone, as, for example, when the therapist has been forewarned that the teenager is likely to be extremely resistant and wishes to immediately begin building rapport before collecting information.

In seeing family members alone, however, the therapist risks suspicions about "secret information" and alliances, which may damage rapport with the parents or the adolescent. Confidentiality problems may arise as well, as when a teenager confides major drug use about which the parents are unaware. These dilemmas are serious enough to warrant judicious consideration of how to structure the initial interview. To avoid later difficulties, the therapist who interviews individuals alone should inform the parents and adolescent about his or her stance regarding confidentiality (Margolin, 1982). This stance can range from telling family members that disclosure of information from individual sessions is up to the therapist, to informing them that such information will not be revealed without their oral or written consent. We prefer two intermediate positions. In the first, family members are told that information will be shared at the therapist's discretion, but that the therapist will respect members' wishes about what should not be disclosed unless this secrecy interferes with progress, and will discuss sharing of sensitive information with them in advance. In the second, members are told that they will be able after the individual interview to inform the therapist as to which information should be treated as confidential, and the therapist will respect these wishes. In selecting a position about confidentiality, it is important for the therapist to investigate professional guidelines and state laws, particularly those related to the confidentiality of information given by an adolescent minor, as these vary from state to state.

Several snags can occur when the therapist elicits family members' perceptions of what they think will transpire during the initial sessions of assessment and therapy. The following annotated dialogues illustrate some of these, with samples of recommended responses for the therapist.

Example 1.

BILL: My mom said we were going to the doctor, not to see a psychiatrist.

THERAPIST: Well, I'm not exactly a doctor, but I'm not a psychiatrist, either. I'm a psychologist [social worker, etc.]. I don't give shots or medicine or anything like that. I talk with families who want to learn some ways of getting along better. That doesn't mean they're crazy, or that anyone in the family is a bad person—just that they want to find out some new ways of handling things so they can be happier.

Commentary. In this segment, the therapist attempts to correct the teen's misinformation, and debunk the child's belief (implied by the "psychiatrist" comment) that he is "crazy" because he is visiting a therapist. The therapist also labels the intervention as a family process in which the participants learn more productive interactive styles. This implicitly assists in establishing appropriate expectations for treatment.

Example 2.

MR. JOHNSTON: Actually, this was my wife's idea. To be perfectly honest, I'm not sure why I'm here. The problem has always been between her and Bill. She simply is too soft on him.

THERAPIST: So to you, the problem is with Mrs. Johnston and Bill, and you're not sure what role you should play in this whole process *(Mr. Johnston nods)*. I can understand your feelings, and appreciate your taking the time to come in this afternoon. One of the things we'll try to figure out today is whether or not you do fit into their conflicts. It's possible, too, that even if you aren't directly involved, you could be a big help in assisting them to get along better. Probably this will all get sorted out as we go along, though, and we'll be able to figure out better whether and how your family can best benefit from my help once I know a little bit more about you. Does this seem reasonable?

Commentary. In this segment, the therapist wishes to establish rapport with the father and therefore reflects Mr. Johnston's feelings, acknowledges his point of view, and provides information about how his concern will be addressed during the course of the session. The therapist also sidesteps siding with one parent against the other, despite the father's attempts to enlist him/her as an ally.

Example 3.

SUSAN: I don't know why my parents brought *me*. We get along OK.

THERAPIST: It sounds like you're not sure you should be here. *(Susan shrugs)* Did you want to come?

SUSAN: No.

MRS. BROWNING: We had quite an argument about it this afternoon.

THERAPIST: *(To Susan)* So coming here wasn't exactly your choice.

SUSAN: No.

THERAPIST: I appreciate your coming even though you didn't want to. One of the things I want to do today is for all of us to consider whether there is anything that any of you can get out of working with me. It doesn't mean that you are here for good. In fact, I don't want you to keep coming after today if you really don't think you and your family can get anything out of this.

SUSAN: I don't think it will do any good.

THERAPIST: Right now you're not sure it will help. And I don't want you to be here unless you can get something out of coming. *(To the family)* That's true for all of you. *(To Susan)* And maybe you're right. But I'd like for us to wait to make that decision until later on. And if at the end of the session it seems like this isn't for you or your family, then you don't have to come back. OK?

Commentary. The therapist's statement that Susan is not yet committed to returning is made in order to establish rapport with Susan and increase the likelihood that she will participate instead of resisting the therapist's questions throughout the assessment. Hopefully, permitting Susan to contribute to the decision to return will buy the therapist enough time to help Susan see the potential benefits of further treatment. The therapist risks, of course, losing her subsequent participation. In our experience, few adolescents we interview refuse to come back, at least for a time-limited course of intervention.[1] In cases where the teen's participation is mandated (e.g., by the court or by a physician, as in a case of a life-threatening condition such as anorexia nervosa), the therapist can elicit and reflect the adolescent's concern about therapy, tell the teenager that s/he unfortunately does not have a choice about whether or not to be there but does have a large voice in how therapy will proceed, and encourage the adolescent to use that infuence in order to make therapy a beneficial experience for him/her. With either approach, the therapist's remarks approach Susan as a young adult, capable of making important choices.

Information Gathering

The bulk of clinical interviewing revolves around information gathering. Two kinds of information collected during this phase form the basis for later hypotheses about functional relationships among family interactive behaviors: (1) information about the content of family discord and (2) information about the process by which disagreements are resolved or left unsettled. The interview provides two sources for collecting this information. One comes from the content of family members' responses, while the other is based on therapist observations of family process during the session, which supplement and corroborate the content the family provides verbally. Questionnaire and observational measures also assist this information gathering, and are discussed in Chapter 5.

Although we have broken down the information to be collected into content and process categories, in practice the therapist's questions integrate the two areas. As mentioned previously, when family members appear reluctant or anxious, a useful rule of thumb is to begin the interview with more general questions, then lead into more focused and specific probes about conflict resolution and communication patterns. A good way to begin is to gather demographic information (age and occupation of parents, names and ages of siblings, etc.), then to inquire briefly about the factors that prompted the family to request intervention. These factors establish in preliminary fashion the treatment goals of at least some family members, and may indicate the respondent's view of who is responsible for the problems—adolescent, parent, or family. In general, more accusatory statements of reasons for referral will require more relabeling and explanation from the therapist for family intervention to seem relevant to the individual making the statement. The therapist short-circuits lengthy tirades and minute explications of particular troublesome incidents at this point, as these are often accusatory and anger-provoking, and/or their relevance does not justify the time required for the family member to describe the episode.

It is prudent to ask family members about their perceptions of reasons for referral, particularly when opening remarks by one member provoke a negative response from someone else. This reaction may be expressed overtly, by contradicting the speaker, or more covertly, by nonverbal mannerisms such as frowning, turning away slightly, or sighing. The goal of the therapist in requesting other opinions is to establish a pattern of acknowledging all points of view without allowing an argument to ensue.

   Example.

THERAPIST: To start out, I'd be interested in briefly hearing your reasons for coming in today.

MR. WEAVER: Well, we've been having problems with Matt. He never used to talk back—he was a real good kid—but now he's got a smart mouth. *(Matt rolls his eyes)* We thought it was getting out of hand, and some friends suggested that we get some help.

THERAPIST: Then you've been concerned about what you see as Matt's backtalk? Sassiness?

MR. WEAVER: Backtalk and swearing.

THERAPIST: *(Nods)* OK. *(Turns to Matt)* Matt, when your father was talking, you looked like you didn't agree with something he said.

MATT: No. I guess I agree. I just don't like it when he talks about me like that.

THERAPIST: So you rolled your eyes because you didn't like how your dad talked about the backtalk.

MATT: Right.

THERAPIST: How often does Matt roll his eyes at home?

MR. WEAVER: All the time. Whenever he disagrees with us.

THERAPIST: How does Matt's eye-rolling affect you?

MR. WEAVER: It annoys me. If he has something on his mind, he should say it.

THERAPIST: Matt, do you think you backtalk?

MATT: No, not really. But I've got a good temper, and I let them know when I'm not happy. Which is a lot.

THERAPIST: So you, Matt, sometimes express your opinion when you're not pleased about something, and you, Mr. Weaver, don't like the way he does it and see it as backtalk. *(Both Mr. Weaver and Matt nod)* Mrs. Weaver, how do you see the situation?

Commentary. The therapist collects information from all family members in turn, succinctly reflecting relevant content (note that Matt's overgeneralized statement, "Which is a lot," is ignored). By observing and responding to nonverbal as well as verbal cues, the therapist models and establishes a pattern of listening to, clarifying, and acknowledging divergent points of view without taking sides. The therapist also assesses the generality of Matt's in-session eye-rolling behavior by inquiring about its frequency of occurrence and environmental consequences at home.

In the example presented above, the family's reasons for referral are clearly specified and are unambiguously related to their patterns of interaction, and the parents and teen participate in the interview without signs of excessive anxiety. In these cases, the therapist can use the content expressed in the reasons for referral as a springboard for discussion of topics directly related to family interaction. In other cases, the reasons for referral may not seem directly related to family interaction. These include court referrals for delinquent or pre-delinquent behavior, school problems, psychosomatic illness, suicide attempts, and drug abuse. In these cases, a transition statement can help the family to understand better the purpose of the questions about family interaction that will follow. The therapist might begin, "I'll come back to your reasons for coming in later on today. But now, to better understand your situation, I'd like to spend some time talking about how the family as a whole gets along—what you do together, the things each of you likes and dislikes about the family—those sorts of things." Families with obviously anxious members can be asked to discuss positive feelings and behaviors first, as this generally reduces anxiety.

After the interviewer has determined that family members are comfortable discussing their interactions, more specific questions about the content and process of family disagreements can be asked. Below are sample questions that can be used to help family members pinpoint and describe their interactions in specific terms.[2] Note that descriptions of private events (i.e., thoughts and feelings) are elicited along with descriptions of observable behaviors. These are important in deriving functional analyses of family problems and will be discussed further in Chapter 6.

Content-Focused Questions

- What do you like [dislike] about your family [mother, father, son, daughter]?
- If you could choose three things never to discuss [argue about] again, what would they be?
- When you have arguments with your parents [son, daughter], what are they most often about?
- Think about the last time you had a good talk [an argument]. What did you talk [argue] about?
- If you wanted to make your parents [child] really mad, what would you do? Do you ever do that?
- Do you ever feel like you are "nagging"? What are the things you find yourself reminding others about?

Process-Focused Questions

- Think of the last time your family had an argument. Describe what I would have seen if I'd been there. Is this typical?
- How do you let your child [parents] know when you are angry with him [her, them]? (When you are happy with him [her, them]?) How does he [does she, do they] react?
- What do you do when your mother [father, child] gets angry? How do you feel? What do you think about?
- Do you ever try to talk problems over calmly? If so, what happens? How are the times you resolve things different from the times you argue?
- *(To parents)* How often do you find yourself yelling at your child? When are you most likely to yell? What is the effect?
- I'd like to get a general picture of what your family life is like. Could you describe for me a typical day? Start from the time you get up, and tell me about when you see each other, the kinds of things you do, and so forth.

- What would you most like to change about the way you and _____ get along? What is it about the way _____ acts that makes you say that? What is it about that behavior that particularly bothers you?
- What things about yourself could you change to help improve the way you get along with _____ ?
- How do arguments in the family end?
- What would the ideal family be like for you? How is your family like and not like this? What specific things about your family make you say that?
- What is it about _____'s behavior that makes you say he [she] is [trait label]?
- If you wanted to get _____ to change something about her [his] behavior, how would you go about it? How do you think she [he] would react? How would you feel [think] about that?
- How can you keep from getting into arguments? What happens when you do that?
- *(To parents)* How often do you agree on decisions involving your son [daughter]? How do you handle disagreements? How does this influence the way each of you gets along with your son [daughter]?
- *(To adolescent)* Which of your parents do you get along with better? What are the differences between your mom and dad that make you say that? Who is stricter? More lenient?
- *(To adolescent)* When you want something (a privilege, a favor, etc.) from your parents, how do you try to get it?
- Do you have any family rules or routines? What are they? Do people stick to them? If not, what happens? Do you see this as a problem?

An important part of assessing family problems is the informal observation of the ways members interact during the session. Noting consistent, salient verbal and nonverbal exchanges assists in pinpointing communication excesses and deficits and in determining the antecedents and consequences of these patterns. Looking for patterns of influence permits the therapist to begin to formulate structural hypotheses. Checking the congruence between what family members say they do and what they actually do in the session helps the therapist estimate the accuracy of family members' self-reports. The following series of preliminary questions offers a guide to the therapist's observations of family process in sessions.[2]

- What sequences occur in interaction behaviors?
- Under what circumstances and how does communication vary?
- Which family members listen to each other?
- When are they inattentive, and what stylistic features communicate this inattentiveness?
- When do interruptions occur? What form do they take? What happens as a consequence?

- Does the family stay "on-task" when answering a question, or must the therapist exert a great deal of redirection to keep the topic focused?
- How are problems described—in vague, general terms, or more specifically?
- Which topics lead certain family members to clam up, become angry, or change the topic? At which point in the discussion does this occur? How do others respond?
- How does each member respond to similar and divergent opinions? To expressions of positive and negative affect? What reactions are provoked by these responses?
- Does the communication change if parents and adolescents are interviewed separately? How?
- Does one parent intervene and attempt to "make peace" if the other parent and the teenager disagree?
- Does the teenager interfere in parent–parent or parent–therapist communication with interruptions? Other distractions?

While in-session observations may be valuable for generating clinical hypotheses, such hypotheses are best viewed as tentative and subject to verification. There are several reasons for this. One involves generalizability of in-session observations. As systems family therapists point out, the therapist working with a family becomes part of the system, thus changing its structure (Haley, 1976). Put behaviorally, the interview may be reactive: Interactions generated in the therapy environment may differ markedly from those occurring regularly in the home. One way to assess this generalizability informally is to ask the family at the end of the session to describe how their interaction did and did not resemble their discussions at home. This assumes, however, that family members are able to observe, label, and veridically report their behavior.

A second concern about informal in-session observation relates to its status as an assessment device. As such, it should be subjected to the same scrutiny given other assessment instruments. Yet the reliability and validity of unsystematic participant observation have been given little attention. In the absence of such evaluation, therapist observations should perhaps be viewed as one source of potentially biased data that can be added to other assessment sources to produce a tentative composite picture of the family and its interaction.

Feedback and Description of Treatment

The therapist provides summary feedback regarding the family's difficulties and a description of the proposed treatment toward the end of the assessment session(s). This should be a natural outgrowth of the interaction between the therapist and family members up to that point. Throughout the assessment, the therapist labels the information provided by the family in ways that lead the family to see that the treatment strategy is relevant to their particular problems and interaction styles. By rephrasing the family's comments or juxtaposing pieces of information in a novel way, the therapist shifts the family's perceptions of their interactions. Behaviorally oriented clinicians call this relabeling procedure "attributional training" (Valins & Nisbett, 1976), while strategic family therapists use the term "reframing" (Minuchin, 1974). During the assessment session(s), the therapist shapes the members' perceptions by (1) eliciting and reflecting descriptions of their interactive styles, (2) establishing a link between these styles and their presenting problems, and (3) describing how the treatment strategy fits these styles and problems.

The first of these steps involves focusing discussion on family interaction patterns. In part this is accomplished by asking questions like those presented above. Equally important are therapist summaries of family members' responses to these questions. These are the building blocks by which the therapist reconstructs the information, using it to describe for the family the sequences of interactions that transpire among them. As the family members' interaction patterns are fed back to them in this fashion, they are often able to follow the therapist's line of reasoning and to begin to identify problem areas in their interactions that prevent constructive conflict resolution.

Example: The Simpsons (Part 1).

THERAPIST: I'd like to hear more about what you, Bob, mean when you say you don't think your dad understands you.

BOB: Well, it's like he doesn't listen to what I say.

THERAPIST: Can you give me an example?

BOB: Yeah. Yesterday he wanted me to mow the lawn. I started to tell him that I had to go down to Stuart's to help on his car, but he just interrupted and told me to cut the lip and do my job.

THERAPIST: *(To Bob)* And then you felt like he didn't understand you. *(Bob nods)* *(To Bob's father)* From your point of view, is Bob's description accurate?

MR. SIMPSON: Pretty much, except that I had told him earlier in week not to plan anything for yesterday afternoon. And after I told him to mow the lawn, he stomped off and did such a lousy job I had to have him redo it.

THERAPIST: How did you feel about that?

MR. SIMPSON: Oh, a little upset, but I've gotten used to it. Bob always has something else to do when chores roll around.

THERAPIST: OK—let me see if I have this straight so far. Mr. Simpson, you asked Bob to leave Wednesday afternoon free for mowing the lawn. Bob, you agreed to help Stuart with his car on Wednesday?

BOB: Yeah. It was the only day he could borrow his brother's dwell tack.

THERAPIST: Oh, I see. Did you remember what you dad had said?

BOB: Yeah, but I thought he wouldn't care if I waited 'til Saturday.

THERAPIST: So then Wednesday came, and you, Mr. Simpson, reminded Bob to do the lawn. You, Bob, started to tell him about the car, and then you *(looking at Mr. Simpson)* thought to yourself something like "Another excuse," and told Bob to get busy. You, Bob, thought your dad wouldn't listen. How did you feel?

BOB: Real mad.

THERAPIST: So you were mad, and so you did the lawn really fast, without doing a very good job?

BOB: Well, yeah. Also, I wanted to get to Stuart's.

THERAPIST: You were in a hurry, too. How did it end up?

BOB: A mess. I didn't get to help Stuart at all.

MRS. SIMPSON: And both of them were in bad moods all evening.

THERAPIST: And how did that affect you?

MRS. SIMPSON: Well, I never know what to say or do when they are like that.

THERAPIST: So you felt awkward?

MRS. SIMPSON: Yes.

THERAPIST: And what do you do when that happens?

MRS. SIMPSON: Oh, I stay out of their way!

THERAPIST: So all in all, the situation wasn't good for anyone. Bob, how would you rather see things happen when you don't want to do your chores at a particular time and have what seems to you like a reasonable reason?

BOB: Well, I'd like to be able to just say, "I'll do it on Saturday," or something like that.

THERAPIST: So you'd like to be able to work out some other plan and feel like your dad is listening to you, too, I would guess. How would you feel about talking about it that way, Mr. Simpson?

MR. SIMPSON: Well, I like Bob to stick to a schedule, but I'd be willing to talk, sometimes anyway. As long as it doesn't happen too often.

THERAPIST: So both of you think it would be better to work something out calmly. But when it comes up now, a lot of the time that doesn't happen. And you, Mr. Simpson, wind up thinking Bob is lazy, and you, Bob, wind up thinking your dad doesn't understand you. And you, Mrs. Simpson, wind up feeling like you're walking on pins and needles.

Commentary. The therapist uses the description of this incident to collect information about family interaction styles. S/he reflects and integrates information to accentuate the interactive nature of the situation, and then switches the focus to positive goals by asking what Bob and Mr. Simpson would rather see happen in similar situations. The therapist probes the mother's role in the sequence, even though Mrs. Simpson is not mentioned in the description provided by Mr. Simpson and Bob. By contrasting the benefits of resolving difficulties verbally with the disadvantages of their current methods, the therapist sets the stage for a later summary and presentation of a possible treatment program.

Throughout the assessment interviews, the therapist integrates the information the family provides without offering interpretations, that is, discussions of the "meaning," historical role, or metaphorical significance of behaviors. We avoid interpretive comments, principally because they distract from the emphasis on the nature and interdependence of current interaction patterns essential to our approach. In addition, parental interpretation of a teen's behavior is often a target for modification, particularly with psychologically sophisticated parents, who tend to stray from solution-oriented discussions in favor of interpretive speculation.

Another step in this phase of assessment involves juxtaposing the information about problematic conflict resolution styles with the presenting problem. With families who present interactional problems per se, such as arguments, compliance, and backtalk, the therapist can present a relatively straightforward summary. The summary frames the presenting problems in terms of the specific interactive components of these problems.

Example: The Simpsons (Part 2).
THERAPIST: Let me summarize what we've talked about so far. You, Mrs. Simpson, would like to see Mr. Simpson and Bob get along better. You see yourself and Bob having a good relationship most of the time, but sometimes feel you are in the middle when Bob and his father are upset with each other. Also, you have a hard time following through on the decisions you and your husband make because you sometimes think he's too hard on Bob. Right?

MRS. SIMPSON: Yes. That's pretty accurate.

THERAPIST: And you'd like for you and your husband and Bob to have more workable agreements, so you don't have to do as much enforcement. *(She nods)* You, Mr. Simpson, feel that Bob doesn't live up to his responsibilities and that you have to keep on him. And you, Bob, feel like your dad doesn't allow you enough say, so you get angry and goof off all the more. And then dad gets tougher. So the two of you get into a vicious circle and don't enjoy each other very much. Have I got it fairly well so far?

MR. SIMPSON: I'm afraid so. But I don't want to let up on Bob for fear he won't do anything at all if I do.

THERAPIST: Yes. *(To Bob)* Did what I said sound right to you?

BOB: Uh-huh.

THERAPIST: Now, you have all said that you'd rather not be locked into this pattern of getting along poorly. But you, Mr. Simpson, are afraid that if you let go all at once, things will just get worse.

MR. SIMPSON: That's right.

Commentary. Throughout the summary the therapist elicits feedback regarding the extent to which the formulation makes sense to family members. The summary is modified when members mention omitted information. Revising the problem formulation highlights the importance of collaborative interchange between the therapist and all family members: The treatment approach is adapted to fit the family's difficulties, and not vice versa.

If the presenting problem is not initially described by the family in interactional terms, the therapist should spend a portion of the interview exploring the functional relationship between that problem and family interaction. Assuming that family interaction patterns are related to the presenting problem, the therapist can use mini-summaries throughout the session to emphasize the mutual interdependence of family behavior and the presenting problem, thus reframing the presenting problem as a family interaction difficulty. The following vignette illustrates how a seemingly noninteractional presenting problem is linked to an interactional framework.

Example.

THERAPIST: Let me summarize my understanding of the problem. Andrea, you get really bad headaches, and the doctors haven't been able to find a medical reason why. Right?

ANDREA: Right.

THERAPIST: But the headaches are very real. And Mr. and Mrs. Jones, you are puzzled by Andrea's headaches. Now you also told me that there have been a lot of hassles around the house since you discovered Andrea was sexually active with boys.

MR. JONES: You bet. A 15-year-old girl is too young to be involved with boys. She doesn't know her own mind at that age. . . .

ANDREA: *(Interrupting)* Yes I do. I've told you I want birth control pills but you won't let me get them. You want me to get pregnant.

THERAPIST: How are you feeling right this minute, Andrea?

ANDREA: Mad!

THERAPIST: And how does your head feel?

ANDREA: Beginning to hurt a little.

THERAPIST: How often do you get headaches when you're mad at your parents?

ANDREA: A lot! I can't stand it when they treat me like a baby!

THERAPIST: They give you a pain in the head. And when else do you get headaches?

ANDREA: Whenever they get on my case.

MRS. JONES: Now she is going to say the headaches are our fault, like everything else that doesn't go her way!

THERAPIST: It may seem like you are being blamed, Mrs. Jones, but I'm really not interested in deciding whose fault things are. Bear with me for a moment. What do the two of you do when Andrea gets a headache?

MR. JONES: We tell her to take an aspirin and go lie down.

THERAPIST: So what happens when she gets a headache during an argument over boys?

MR. JONES: She goes and lies down.

THERAPIST: When does the disagreement get resolved?

MRS. JONES: Never. It's really frustrating. That's why we're here.

THERAPIST: Let me understand what I hear the three of you saying. Andrea, you want birth control pills and your parents are opposed to this. Mr. and Mrs. Jones, you feel she is too young to be messing around with boys. The three of you get into an argument about this issue. Sometimes, Andrea, you get so angry that you get a bad headache during the argument. When this happens, your parents tell you to take an aspirin and lie down. Then the argument stops, but the problem never gets solved. When headaches start, arguments stop. Right?

MRS. JONES: Well . . . I guess so. . . .

MR. JONES: We never thought of it that way.

Commentary. The therapist summarizes the somatic presenting problem of headaches and the interactional pattern of arguments over Andrea's sexual behavior, looking for a way to test the hypothesis that the two are related. When the family begins to display the interactional pattern of parental accusations followed by angry adolescent rebuttals during the interview, the therapist takes the opportunity to probe whether Andrea is beginning to get a headache. Her affirmative answer tentatively confirms the hypothesis and permits the therapist to link headaches and arguments directly in the summary at the end of the example. Note how the therapist integrates and utilizes the content of the information provided by the family and observation of the interactive process that transpires during the session.

If this reframing fails to convince some of the family that their behavior is related to the presenting problem, the therapist can resort to authority and indicate that in his/her professional judgment, therapy is most likely to be successful if parents and adolescent are seen together. In addition, reluctant participants are sometimes willing to attend a few family sessions and then to reevaluate the need for their attendance with the therapist.

As the final step before establishing a treatment contract, the therapist presents a treatment proposal that fits the problem formulation. When problem-solving communication training is an appropriate treatment, the description should be adapted to emphasize the components that fit the specific nature of the family's problems.

Example: The Simpsons (Part 3).

THERAPIST: So what you need is a better way of working things out—so that you, Mr. Simpson, feel more confident that your son will follow through on responsibilities and you, Bob, feel like your point of view gets heard, and you, Mrs. Simpson, don't feel caught in the middle and tense.

MRS. SIMPSON: It sounds ideal.

THERAPIST: Yes, it does, and I think it's possible to get there, with some work from each of you. Here's how I'd like to go about it. First of all I'd like for us to work on the ways you discuss problems with each other, since the ways you are using right now most often wind up in arguments. While we do this, I'll be teaching you some specific ways to talk about disagreements that will satisfy all of you and work well. In this case, that means that Bob feels like his ideas have been considered, and both of you feel confident that there's a good chance that Bob will follow through on his part of the solution. I'll also work with you on any parts of your communication that get in the way of reaching agreements. To do this, we'll work with topics that cause arguments at home, starting with easier ones, working with harder ones later on. I'll also ask you to try out some of the things you learn here at home so that you can eventually work things out without me. How does that sound so far?

MR. SIMPSON: I guess it's OK.

THERAPIST: You sound like you have some reservations.

MR. SIMPSON: Well, I'm not sure I believe Bob will change just by talking about problems.

THERAPIST: You've tried talk before and it hasn't worked?

MR. SIMPSON: No.

THERAPIST: What is it about your talks that hasn't worked?

MR. SIMPSON: Well, even when we reach an agreement it doesn't seem to work well.

THERAPIST: So you have problems not only with agreeing, but also with coming up with solutions that will work.

MR. SIMPSON: That's right.

THERAPIST: You know, solving problems together is like driving a car. If no one ever teaches you how to do it, you might occasionally figure out how to turn the key and move the steering wheel and pedals. But that doesn't guarantee you'll be able to get to where you're going. It sounds like you frequently can't start the car and even when you do, you don't like where you end up.

MR. SIMPSON: *(Laughing)* I guess not.

THERAPIST: I want to teach you how to drive the car—in other words, solve problems—the right way. I think that if you learn how to do that correctly, you'll be happier with your destinations.

MR. SIMPSON: I guess I can see that.

THERAPIST: Bob, how does it sound to you? Willing to give it a try?

BOB: Well, OK. I guess so.

THERAPIST: Mrs. Simpson?

MS. SIMPSON: It sounds ideal to me. I just hope we can do it.

THERAPIST: I think you can, but, as I said, everyone will have to put in some effort. Let me tell you a little bit more about arrangements. . . .

Commentary: The therapist presents an overview of the treatment strategy, then checks whether the rationale is acceptable to the family. Verbal and nonverbal cues of reluctance should be directly addressed to promote maximum commitment to treatment. In this case, the therapist uses the "learning a skill" metaphor to overcome the father's concern and gain his cooperation. With the teenager, frequently the most reluctant to return, the therapist elicits a general commitment when the benefit of continued sessions for the teen seems most salient.

At this point, the therapist informs the family about treatment logistics and the family and therapist begin to formulate a treatment contract. The purpose of this contract is to make explicit what the family can expect from the therapist and what is expected of them, and to increase their cooperation with therapeutic directives. Table 4-1 summarizes key points covered in the contract.

TABLE 4.1 Key Features of the Therapeutic Contract

Establishes goals of therapy

Outlines therapist responsibilities
  Nature of treatment
  Who will provide treatment
  Confidentiality

Outlines family responsibilities
  Attendance and cancellations
  Which family members will participate
  Fees and payment
  Homework assignments
  Completion of assessment data

Specifies other administrative details
  Length of sessions
  Location of sessions
  Audio or videotaping of sessions
  Probable duration of therapy

In addition to logistic details, the contract should clarify the implicit two-way commitment between the therapist and the family. The therapist will do all in his/her power to help the family change, using whatever procedures are likely to be effective. The family will be expected to describe problems honestly and openly and to complete assignments at home. A description of the treatment procedures can be given in terms reflecting the earlier presentation of the treatment approach. It is often helpful to state that the arguments described by family members reflect "bad habits" of long-standing duration; therapy will be designed to help them learn better habits for communicating. As in any learning process, there will be instructions, practice, and feedback.

While drawing up the contract, special attention should be paid to the adolescent, who is most likely to be resistant to participating in sessions and completing assignments between sessions. The needs of the adolescent and the ways in which therapy will help to meet these needs should be clearly articulated. The issue of assignments should be discussed in a way that makes it clear that tasks will not resemble academic homework and will not interfere with the adolescent's recreational activities. In fact, it is helpful to look at and face the adolescent while presenting the contract. Parents of resistant adolescents readily sense and appreciate that the therapist is trying to "win over" their son or daughter.

Duration of therapy may vary from 7 to 17 sessions, depending on the severity of the presenting conflicts, but a tentative time limit is always established at the end of the assessment phase. In our experience, time-limited contracts are preferable to open-ended contracts. When family members know the termination date in advance, they may maximize their use of therapy time. In addition, adolescents who are less than enthusiastic about participating in therapy are more likely to commit themselves to a set number of sessions. In our research studies the duration of therapy has been nine sessions (including pre- and postassessment sessions), a comfortable number for mildly to moderately distressed families.

Mutual goals should be clearly established by this time. It is frequently helpful to ask family members to write down any goals they have other than those that have been articulated in the assessment summary. These can then be reviewed during treatment and as therapy nears its time limit to determine whether additional sessions are needed. Attainment of goals can be subjectively estimated by the family member who established the goal, and used as a social validation measure (Kazdin, 1977; Wolf, 1978). More rigorous systematic goal attainment scaling methods are described by Lloyd (1983).

Goal setting and establishing a treatment contract also provide a convenient means to end the session on a positive note. Family members have voiced expectations of positive change, formulated positive goals, and committed themselves to working on a joint task: improving their interaction. This process hopefully enhances the likelihood of future cooperation with treatment and contributes to what Jacobson and Margolin (1979) term a "collaborative set."

Relationship Factors in the Interview

The therapist–client relationship provides the context for successful therapy. In fact, Alexander, Barton, Schiavo, and Parsons (1976) found that supervisory ratings of therapist characteristics taken immediately after family therapy training accounted for approximately 60% of the outcome of their behaviorally oriented treatment for parents and delinquent adolescents. Correlations among the different ratings suggested two separate dimensions of therapist attributes, each of which contributed to predicting outcome. One they labeled a "relationship" factor, represented by the mean of ratings on items labeled "warmth," "humor," and "affect–behavior integration" (i.e., verbally reflecting the relationship between affect and behavior in ongoing family interactions). The second dimension, "structuring," was obtained by averaging ratings of "self-confidence" and "directiveness."

Unfortunately, this study explored only supervisor perception of therapist behavior rather than the behavior itself. The results do, however, indicate that the authors' structured family therapy was not uniformly effective and suggest the importance of exploring actual therapist behaviors in greater empirical detail. In the absence of more detailed evidence, we spend the remainder of this section discussing therapist behaviors that may contribute to each of these two dimensions during family assessment interviews. Based on the work of Alexander *et al.* (1976), we divide these into *directive skills,* which function to guide the interview and to prevent unnecessary distraction and disruption, and *rapport-building skills,* which enhance the therapist's influence with family members.

Directive Skills

A major task of assessment interviewing is to collect information from family members. To accomplish this, the therapist must manage the session by keeping the family focused on relevant topics of discussion, ensuring that each person has the opportunity to speak and avoiding or defusing major arguments among family members.

Sticking to specific topics increases the amount of information the therapist can collect. This process requires a certain amount of balance between the therapist's and the family's agendas for the session: family members on occasion enter therapy with a particular incident or set of ideas to communicate to the therapist and respond inadequately to the therapist's questions until they have "had their say."

Directing the interview involves providing both verbal and nonverbal signals that guide the session. Providing a verbal overview of the session gives the family a general sense of relevant and irrelevant material. Verbally redirecting the conversation soon after the therapist notices that a family member is off-task can establish a pattern of topic-relevant discussion. This can be done with comments like "Excuse me. I'm not sure I understand how this fits in with what we were discussing" or "Let me stop you for a moment and go back to what we were discussing earlier." If the family member seems reluctant to do this, the therapist can suggest that they return to the topic later in the session if there is time.

Allowing each participant to speak involves inviting participation and intervening to reestablish that participation if the speaker is interrupted. This intervention has two goals. First, it allows the therapist to hear from all involved parties. Second, interruptions are prevented from functioning as punishers, which in some families eventually reduce an interrupted speaker to silence. The following illustrates one way this can be done:

Example: The Simpsons (Part 4).
THERAPIST: Bob, how would you like your mother to be different?
BOB: Well . . .
MRS. SIMPSON: I think he'd like me to be less . . .
THERAPIST: Just a second, Mrs. Simpson. I'd like to hear from Bob right now. I'll give you a chance in a minute.

Commentary: Interruptions such as Mrs. Simpson's may interfere with information collection and rapport building while simultaneously providing a sample of an important family interaction pattern. In some families, interruptions indicate deficits in listening skills. In others, they reflect genuine knowledge of the other's thoughts and feelings, but may be part of a general pattern of enmeshed overinvolvement that prevents the adolescent from achieving age-appropriate autonomy.

Preventing excessive arguments during the interview has several rationales. First, bitter arguments are frequently unproductive and time-consuming. Second, the level of anger and distress aroused by serious arguments often requires that the therapist "calm the family down" before proceeding with the assessment. Finally, although arguments provide an in vivo behavior sample of conflict, they can also contribute to negative client expectations that therapy will simply rehash old problems with no new solutions. Several clients have told us they dropped out of earlier attempts at family therapy after one session because "all we did was argue, just like we do at home." An early experience that demonstrates that therapy will not simply recreate pointless arguments increases the likelihood that clients will return with positive expectations about prospective sessions (cf. Jacobson & Margolin, 1979).

While discouraging excessive arguments, the therapist may want to permit some negative interchanges to continue long enough to observe the family's patterns, then intervene to prevent further escalation. At times, negative interactions can help the therapist confirm clinical hypotheses or to point out functionally related behavior patterns to the family, as in the example of Andrea's psychosomatic headaches described earlier. Later in therapy, the therapist may deliberately bring up conflictual topics in order to teach the family to modify their ways of expressing anger. Nonetheless, these uses of family conflict in the session require careful attention to preventing counterproductive hostility, particularly in early sessions.

Preventive strategies can reduce the probability of excessive arguments. Reflecting all parties' points of view, allowing everyone to speak, and collecting specific behavioral descriptions all assist in avoiding arguments. The judicious use of humor sometimes defuses the anger kindled by a provocative comment. If the therapist suspects a topic will be particularly explosive, prefacing a question with a comment like "I realize this may be a touchy issue, but it's important that I ask you about it. I'd like us all to try to discuss it as calmly as possible" can help keep the ensuing portion of the interview under control.

Despite these efforts, angry disputes will sometimes arise. Accusations, grocery lists of past wrongs, and negative trait labels and attributions may all surface when discussing conflictual topics. These can prompt one or more family members to "tune out;" to stop participating; to produce more active contradictions, sarcasm, and bickering; or, in the extreme, to storm out of the session. The therapist who is aware of nonverbal anger cues can often catch incipient arguments early and redirect the conversation to a less argumentative but equally relevant topic.

Example: The Simpsons (Part 5).

MR. SIMPSON: Bob never seems to do what I say.

BOB: *(Sarcastically)* That's because everything you say is stupid.

MR. SIMPSON: Don't talk to me like that, young man.

THERAPIST: Hold on! What's starting to happen?

BOB: I'm starting to get mad.

THERAPIST: Yes. I noticed. *(Bob grins)* What would have happened if this had gone on?

BOB: Well, I probably would have gotten madder.

THERAPIST: What about you, Mr. Simpson?

MR. SIMPSON: Well, when he talks that way, I get angry too.

THERAPIST: So you both would have gotten angrier, and the discussion would have. . . ?

MR. SIMPSON: Gotten nowhere.

THERAPIST: Yes. Let's go back, then, to the original point, about Bob's following directions. Bob, I'll ask for your side in a minute, so I'd like you to try to keep cool, even if you don't like what your dad is saying. OK?

Commentary. The therapist changes the topic by labeling the interaction that just occurred and interjecting a remark designed to lighten the tension ("I noticed").

S/he then provides a rationale for why an argument would prove counterproductive and gives instructions designed to reduce the incidence of angry outbursts.[3]

In directing the session, the therapist must avoid becoming overly embroiled in the family's interaction. Overinvolvement can cause several problems: The therapist's objective observations of family interactions may disappear and the therapist can find himself/herself inadvertently controlled by, instead of directing, the interview process. Families who react to each other quickly and spontaneously and who interrupt loudly can easily steal control of the interview from the unassertive therapist. Unwary clinicians can also be sucked into complex family interaction chains, particularly when the parents are highly articulate and their statements appear quite reasonable.

Several cues should alert the therapist that s/he has lost control of the session. A discussion that has strayed far from its original topic, a feeling of discomfort, and a thought like "Oh, no—what's happening and where am I going?" are good clues that redirection is needed. The therapist who cannot get a word in edgewise or is interrupted with regularity also needs to become more directive with the family.

Example.

MR. CAMPBELL: Sally is just too young to be out at night with boys.

SALLY: Dad, I'm not.

MRS. CAMPBELL: It's not a question of maturity, it's . . .

SALLY: It *is so.*

MRS. CAMPBELL: Sally, be quiet. Dear, it is a question of her growing up. As I've told you many times, it's a different society nowadays. . . .

THERAPIST: I think . . .

SALLY: She's right, Dad.

MR. CAMPBELL: Sally, be quiet.

MRS. CAMPBELL: Let her talk. She has a right to be heard.

THERAPIST: Excuse me . . .

MR. CAMPBELL: I think this decision is ours, not hers.

Commentary. After allowing negative interaction for a few minutes, the therapist's attempts to regain the floor are ineffective. Sally and Mr. Campbell's interruptions should signal that the session may be moving too fast.

Several strategies can help to extricate oneself from a runaway interview. When the therapist feels completely lost, s/he can actually stop the session for a few moments to plan a new course of action, saying something like, "Hold on! Everyone stop for a moment, please. This discussion is moving very fast and I would like to think over what you are saying for a few minutes." A variant on this approach involves calling "time out" for a few seconds, then asking direct questions of family members. The therapist may have to be loud, emphatic, or use noticeable gestures initially to get family members' attention. When a family member regularly interrupts the therapist, the interviewer can ask the intruder to wait for a moment before speaking. Alternatively, s/he can label interruptions as a problem and make a rule that only one person at a time may speak in the session. Below, we replay a more effective example of therapeutic redirection with the Campbell family.

Example.

MRS. CAMPBELL: Dear, it is a question of her growing up. As I've told you many times, it's a different society nowadays. . . .

THERAPIST: *(Leaning forward and raising one hand)* Let me interrupt here.

SALLY: She's right, Dad.

THERAPIST: Excuse me, Sally. I'd like to stop talking about this topic for a minute. . . .

MR. CAMPBELL: *(Interrupting)* Yes, the doctor is right. Sally, be quiet.

THERAPIST: Hold on! We have a problem here. Everyone wants to have their say, and we all seem to be interrupting each other a lot. I am finding it hard to get the information I want from you. For the next few minutes, I would like to ask each of you some questions. My job will be to ask, yours will be to answer. If you disagree with what someone else says, please be patient and try not to interrupt. I'll give you a chance in a minute.

Commentary. The therapist uses forceful verbal and nonverbal communication to gain the family's attention. When Sally interrupts, the interviewer immediately retakes the floor and tries to cut off the previous discussion. Mr. Campbell then interrupts and attempts to side with the therapist. The therapist sidesteps this alliance by targeting interruptions as a problem for everyone and announces a plan to redirect the session and hopefully reduce interruptions.

Rapport-Building Skills

Establishing rapport with all family members facilitates intervention by setting the stage for collaborative effort among therapist and family members. A family that regards the therapist's opinions as the views of an expert who understands each of their vantage points will be more likely to participate openly in sessions and to comply with directives than a family where one or more members see the therapist as "on the other person's side." This in turn implies that the therapist must simultaneously communicate understanding to all family members while remaining unaligned with particular individuals.

Involving All Family Members

Several therapist behaviors can help family members to feel equally involved. Eye contact, body orientation, and questions can be distributed equally among mother, father, and adolescent. The therapist should also ensure that everyone has an opportunity to speak and try to keep any single individual from dominating the session. Genuine, nonjudgmental interest in each participant's experience also communicates therapist involvement with the family. Frequent reflection, paraphrasing, and summaries of information in the interview, punctuated by requests for feedback from the family, can establish a pattern where corrective feedback and alternative viewpoints are acknowledged, not punished.

In our experience, the adolescent is the most difficult family member with whom to establish rapport. In extreme cases, teenagers feel that they have been "dragged in" and blamed as the source of the problem. Consequently, teens may generalize to the therapist the expectations they have of other adults such as parents, teachers, and officials who lecture, accuse, and use aversive control. Therapists, too, may have more difficulty understanding the thoughts, feelings, and behavior of the teenager than they do those of the parent. Thus we find it wise to attend particularly to adolescents and to attempt to "hook" them during the initial interview.

We have already given several suggestions for doing this: informally conversing with adolescents about their interests, allowing teenagers to verbalize concerns about coming to therapy, eliciting and acknowledging adolescents' viewpoints. Reframing problems as vicious interactional circles may defuse the hostility some teens experience if they judge themselves to be unjustly blamed for family conflict. Adolescents appreciate being addressed as adults, and most respond well to being given choices and to discussing issues with the same interactional style used with their parents. The therapist should avoid elaborate vocabulary and sentence structure and resist the temptation to give long-winded pronouncements during which the adolescent is likely to tune out. Finally, the therapist may wish to ask the parents to give the teen explicit permission to say whatever s/he wishes, without fear of parental retribution at home after conclusion of the session.

Parents can sometimes interfere unintentionally in rapport building with the teenager by talking as though the child were not present and/or attempting to engage the therapist in conversation about abstractions, which the adolescent may not be able to follow. Redirecting the topic to one in which the adolescent can participate will often help regain lost attention.

The therapist also should be particularly sensitive to the feelings and participation of quieter adolescents, and intervene if parental complaints become hostile. It is frequently helpful to prompt teens for their honest opinions. The therapist can then acknowledge these opinions, demonstrating that honesty will not be punished during therapy.

Example 1.

MRS. VAN GUILDEN: I think the real problem is that Sara is just immature. She is unwilling to do anything around the house, and . . .

THERAPIST: Let me stop you for just a moment. You said that you see Sara as unwilling to do anything around the house.

MRS. VAN GUILDEN: Yes.

THERAPIST: Sara, what's your opinion?

SARA: I dunno.

THERAPIST: *(Exaggerating, without sarcasm)* You mean you agree that you're *completely* unwilling to do a single thing anywhere in the house at any time?

SARA: Well, no. I'm willing to do a reasonable share.

THERAPIST: You are willing to do some things if you think your part is reasonable. What would be reasonable to you?

Example 2.

MR. BAXTER: I hate to say this, but I'm afraid that Joe is just going to turn into a bum, like his brother. *(Joe turns away)*

THERAPIST: Joe, you look like you didn't like what your father said.

JOE: No, I'm used to it.

THERAPIST: Well, it seems to me that if *my* dad said he thought I'd turn out to be a bum, I'd be upset and want to say what I thought. Do you think you'll turn out to be a bum?

JOE: No. I just wish Dad wouldn't say that all the time.

Commentary. In the first case, the therapist uses exaggeration and humor to prompt the adolescent. In the second, the intervention relies on self-disclosure of what the therapist's own feelings might be in the situation.

With reluctant adolescents, the therapist should make sure to highlight the potential benefits the adolescent can derive from therapy before attempting to elicit a treatment agreement. In addition to increased privileges, most adolescents do not enjoy family conflict and would like to get along better with their parents, to decrease parental yelling and nagging, and to feel that their parents understand them. Some may feel very guilty about their role in family problems. Eliciting positive family goals and helping the teenager to see that they may be attainable (without promising an unrealistic world of neverending permissiveness) can enhance the adolescent's commitment to therapy.

Remaining Unaligned

Remaining unaligned is important both to rapport building and to session control. When individual family members draw the therapist into a coalition, they manipulate the therapist into supporting their goals rather than permitting the therapist to guide the family. Occasionally during the course of treatment the therapist may choose to align temporarily with an adolescent or a parent to accomplish a particular goal, but planned coalitions are quite different from the unplanned variety.

One way to avoid one-sided discussion involves equitably distributing therapist attention within the family. In addition, the therapist should avoid stating or endorsing statements of blame or opinions that polarize family members. One way to avoid accusatory attributions or maladaptive attitudes involves acknowledging the speaker's opinion but reflecting it as a thought or an opinion rather than as "truth."

MR. JOHNSTON: It's really Billy's fault that he and his mother argue, because he just doesn't listen.

THERAPIST: Then it's your opinion that Billy doesn't listen and that this contributes to his arguments with his mother. What is it about Billy's behavior that lets you know he's not listening?

Another way to avoid endorsing accusatory statements is to summarize an interaction so that the negatively labeled behavior is reframed as motivated by a positive intent. Parents who interpret a teenager's arguments and backtalk as a lack of respect or love will sometimes be more tolerant if the therapist relabels these behaviors as signs of a "natural desire for independence," expressed in an unskilled fashion. Parental restrictiveness can be framed as an expression of love and concern about the adolescent's well-being, rather than a desire to see the teen rejected by peers. The uncommunicative behavior of some teenagers will prompt fewer parental attacks if viewed as motivated by "fear of parental condemnation" rather than malevolent intentions.

Parents are sometimes less than subtle about trying to form an alliance with the therapist and may directly request that the therapist corroborate their opinions. These opinions may have been voiced repeatedly to the adolescent, with little or no result. In these cases the therapist can acknowledge the parent's comment, then reframe it or sidestep the question by rephrasing the issue.

Example 1.

MRS. BANCROFT: After all, Sara, it's your responsibility as part of the household to help out. *(To the therapist)* Don't you agree?

THERAPIST: Certainly many parents share your opinion. But here I think the issue really is that you want Sara to take more responsibilities. Isn't that correct?

Commentary. The therapist sidesteps the inquiry, then reframes the mother's general statement as a specific wish. This allows the therapist to pursue this issue rather than a vague discussion of what children "should" do.

Example 2.

MRS. WILLIAMS: I punish Walter regularly. It's a parent's responsibility to discipline a child, and I try to be a responsible parent. Don't you think that parents should discipline their children, Doctor?

THERAPIST: I think the most important issues are whether or not all of you are satisfied with the discipline and how it's working. If discipline is working, eventually you don't need to use it. But in your case, you seem to be having to punish Walter over and over for the same things. And Walter doesn't like to be punished—right? So it looks like in your case, you need a more effective way of handling things with Walter.

Commentary. Again, the therapist avoids endorsing the mother's problematic punishment patterns by redirecting the conversation to the effects of the mother's attempts at discipline. When given a choice between being right and being effective, most parents will sacrifice the former for the latter.

As an alternative for handling alliance attempts, the therapist can explicitly label the parents' attempts to draw him/her into an alliance against the teenager as a ploy to assess the degree to which dyads within the family form alliances against a third member at home.

Example 3.

MRS. JONES: I object to the whole idea of Bill smoking marijuana. His dad and I have talked this over extensively, and we feel Bill is ruining his health by smoking that stuff. Doctor, isn't that what medical research has shown?

THERAPIST: I feel put on the spot. If I say "yes," I side with the two of you against Bill. If I say "no," I side with Bill against the two of you. Either way I lose. I've noticed this kind of thing happening several times during our session. How much of the time does one of you try to get a second to side against the third at home?

Commentary. Instead of responding substantively, the therapist labels the effect of the family's behavior on him/her and takes the opportunity to assess whether alliances occur at home.

More insidious attempts to draw the therapist into a coalition are more indirect. Parents may make a general, preaching statement to their adolescent, the content of which presumes a "united front" with the therapist. Female adolescents may attempt to use physical attractiveness as a means of winning a male therapist over to their side. Therapists should dissociate themselves from presumed united fronts, for example, by saying something like "I'm sorry—I must not have made myself clear on that issue," then indicating how their opinion differs from that attributed by the parent. Similarly, seductive overtures must be declined. One of us can recall an attractive 15-year-old client who wrote on the back of her Issues Checklist, "You big handsome brute." The comment was ignored.

It is also crucial to rapport to be aware of any cultural and ethnic differences between the therapist and the family. Acceptable interaction patterns vary from culture to culture, and a therapist ignorant of culturally appropriate behavior may inadvertently drive one or more members away from treatment. For example, Bernal and Flores-Ortiz (1982) suggest that therapists should begin a family interview with Latino families by asking the father to describe the problem, thus recognizing his authority in the family. It is also important to attend particularly to the structural organization of family interaction that predominates in the client's culture and consider these factors in planning and discussing with the family the treatment approach to be used.

RESEARCH ON THE CLINICAL INTERVIEW

There are two possible sources of unreliable data in the behavioral interview: client inconsistency in providing information and therapist inconsistency in evaluating it. Each of these has been examined with parents and children interviewed separately using structured and semistructured interviews.

Client consistency can be examined over time (test–retest reliability), across interviewers, or across family members. Rutter and Graham (1968) found only poor to fair test–retest correlations between ratings of specific symptoms based on interviews with children and with mothers. Unfortunately, data were based on interviewer ratings and semistructured interviews, and poor reliability could have been due to differences in questions asked by interviewers, scoring judgments, or client report.

A study by Edelbrock, Costello, Dulcan, Kalas, and Conover (1985) has fewer interpretive difficulties, since their interview was more structured and therefore any unreliability should be more closely related to differences in client reports over time. Test–retest correlations over a median of 9 days, based on summary scores derived from interviews with parents and clinic-referred children (ages 6–18), averaged .62 for children and .75 for parents. Interestingly, children's reports of behavior and conduct problems showed higher test–retest correlations than scales based on affective and neurotic items, and reliability of child reports improved significantly with age. Parents of children of different ages did not show these patterns, however. Children reported on average 23% fewer symptoms on the second interview, a highly significant drop. Parent report of symptoms dropped as well, but only 5%.

Agreement on the information clients give to different individuals at the same point in time has not to our knowledge been examined with parents and children, but Hay, Hay, Angle, and Nelson (1979) found that the information adult drug-use clients provided to different interviewers agreed on average 86% of the time. Comparisons of whether child and parent reports agree have yielded mixed findings. Herjanic, Herjanic, Brown, and Wheatt (1975) compared children's and parental responses to yes/no questions tapping various child symptomatology. Mean agreement was 80%, but this figure dropped considerably when only reports of the occurrence of problem behaviors were considered and agreement was corrected for chance agreement (mean kappa = .22; Herjanic & Reich, 1982). Weissman, Orvaschel, and Padian (1980) found no relation between mothers' and childrens' reports of depressive symptoms.

A second source of unreliable data lies in clinicians' judgments and/or reports of the interview. In general, interviewer agreement figures on information collected in structured and semistructured interviews appear to vary with the interview employed (see Edelbrock & Costello, 1984, for a review).

These studies, however, do not directly address the kinds of information and decision making common to behavioral interviewing. Two studies conducted by Nelson and her colleagues examine these issues. The first (Hay et al., 1979) assessed the reliability of problem identification. Each of four behaviorally trained, advanced graduate students first was instructed to identify as many problem areas as possible, then interviewed four different adult clients and dictated a summary of the client's problems after the session. The problems identified by different interviewers during the interviews per se and in dictated session summaries were compared. Based on the interviews, agreement averaged 55% for general problem areas and 40% for more specific items comprising the problem areas. Session summaries yielded a mean agreement of 48% for general areas. An average of 28% of the problem areas mentioned in the interview were not reported in the summaries. Interviewers also failed to agree on the questions they asked, in terms of both general problem areas (mean overlap in questions = 62%) and specific items comprising these areas (mean overlap = 29%). Clients, however, were very consistent (86%) in reporting information.

Felton and Nelson (1984) reported comparable findings from a similar study in which assistants role-played actual clients in an investigation of agreement among interviewers' descriptions of stimulus, organismic, and consequence factors related to client problems, essential components of the functional analysis. Interviewers agreed, on average, on only 41% of the controlling variables they derived from interviews. Augmenting interviews with role-play and questionnaire data made no difference in reliability. As in the Hay et al. (1979) study, information clients provided to interviewers was very consistent (97%), but interviewers' questions only overlapped 33%. Agreement on treatment plans exceeded agreement on controlling variables, averaging .61. Together, these studies indicate that therapists' identification of problem areas and controlling variables may be remarkably unreliable and appears to be associated with differences in the content of their questions.

Berg and Fielding (1979) examined another sort of reliability—the reliability of interviewers' global appraisals of enuretic children's behavior during a psychiatric interview. One interviewer spoke with the children; the second was present but did not participate. After the session, the interviewers rated the children on categories such as "anxious," "tense," and "poor rapport." Ratings were then collapsed into dichotomous occurrence–nonoccurrence ratings. Interviewer agreement was not presented using standard coefficients of agreement, but percent agreement (agreements/[agreements + disagreements]) could be computed from the data presented in the study. Overall agreement was 60% or higher for all 10 categories. However, agreement based solely on occurrence dropped to an average of 44.5% (range, 11.2%–73.0%).

The evidence thus far, albeit limited in scope, indicates that clients respond with varying reliability to interview questions. Clinicians, too, are fallible and may differ in the questions they ask, the problems they identify, and the global appraisals they make about the client's behavior in unstructured interviews.

Because most interviews investigated in research have been devised for screening or diagnostic purposes, validity-related examinations have generally focused on concurrent and discriminative validity questions related to these purposes. Several structured interviews yield data that discriminate clinic-referred from nonreferred populations (e.g., Herjanic & Campbell, 1977; Hodges, Kline, Stern, Cytryn, & McKnew, 1982; Rutter & Graham, 1968) and correlate with other measures of child deviance (e.g., Hodges et al., 1982).

More important for the behavioral assessor are questions of the accuracy of information provided during the interview and the generalizability of behavior displayed during the interview to other settings and situations. Haynes, Jensen, Wise, and Sherman (1981) provided data from marital interviews addressing the first of these issues. Distressed and nondistressed couples were interviewed either together or apart. Their responses to questions regarding marital satisfaction and assertiveness were compared with responses to similar questions on questionnaires completed later, which served as one criterion measure. In addition, couples' reports of which spouse was more positive and which more negative in their conversations were later contrasted with observational data based on couple discussions of marital problems. Correlations between questionnaire and interview report were significantly higher for separate then joint interviews for a majority of questions related to marital satisfaction, with greater discrepancies associated with more sensitive interview questions. Similarly, spouses were more accurate about their communication patterns when interviewed separately. Spouses agreed more closely with each other in their evaluations of their satisfaction and communication when interviewed together, suggesting that the presence of the spouse elicits greater conformity in verbal reports.

Berg and Fielding (1979), in a study described earlier, addressed the generalizability of child behavior in the interview by correlating clinicians' judgments of children's behavior during the interview with global ratings of child behavior problems based on maternal interview and with scores on the Rutter Scale B questionnaire assessing school adjustment. None of the correlations approached significance. Unfortunately, the behaviors rated during the interview were very different from the behaviors rated by mothers, and therefore should not necessarily be expected to be related. A more interesting question, the generalizability of observations of the *same* behavior from the interview to other settings, has not been examined.

The studies cited thus far (with the exception of Haynes *et al.,* 1981) have explored interviews of individuals, not families, and have only begun to examine the psychometric characteristics of the interview as an assessment tool. These characteristics may vary according to the format of the interview (e.g., structured vs. unstructured) as well as the types of information collected. Continued reliability and validity research should address three separate aspects of the family interview. The first is the *content:* Are the domains assessed relevant to distressed families? Which dimensions of interactive behaviors (e.g., frequency, intensity, sequence) are important? Most important, does the client report provide an accurate description of actual behavior? The second area lies in observations of family *process:* Again, are these dimensions relevant to family distress? To what extent may they be generalized to behavior at home? Finally, the clinician's *appraisal and use of information* from the clinical interview should be further assessed: Do clinicians reliably observe and report family interaction patterns? If biases occur, what are they and what are their effects? Finally, does the treatment plan derived from the interview data enhance the outcome of therapy—that is, is it useful?

The questions and issues posed thus far relate to the initial interview as an assessment device. It is important to recall as well that we emphasize its role as the preliminary stage of treatment. We have postulated several functions of the assessment interview, including rapport building, expectation setting, and enhancing later treatment effects. Certainly these hypotheses, too, warrant further empirical consideration.

SCREENING THE FAMILY

The problem-solving communication training approach is designed for families whose problems appear to be maintained or exacerbated by faulty parent–child interaction styles. It is not the treatment of choice for certain other sorts of families. In the first of these, parents and child report a good relationship inside the family, but the child experiences difficulty outside the home, such as learning problems or poor peer relationships. Such families require individually oriented interventions aimed specifically at remediating the child's learning problems or teaching the child appropriate social skills. The second type of family demonstrates problematic interactive styles, but these styles prove to be a function primarily of marital problems or of individual psychopathology. If individual or marital problems would interfere with problem-solving treatment, family therapy might not be appropriate unless these problems are also addressed.

Example 1. Mr. and Mrs. Matteson brought their daughter Tina for therapy. Initial interviewing revealed that the parents had very different styles of discipline. Tina regularly asked her father's permission for privileges when he was at home; he regularly granted her requests. The mother, who strongly opposed what she perceived as her husband's permissiveness, often refused to give Tina even minor privileges, in order to compensate for her husband's laxity. However, Mrs. Matteson rarely voiced her feelings to her husband, but instead occasionally became extremely angry when Tina made a request for a privilege. Mr. and Mrs. Matteson in fact rarely discussed any of their marital disagreements with each other, but both acknowledged that marital problems were present, and they characterized their relationship as emotionally unsatisfying but relatively conflict-free. Tina naturally followed the permissive rules sanctioned by her father. As a consequence, she became embroiled in disagreements with her mother. During these disagreements, her mother seemed to be arguing with Tina to "punish" her father for his lax discipline. Her father seemed to enjoy subtly "needling" his wife by encouraging Tina to disobey her stringent regulations.

Commentary. The mother–daughter conflict in this case appears to be a consequence of parental disagreement concerning child rearing and discipline, which overlays a spouse relationship characterized by indirect conflict. The parents engage in a reciprocal exchange of punishment through the medium of their daughter's behavior. Before the mother–daughter conflict can be resolved, we hypothesize, the spouses must resolve or at least acknowledge and begin to discuss their disagreements. Behavioral marital therapy, prior to or concurrent with problem-solving communication training, would be the treatment of choice.

Example 2. Mrs. Lipinski and her son Martin self-referred for therapy, stating as a principal reason Mrs. Lipinski's inability to discipline Martin. Comments from both mother and son indicated that the mother was erratic in enforcing rules and attributed this to "nerves." Further interviewing revealed that Mrs. Lipinski experienced severe bouts of depression during which she substantially decreased interaction of all types with her son, missed work, and failed to complete her household responsibilities. These episodes appeared to be independent of her relationship with Martin.

Commentary. In this case, individual therapy for depression would be preferable to problem-solving family therapy at this time. Although it is not certain that the problems with Martin would clear up if Mrs. Lipinski's depression lifted, it is equally unclear whether she currently has the requisite abilities to follow agreements reached during problem-solving sessions. Should the family problems persist when Mrs. Lipinski is no longer depressed, problem-solving communication training would be appropriate. Again, note that if her depression appeared to be functionally related to conflict with Martin, problem-solving therapy might be appropriate.

Problem-solving communication training is also probably not the treatment of choice for families with older adolescents who are having difficulty leaving home. We refer here to persons in their late teens who behave in atypical ways as the time to leave home approaches (Haley, 1980). These older adolescents often become embroiled in bitter conflicts with their parents over failures in areas such as graduating from high school, obtaining and maintaining a job, staying out of trouble with the police, living independently, or taking drugs. Haley hypothesizes that the parents in these families are unable to function as a viable dyad without their offspring present to detour conflict. The young person's failures and misbehavior provide a reason for remaining at home, thus stabilizing the family and preventing marital distress from escalating. In essence, "leaving-home" problems are a variation on the theme of the occasional interdependence of marital and parent–teen problems.

The intervention for these families proposed by Haley involves a strategic–structural approach, reestablishing the parents as agents of control for their adolescent and forcing them to work together to get the youth to act normally. The adolescent's "failing" behavior is reframed as "rebellion," and the parents are called upon to act consistently as "disciplinarians." When successful, this approach unites the parents in the common endeavor of helping their son or daughter to begin to live independently and to become free of the need to protect the parents' marriage from disintegration. Afterwards, the parents may be helped to resolve their conflicts directly without involving the adolescent. A problem-solving communication training approach would be inappropriate for such problems because it relies upon a strategy of democratic conflict resolution. With leaving-home problems, the parents work instead to take an authoritarian stance with their offspring. By working together, they hopefully reestablish an appropriate hierarchy within the family and free the youth from parental problems.

Finally, problem-solving communication training is probably doomed, at least as an initial intervention, in a family where the teenager actively refuses to participate and creates intense disruptions during family sessions in order to escape from therapy. The majority of reluctant teens express their reluctance early in the initial session but generally agree to participate by the end of the assessment session(s). On rare occasions, however, the child's behavior completely disrupts the interview and the child fails to respond to therapist interventions designed to halt the disruptions and "hook" the child. In these cases, the family is better treated initially either individually or via a family intervention specifically tailored to the in-session disruption.

Assessment of individual and marital difficulties should be conducted with a great deal of tact. Parents who attribute their presence in therapy solely to their child's problems may feel startled, annoyed, or awkward if the therapist questions directly their marital and individual adjustments with the adolescent present. For that reason, we often collect preliminary screening information via paper-and-pencil measures, such as the short form of the Locke–Wallace Marital Adjustment Test (Locke & Wallace, 1959), an easily administered and scored questionnaire used extensively in marital therapy research. Problems related to individual adjustment can be collected by embedding questions into a fact sheet with demographic information. These include:

- Has anyone in your immediate family ever been hospitalized or sought mental health services for reasons related to their moods, thought patterns, or behavior? If so, when? What was the reason?
- Are you or your spouse ever bothered by

excessive drinking or use of drugs?	yes/no	you/spouse
spells of depression?	yes/no	you/spouse
hallucinations?	yes/no	you/spouse
anxiety or panic attacks?	yes/no	you/spouse

If answers to these questions, together with the information gained from the family interview, suggest that individual or marital therapy should be considered, the therapist may wish to interview the parents alone to explore the issue further. Usually it is best at this point to raise the topic directly as one requiring additional assessment, rather than pronouncing to the parents that they need marital or individual therapy. Reflecting information during this discussion using the same therapeutic strategies discussed earlier in the family interview section can help the parents to reframe their notions of the problem and to see that individual or marital treatment is more appropriate than family therapy, if in fact the individual interview indicates this is the case. After the parents accept an alternative approach, necessary referrals or revised treatment contracts can be made.

This chapter has highlighted goals and strategies common to assessment interviews. Problems in interviews are best handled by early intervention. More persistent problems in managing sessions will be discussed in Chapter 12.

NOTES

1. This statement is based on our experience with treatment outcome studies and in psychology department and university medical center clinics. Rates of adolescent refusal may be different in different settings.

2. This material is adapted from Robin and Foster in *Adolescent behavior disorders: Foundations and contemporary concerns,* P. A. Karoly & J. J. Steffen (Eds.), 1984, Lexington, MA, D. C. Heath. Copyright 1984 by D. C. Heath. Adapted by permission

3. Had this happened in a later session, the therapist would probably have used a more change-oriented approach, helping Mr. Simpson and Bob identify the interactive behaviors and cognitions that elicited feelings of anger from each of them, instructing them in more effective ways of communicating their viewpoints, and replaying the episode with the new behaviors. While this strategy can be used during the assessment session, it is more time-consuming than simple redirection and involves active intervention prior to establishing a treatment contract.

CHAPTER FIVE

Questionnaire and Observational Assessment

Questionnaires, home report measures, and direct observation supplement the interview as methods of gaining information about family functioning. Although numerous measures are available (see Filsinger, 1983, and Foster & Robin, 1988, for reviews), this chapter focuses primarily on procedures developed in our laboratories specifically for assessing parent–adolescent conflict.

PAPER-AND-PENCIL MEASURES

Descriptions and Clinical Uses

Paper-and-pencil measures have several advantages as assessment methods. They require little therapist time to administer and score. They provide information on family members' perceptions of the nature and severity of their difficulties. When questionnaire items are specific and anchored in discrete events, they also encourage family members to focus on specific behaviors rather than broad, vague complaints.

However, even when anchored by descriptions of discrete events, questionnaire items reflect perceptions of behavior at another time and another place (Cone, 1979). Unless family members' reports on an inventory have been empirically demonstrated to mirror the behaviors they are assumed to reflect, the therapist cannot legitimately infer that a family's responses accurately describe actual behavior. Extraneous factors can also affect retrospective verbal report, thus producing misleading data. Problems sometimes associated with self-report include social desirability and idiosyncratic personal biases, faulty recall, and susceptibility to demand characteristics of the assessment situation.

In our clinical and research work with families, we routinely administer self-report inventories assessing the major dimensions of parent–adolescent conflict: issues of dispute, skill deficits, faulty cognitions, and functional/structural problems. At first, our approach was to create individual measures for each dimension; more recently, we have moved towards developing multidimensional instruments assessing all of the relevant content domains. We will review samples of both types of instruments, first describing the instruments and their clinical utility, then summarizing data on their psychometric properties.

Family members complete these questionnaires retrospectively, giving ratings of their perceptions of the target events. For most measures, both parents complete the questionnaires, and the adolescent completes two sets of questionnaires, one for relations with each parent. The family may also be asked to complete some home data collection task. In addition, we often administer a marital questionnaire (e.g., Locke–Wallace Marital Adjustment Test, Dyadic Adjustment Scale, or Marital Satisfaction Inventory) and a child problem behavior checklist (e.g., Child Behavior Checklist). The information is used (in coordination with observational and interview information) to plan treatment. Questionnaires can also be readministered at periodic intervals throughout treatment, as well as after termination, to assess progress.

Conflict Behavior Questionnaire

The Conflict Behavior Questionnaire (CBQ) is a measure of perceived communication–conflict behavior at home (see Appendix A). It gives a general estimate of how much conflict and negative communication the family experiences. Parents and adolescents complete parallel versions of the CBQ, retrospectively rating their interactions over the 2 or 3 weeks preceding the assessment session. They are asked to read and decide whether each item is "mostly true" or "mostly false" for their relationship, and to endorse it by circling the word "true" or "false." The parent version contains 75 statements, 53 regarding the parents' appraisal of their adolescent's behavior (e.g., "My child sulks after an argument") and 22 regarding their perceptions of their interaction with the adolescent (e.g., "We joke around often"). Each group of items yields a separate score ("appraisal of the adolescent" and "appraisal of the dyad"). The adolescent version contains 73 items, 51 regarding the adolescent's appraisal of the parent (e.g., "My mom doesn't understand me") and 22 identical to the parent form, tapping the adolescent's perception of interaction with the parent. Item content reflects positive and negative interactive behaviors drawn from nonconflictual discussions and argumentative exchanges. The items are counterbalanced such that in some cases a "true" response corresponds to a negative perception and in others to a positive perception. Scoring is readily accomplished by constructing transparent overlays following the item key (see Appendix A), with high scores representing negative perceptions.

The CBQ was based on an item pool initially generated by eighth-grade students, clinical psychologists, and research assistants. It was refined based on responses of college students (recalling their relationships as young adolescents with their mothers) and mothers with teenage children. Mothers and college students completed pilot versions of the CBQ and also rated the overall quality of the relationship they were evaluating. Items reported by significantly different numbers of subjects in positively versus negatively rated relationships formed the final versions of the CBQ (Prinz, 1977).

Two shorter versions were subsequently developed. A 44-item form (the

CBQ-44) retains the two scales of the original questionnaire, and was created by Ronald J. Prinz by extracting those items that best correlated with scale totals in the sample of distressed and nondistressed mothers and adolescents used to validate the longer version (Prinz et al., 1979). These scales correlate .98 or higher with long-form scores. A 20-item form (the CBQ-20) has also been developed and retains the items from the CBQ that maximally discriminated distressed from nondistressed families in a larger sample that included fathers. This form yields a single summary score which correlates .96 or more with scores from the long form of the CBQ (see Appendix A for CBQ-44 and CBQ-20). The CBQ-20 is particularly useful because it can be completed in about 5 minutes. By modifying the instructions and asking family members to report on the last week only, the CBQ-20 can be completed in the waiting room before sessions and used to monitor therapeutic progress systematically.

The CBQ is perhaps best used as one indicator of the level of distress family members experience related to their interaction patterns. The tables in Appendix A convert the CBQ summary scores to *t* scores for the long form of the CBQ, computed using data from 205 families. These tables allow the clinician to determine roughly how distressed the family is with respect to normative distressed and nondistressed samples. For example, a mother who complains of communication problems with her son, whose appraisal of her son and appraisal of the dyadic relationship are 30 and 17, respectively, receives standardized scores of 55 and 66, based upon the norms for distressed dyads. Since these scores are close to the mean for distressed dyads, the mother reports average to above average relationship distress relative to other clinical families. On the other hand, if her appraisal of her son is 8 and the dyad 2, her standardized scores relative to distressed families are extremely low (30 and 33). In this case, it is possible that the mother has misrepresented the source of her difficulties, has extremely high expectations for her relationship with her son, or is extremely inaccurate in her report—all possibilities that require further assessment prior to determining a treatment strategy. Of course, conclusions based upon these tables must be tempered by the possible limitations of the normative data, which were from a predominantly lower middle– to upper middle–class, white population.[1]

A final cautionary note: Because individual CBQ responses have never been compared with their behavioral equivalents, inferences that individual items correspond directly with specific behaviors are tenuous at best. In addition, the forced-choice format of the questionnaire does not permit estimates of more subtle changes in the magnitude or quality of interaction behaviors described by the items. Thus, the CBQ is probably best used in conjunction with the interview and observational measures of interactional behavior.

Issues Checklist

The Issues Checklist (IC; see Appendix A) consists of a list of 44 issues that may lead to disagreements between parents and adolescents. It is modified from an instrument developed by Robin (1975). The IC assesses both conflictual issues and the perceived anger intensity of disputes over these issues. Parents and adolescents complete identical versions of the IC by recalling discussions of issues such as curfew, chores, and drugs. For each topic, the respondent indicates whether the issue has been broached during the previous 4 weeks. For each topic endorsed as having occurred, the respondent rates the anger intensity of the discussions on a 5-point scale ranging from calm to angry and estimates how often the topic arose.

The IC yields three scores for each respondent: (1) the quantity of issues, obtained by summing the number of issues circled "yes"; (2) the mean anger-intensity level of the endorsed issues, obtained by averaging the anger-intensity ratings for all of the endorsed issues; and (3) the weighted average of the frequency and anger-intensity level of the endorsed issues. This is obtained by multiplying each frequency estimate by its associated intensity, summing these cross products, then dividing by the total of all of the frequency estimates. This gives an estimate of anger *per discussion*, whereas the intensity score reflects merely the average anger *per issue*, regardless of the frequency with which the issue was discussed.

Clinically the IC is useful for pinpointing sources of conflict and surveying which topics are perceived as promoting greatest anger. These topics ordinarily include the family's presenting problems and warrant further assessment in the interview. The therapist can also use the IC to sequence problem-solving communication therapy so that early intervention sessions focus on less intense conflicts and later training sessions address more intense problems. Striking discrepancies between parent and teen reports can be explored further with follow-up questions. However, the fact that discrepancies occur emphasizes the potential inaccuracy of IC reports and indicates that the IC should not be used as the sole measure of conflict in the family.

Family Beliefs Inventory

The Family Beliefs Inventory (FBI) assesses distorted cognitions and unreasonable beliefs in parent–adolescent conflict. (The FBI is reproduced in Foster & Robin, 1988.) The FBI taps adherence to 10 unreasonable beliefs, discussed in Chapter 2. For the parents, these include ruination, obedience, perfectionism, approval, self-blame, and malicious intent; for adolescents, the beliefs are ruination, autonomy, approval, and unfairness. The FBI consists of 10 vignettes, each describing a typical parent–adolescent conflict, such as choice of friends and spending money. Topics were selected based upon issues a large number of families reported frequently on the IC. Following each vignette is a series of statements (one for each belief). Each is rated on a 7-point Likert scale indicating how much the respondent agrees with the belief. Two statements reflecting less extreme, more rational beliefs are intermingled to reduce response bias, but are not scored. Parents and adolescents complete different versions of the FBI, with vignette descriptions and beliefs slanted toward the perspective of the respondent. Scores are obtained for each belief by summing across the 10 vignettes and range from 10 to 70, with higher scores representing more extreme beliefs. A summary score may also be obtained for the entire inventory.

The FBI can help the therapist formulate hypotheses about the nature, source, and extent of distorted cognitions within the family. This in turn contributes to pinpointing how cognitive events interact with communication skills in maintaining the family's interactional problems.

Parent–Adolescent Relationship Questionnaire

The new Parent–Adolescent Relationship Questionnaire (PARQ) (Robin, 1985; Robin et al., 1986) was designed to be a comprehensive family assessment inventory. The parent and adolescent forms of the PARQ contain 428 yes/no items. Items were developed based on existing literature and assessment instruments and the behavioral–family systems theory espoused in Chapter 2. Items are grouped, based on content, into 13 scales: global distress, communication, problem solving, beliefs, warmth/hostility, coalitions, triangulation, hierarchy reversal, cohesion, somatic concerns, conflict over school, conflict over siblings, and social desirability. The general beliefs scale is further broken down on the parent form into subscales assessing ruination, obedience, perfectionism, self-blame, and malicious intent; on the adolescent form, subscales include ruination, unfairness, autonomy, perfectionism, and approval. Coalition and triangulation scales can also be broken down according to who is involved (e.g., mother–father with adolescent in the middle).

The PARQ's major asset is its comprehensiveness: It gathers data on multiple domains of family functioning with a single instrument, thus assessing family dimensions of parent–adolescent problems besides excessive conflict. When sufficient normative data are available, profile analyses should also be possible, allowing the clinician to see the family's scores in an MMPI-type profile relative to parent–adolescent norms. The drawback of the instrument is its length, requiring an average of 45 minutes to complete. It is currently under revision to create a shorter version.

Home Report

The Home Report (HR) consists of a 13-item yes/no checklist completed daily by the mother, the father, and the adolescent (Prinz, 1977). Items pertain to positive and negative interactive behavior of family members and to dyadic exchanges. Negative responses based on 10 of these items are summed to provide an index of family conflict. In addition, family members are asked to rate the overall pleasantness of their conversations that day on a 5-point scale called the "argument ratio." As an addendum, members may be asked to list and rate the anger intensity of specific disputes that arose that day. Each family member is given a set of addressed, stamped envelopes and instructed to complete the HR independently each evening (ordinarily for a week) and to mail it to the therapist the next morning. When all of the HRs have been received, averages can be computed for the daily conflict and argument ratio scores.

The clinician can use the HR to assess the valence of interactions on a daily basis rather than retrospectively. In other content domains, daily reports of events have proven more accurate than retrospective reports based upon longer time intervals between the events and the reporting (Yarrow, Campbell, & Burton, 1970). In addition, daily data can be used during intervention to monitor progress between sessions. However, the HR has to date been used only as an outcome measure, and its sensitivity to ongoing treatment is unknown. In addition, compliance may pose problems for the clinician, particularly after treatment has ended. In one outcome study (Foster, Prinz, & O'Leary, 1983), we required a $10 data deposit, to be refunded after the postassessment session. Prior to intervention, virtually all HRs were returned. After treatment, 11% of the treated participants failed to return even one HR, and a substantially higher percentage completed only a portion of the seven they had been given. Interestingly, all wait-list family members (who were about to begin treatment) completed their HRs. By follow-up, when the data deposit was no longer in effect, 18% of the treated participants returned no HRs. Robin (1980) encountered similar compliance problems.

Family Satisfaction Time Lines

The Family Satisfaction Time Line (FSTL) was originally developed by Williams (1979) for assessing the affective quality of marital interactions on a daily basis, and was modified for parent–teen relationships (Enyart, 1984; Robin, Nayar, & Rayha, 1984). Like the HR, the FSTL is completed each day independently by family members and is mailed in the next day. In its current form (Enyart, 1984), the FSTL requires family members to rate retrospectively at the end of the day the pleasantness of each 15-minute block of time they spent together. The teenager inserts *M* and *F* into the appropriate block to distinguish between time spent with mother and father. Pleasant time together is computed by summing the number of 15-minute blocks marked "very pleasant" or "pleasant"; unpleasant time represents the total number of blocks marked "very unpleasant" or "unpleasant." Additional open-ended questions ask the parent or teen to indicate things that happened (or failed to happen) to make parts of the day pleasant and unpleasant. As a prompt and check on compliance with instructions, other items ask whether the respondent talked with other members about the form, whether others knew the respondent's answers, and what the date and time of completing the form were.

The FSTL assesses positive and negative interactions on a daily basis. Answers to the open-ended questions provide the basis for hypotheses regarding the antecedents and process of problem interactions, and promote family members' attention to specific events. However, some family members may lack the observation, descriptive, and recall skills necessary to pinpoint specific events that occurred during the day. In addition, clinicians using the FSTL may need to take special steps to promote compliance with data collection procedures. In one study employing the FSTL (Enyart, 1984), families readily completed the forms each day, but in this study families were upper middle–class, nondistressed volunteers who were paid for participation only if all FSTLs were completed and who were systematically phoned every 2–3 days to ensure that data collection was proceeding as planned. In a second study, Robin *et al.* (1984) paid families contingent on completion of a portion of the FSTLs and phoned participants only if there were compliance problems. Participants in this study were more erratic in returning correctly completed FSTLs, suggesting that systematic follow-up is necessary to ensure that families provide daily data as instructed.

Various other pencil-and-paper inventories assess family interaction and individual and marital adjustment, but will not be described here. Table 5-1 lists these measures, as well as those described above, with brief descriptions and references.

TABLE 5-1 Questionnaire Inventories for Assessing Parent-Adolescent Interaction

Questionnaire	Assessment Target	References
Conflict Behavior Questionnaire (CBQ)	Communication and conflict behavior	Prinz, Foster, Kent, & O'Leary (1979); Robin & Weiss (1980)
Family Satisfaction Time Lines	Daily pleasant and unpleasant time	Enyart (1984); Robin, Nayar, & Rayha (1984)
Family Beliefs Inventory (FBI)	Irrational beliefs	Vincent-Roehling & Robin (1986)
Home Report (HR)	Daily interaction and arguments	Prinz *et al.* (1979)
Issues Checklist (IC)	Specific disputes	Prinz *et al.* (1979); Robin & Weiss (1980)
Parent-Adolescent Relationship Questionnaire (PARQ)	Multiple dimension of family interaction	Robin, Koepke, & Moye (1986)
Conflict Resolution Tactics Scale	Handling conflict	Straus (1979)
Decision Making Questionnaire	Family decision making	Prinz *et al.* (1979)
Family Adaptability and Cohesion Scales II	Cohesion, adaptability	Olson, Portner, & Bell (1982)

(*continued*)

TABLE 5-1 (*continued*)

Questionnaire	Assessment Target	References
Family Assessment Device	Multiple dimensions of communication and family functioning	Epstein, Bladwin, & Bishop (1983); Miller, Epstein, Bishop, & Keitner (1984)
Family Environment Scale	Multiple dimensions of family interaction	Moos & Moos (1981)
Family Life Questionnaire	Satisfaction and harmony in family interaction	Guerney (1977)
Parent Adolescent Communication Inventory	Communication	Bienvenu (1969)
Parent–Adolescent Communication Scale	Family Communication	Barnes & Olson (1985)
Parental Control Questionnaire	Parental Control	Prinz *et al.* (1979)
Relationship Likes and Dislikes	Liked and disliked aspects of relationship	Prinz, Rosenblum, & O'Leary (1978)
Structural Family Interaction Scale	Family structure	Perosa, Hansen, & Perosa (1981)
Dyadic Adjustment Scale	Global marital adjustment	Spanier (1976)
Locke–Wallace Marital Adjustment Scale	Global marital adjustment	Locke & Wallace (1959)
Marital Feelings Questionnaire	Unexpressed marital feelings	O'Leary, Fincham, & Turkewitz (1983)
Marital Satisfaction Inventory	Multidimensional scales—global and specific aspects of marital distress	Snyder (1979; 1981)
Primary Communication Inventory	Marital communication	Navran (1967)

Psychometric Characteristics of Self-Report Measures

A number of investigations have examined the psychometric characteristics of the CBQ, IC, FBI, PARQ, HR, and FSTL. These characteristics include discriminative and/or criterion-related validity, internal consistency, test–retest reliability, treatment sensitivity, concordance across family members, and construct validity. These studies are summarized here, together with the results of data analyses undertaken specifically for this volume.

Conflict Behavior Questionnaire and Issues Checklist

Three discriminative/criterion-related validity studies (Nayar, 1982; Prinz *et al.*, 1979; Robin & Weiss, 1980) contrasted the questionnaire responses of parents and adolescents referred for treatment of family relationship problems with the responses of family members with no history of treatment for relationship problems and/or self-reports of satisfactory relationships; significant differences between groups on most IC and CBQ scores were consistently found. Table 5-2 presents data from these studies, pooled with the preassessment data from two treatment studies employing the IC and CBQ with distressed families (Foster *et al.*, 1983; Robin, 1981). The adolescents ranged in age from 10 to 18, were male and female, and most families were white and came from lower middle– to upper middle–class socioeconomic groups. In the aggregated data, all CBQ and IC scores discriminated significantly between groups.

TABLE 5-2 Means and Standard Deviations for Distressed and Nondistressed Families on Conflict Behavior Questionnaire and Issues Checklist

	Distressed			Nondistressed				
	n	Mean	*SD*	*n*	Mean	*SD*	*t*	r_{pb}
Conflict Behavior Questionnaire								
Maternal appraisal of adolescent	137	25.6	8.9	68	8.0	5.7	14.84**	.72
Maternal appraisal of dyad	137	9.6	4.5	68	2.4	2.1	12.67**	.66
Adolescent appraisal of mother	137	19.4	11.5	68	6.8	7.3	8.28**	.50
Adolescent appraisal of dyad	137	9.7	4.9	68	4.0	2.3	9.39**	.55
Paternal appraisal of adolescent	65	21.4	8.7	14	11.1	7.1	4.12**	.43
Paternal appraisal of dyad	65	8.8	4.2	14	2.9	1.8	5.25**	.51
Adolescent appraisal of father	65	17.0	11.0	14	6.1	5.2	3.59*	.38
Adolescent appraisal of dyad	65	9.3	4.7	14	4.2	2.4	3.95*	.41
Issues Checklist								
Maternal quantity	123	22.55	7.35	68	17.83	7.07	3.62**	.25
Maternal anger intensity	124	2.42	.46	68	1.70	.45	11.43**	.64
Maternal anger intensity × frequency	123	2.81	.48	68	1.95	.51	12.29**	.67
Adolescent–mother: Quantity	96	20.68	7.59	68	18.46	7.25	1.88*	.15
Adolescent–mother: Anger intensity	96	2.34	.63	68	1.77	.49	6.20*	.44
Adolescent–mother: Anger intensity × frequency	96	2.68	.84	68	2.07	.68	5.08**	.37
Paternal quantity	60	18.38	5.05	38	11.64	4.63	6.61**	.60
Paternal anger intensity	60	2.18	.60	38	1.82	.57	2.93*	.29
Paternal anger intensity × frequency	60	2.39	.64	38	1.94	.59	3.46**	.33
Adolescent–father: Quantity	38	13.60	5.54	14	10.71	4.65	1.71*	.24
Adolescent–father: Anger intensity	38	2.40	.76	14	1.75	.64	2.80*	.37
Adolescent–father: Anger intensity × frequency	38	2.72	.95	14	1.88	.69	2.97*	.39

Note. R_{pb} represents point-biserial correlation between score and group membership (distressed vs. nondistressed). The *t* column gives values of *t* tests comparing distressed and nondistressed samples. Data are reprinted from "Problem-solving communication training: A behavioral–family systems approach to parent–adolescent conflict" (p. 211) by A. L. Robin and S. L. Foster, in *Adolescent behavior disorders: Foundations and contemporary concerns*, edited by P. Karoly and J. J. Steffen, 1984, Lexington, MA: D. C. Heath. Copyright 1984 by D. C. Heath. Reprinted by permission of the publisher.
*$p < .05$
**$p < .001$

Other psychometric characteristics of the CBQ include internal consisten-
cies (coefficient alphas) of .90 and above for mother and teen reports on each
scale. Each CBQ score has also been shown to change in a positive direction
following treatment (Foster *et al.*, 1983; Robin, 1981). Combined data from the
wait-list control groups in the Robin and Foster *et al.* outcome studies provide an
estimate of test–retest reliability for the CBQ over a 6–8-week interval; these are
presented in Table 5-3. *T* tests for related measures showed significant decreases
from pre- to posttreatment for father and mother appraisal of the adolescents, *ts*
(14, 18) = 2.90, 2.49; *ps* <.05. In both cases, the average improvement was
relatively small (3.8 and 2.8 points, respectively) but consistent, with some
improvement reported by 63% of mothers and 73% of fathers. Of course, given
the interval over which test–retest reliability was assessed, these findings could
represent actual improvement in relationships rather than simply a measurement
artifact.

Agreement between parental and adolescent perceptions of the relationship
on the 22 dyadic items common to parent and teen forms of the CBQ, calculated
for each of the 205 mother–adolescent and 80 father–adolescent dyads represented in Table 5-2, indicated that distressed and nondistressed mother–
adolescent dyads differed significantly in the number of disagreements (7.45 vs.
3.60, *t* (203) = 9.53, *p*<.001). Distressed and nondistressed father–adolescent
dyads showed the same pattern (7.09 vs. 3.64, *t* (78) = 4.56, *p*<.001).
Expressed as percent agreement, distressed dyads averaged approximately 66%–
68% agreement compared with 84% mean agreement for nondistressed dyads,
implying that the CBQ may not accurately reflect actual behavior.

Studies using the IC show that anger-intensity and weighted IC scores have
been sensitive to treatment effects (Foster *et al.*, 1983; Robin, 1981). As with the
CBQ, we computed test–retest stability of IC scores over 6–8 weeks with
distressed samples (wait-list control groups from Foster *et al.* and Robin), and

TABLE 5-3 Test–Retest Reliabilities for Distressed Dyads,
Conflict Behavior Questionnaire

	n	*r*
Maternal appraisal of adolescent	19	.57
Maternal appraisal of dyad	19	.61
Adolescent appraisal of mother	19	.37
Adolescent appraisal of dyad	19	.68
Paternal appraisal of adolescent	15	.82
Paternal appraisal of dyad	15	.61
Adolescent appraisal of father	15	.84
Adolescent appraisal of dyad	15	.85

Note. Correlations computed over 6–8-week interval. Data are from wait-list control families in Foster, Prinz &
O'Leary (1983) and Robin (1981) studies.

present these data in Table 5-4. Also included are Enyart's (1984) figures for a 1–2-week interval with a nonclinic, upper middle–class sample of 33 parent–teen triads. Correlations were much higher over the shorter interval, although the families' generally high educational level and nonclinic status may also have contributed to their more temporally reliable scores. With the distressed samples, only anger intensity reported by adolescents in the Foster *et al.* sample changed significantly over the 6–8-week interval, with an average drop of .49, t (8) = 2.80, $p<.05$.

To examine congruence between mother and adolescent responses, Steinfeld, Foster, Prinz, Robin, and Weiss (1980) computed item correlations for occurrence/nonoccurrence, frequency, and intensity for each issue, comparing the mother's responses with the adolescent's responses using IC data from three studies (Foster *et al.*, 1983; Prinz *et al.*, 1979; Robin & Weiss, 1980). These correlations ranged from .10 to .64 with a mean of .28, indicating a low to moderate degree of agreement on most issues.

We also used data from the three studies cited above to compute percentage agreement (agreements/[agreements + disagreements]) on whether mother and adolescent concurred that an issue either had or had not been discussed. Overall agreement averaged 67.6% for distressed dyads (range, 44.2%–86.4%) and 67.5% (range, 38.6%–84.1%) for nondistressed dyads. Occurrence agreement figures were much lower, averaging 47.9% (range, 13.6%–76.9%) and 43.7%

TABLE 5-4 Test–Retest Reliabilities for Distressed and Nondistressed Dyads, Issues Checklist

	Distressed (6–8-week interval)		Nondistressed (1–2-week interval)	
	n	r	n	r
Maternal quantity	19	.65	33	.70
Maternal anger intensity	19	.81	33	.63
Maternal anger intensity × frequency	19	.90	33	.74
Adolescent–mother: Quantity	10	.49	33	.49
Adolescent–mother: Anger intensity	10	.37	33	.47
Adolescent–mother: Anger intensity × frequency	10	.24	33	.80
Paternal quantity	15	.55	33	.80
Paternal anger intensity	15	.66	33	.73
Paternal anger intensity × frequency	15	.40	33	.80
Adolescent–father: Quantity	8	.87	33	.60
Adolescent–father: Anger intensity	8	.39	33	.72
Adolescent–father: Anger intensity × frequency	8	.15	33	.53

Note. Data for distressed mothers and fathers come from Foster, Prinz, & O'Leary (1983) and Robin (1981). Data for distressed adolescents are from Robin (1981). Data for nondistressed families are from Enyart (1984).

(range 21.1%–77.1%) for distressed and nondistressed samples. Enyart (1984) reported similar figures for a nondistressed sample. Together, these findings challenge the accuracy of the IC as an index of actual conflict at home. Lack of congruence in reports could reflect inaccuracies in parental reports, adolescent reports, or both. The true test would involve comparing reports on the IC with observations of actual discussions of IC topics at home—a difficult task that has yet to be performed.

Despite the lack of concordance between mothers and adolescents on individual items of the IC and CBQ, IC anger-intensity and CBQ scores correlated on average −.44 and −.52 with problem-solving communication observed using the modified Marital Interaction Coding System (MICS) during triadic discussions of conflictual issues (Rayha, 1982). IC and CBQ scores also correlated .45 and .55 with the dissatisfaction-with-child-rearing scale of Snyder's (1981) Marital Satisfaction Inventory, a scale tapping parental perceptions of children's misbehavior (Rayha, 1982).

Family Beliefs Inventory

Vincent-Roehling and Robin (1986) examined discriminative validity of the FBI by comparing families in treatment with families recruited by advertisements. Despite no significant differences for mothers, distressed fathers more strongly endorsed beliefs reflecting ruination, obedience, perfectionism, and malicious intent, and distressed adolescents endorsed greater ruination, autonomy, and fairness beliefs than did their nondistressed counterparts. The FBI had moderately high internal consistency, with coefficients generally above .70.

One FBI summary score for each family member was computed by summing all irrational belief scores across vignettes. Correlations between this score and IC anger-intensity and CBQ-20 scores were generally in the .30 range for fathers and teens but uncorrelated for mothers, suggesting that the FBI taps dimensions of parent–adolescent relationships different from those assessed by the CBQ and the IC. Limited evidence exists for the treatment sensitivity of the malicious intent and self-blame scales, which changed in a more flexible direction for parents after an intervention that included cognitive restructuring (Nayar, 1985). Finally, Robin, Koepke, and Hull (1988) found strong positive correlations between the FBI and an independent measure of similar beliefs (the PARQ), supporting the concurrent validity of the instrument.

Parent–Adolescent Relationship Questionnaire

All of the PARQ scales (except triangulation, coalitions, self-blame, and approval) discriminated between distressed and nondistressed parents and adolescents, with internal consistency above .75 in most cases (Robin et al., 1986). Strong evidence exists for the construct validity of many PARQ scales, which correlated with clinical interview and behavioral observation codings of similar content domains (Koepke, 1986). Factor analyses consistently produce three primary factors: skills deficits/overt conflict, extreme beliefs, and structural problems, and normative data have been collected to permit profile analyses. Investigations are underway to determine the treatment sensitivity of the PARQ, as well as its ability to differentiate families presenting with various types of adolescent problems.

Home Report

Prinz *et al*. (1979) found that conflict scores and argument ratios of both mothers and adolescents discriminated distressed from nondistressed dyads. However, neither Foster *et al*. (1983) nor Robin (1981) found the HR to be sensitive to treatment effects reflected in other measures.

Family Satisfaction Time Lines

Like the HR, little empirical work has been done with the FSTL. However, negative time-together scores recorded by fathers and mothers, and those recorded by adolescents on time with mother and father, discriminated 14 families in therapy from 14 nondistressed families (Robin, Nayar, & Rayha, 1984). Similarly, Enyart (1984) found that negative time reported together was a major predictor of mothers', fathers', and teens' (ages 13–16) scores on a relationship satisfaction questionnaire in her sample of 33 nondistressed triads with teens. In neither study did positive time together relate strongly to indices of family satisfaction.

Enyart also examined occurrence agreement for 15-minute time blocks to see whether parent and teen agreed on time together, resulting in a meager average of 42.2% (range, 15.7–82%). When agreement on time spent together and apart was calculated, this figure rose to 85% (range, 62.9%–97.2%). Kappa statistics, which control for chance agreement, were still quite low, though (mean, .48; range, .19–.87).

FSTL negative time and short-form CBQ scores correlated moderately for fathers ($r = .45$), adolescent reports on fathers (.53), and adolescent reports on mothers (.43; Robin, Nayar, & Rayha, 1984). Positive time together correlated negatively with CBQ scores only for adolescent reports on fathers (−.41). Mothers' reports of pleasant and unpleasant time with their adolescents showed no relationship to maternal CBQ or IC anger-intensity scores. These data indicate that FSTL assessments of negative time together are sensitive indicators of family distress, particularly for fathers and adolescents; with mothers, their interpretation is less clear.

Final Comment on Questionnaire Measures

The psychometric studies summarized here would suggest that the clinician can use the CBQ, IC, FBI, and PARQ with a moderate degree of confidence concerning their psychometric characteristics, but that the HR and FSTL should best be reserved for research use until further studies have been conducted.

At present, the dimensions of parent–adolescent conflict not tapped by most existing self-report measures are family structure and function. While the PARQ has scales to assess structure, their psychometric backing at this point is less than perfect. Selected aspects of family structure are also tapped by parts of the Family Environment Scale (Moos & Moos, 1981) and the Family Adaptability and Cohesion Scales II (Olson, Portner, & Bell, 1982), but these measures were not designed specifically for use with parent–adolescent relationship problems. The Structural Family Interaction Scale (Perosa, Hansen, & Perosa, 1981) is conceptually rich but has poor psychometric characteristics in its present form. Especially in light of Robin et al.'s (1986) findings that structural scales of the PARQ fared poorly psychometrically, it remains to be seen whether constructs such as triangulation, coalitions, and cohesions are amenable to valid, reliable self-reports.

To our knowledge, no standardized questionnaires currently available assess the antecedents and consequences of conflictual behavior directly. Probably the most common way of assessing antecedents and consequences of family behavior is via use of A–B–C (antecedent–behavior–consequence) logs completed by one or more family members each day. Such charts typically have columns for specifying a particular behavior, what happened immediately before the behavior occurred, and what happened after the behavior. Respondents can also be instructed to record what they thought and felt during the interaction. While A–B–C home monitoring seems to be widely used clinically, its potential for research has never been exploited and its evaluation as a systematic assessment instrument has been virtually ignored. It is also possible to develop questionnaires that assess family members' perceptions of antecedents and consequences of conflict in the home.

DIRECT OBSERVATION SYSTEMS

A direct way to assess parent–adolescent interaction is to observe parents and adolescents in conflictual situations. This is ordinarily accomplished by asking families to perform a task requiring interaction among members, while the therapist leaves the room in order to minimize reactivity to the therapist's presence. The discussion is audio- or videotaped and later analyzed, either formally by trained observers or less formally by the therapist. This process provides a sample of the family's interaction style under controlled or semicontrolled conditions, and can help the clinician pinpoint deficits in problem-solving communication behaviors and hypothesize variables related to positive and negative communication on a molecular level.

Obtaining an Interaction Sample

Several types of tasks for eliciting family discussion have appeared in the literature (see Cromwell, Olson, & Fournier, 1976). The family can be asked to (1) play a game or complete a task that requires members to work toward a specific goal, such as consensus on a story or plan (e.g., Barton & Alexander, 1979; Zuckerman & Jacob, 1979); (2) talk with one another about nonconflictual topics (e.g., Guerney, 1977); or (3) discuss an issue about which members disagree (e.g., Prinz et al., 1979). We prefer the last of these since it directly samples problem-solving communication behaviors in conflictual situations.

There are two general methods of establishing a problem-centered discussion. With the first method, the family is given a standard "hypothetical" problem to solve. Each person is provided with background information about the problem, prior to the discussion. In some cases, this is a vignette (Robin, Kent, O'Leary, Foster, & Prinz, 1977). Other investigators require each family member to complete a questionnaire independently, then ask the family to discuss questions for which their answers disagreed (e.g., Zuckerman & Jacob, 1979). In one variant of this approach (Olson & Ryder, 1970), family members are given incongruent information in order to exacerbate the conflict when they interact. With the second method, a current disagreement is selected for discussion. Either the members are asked to suggest a disagreement that one or all of them wish to see resolved, or the ICs are scanned for topics high in intensity and frequency. In much of our research, the topics with the highest intensity by frequency product scores on the parental and adolescent ICs are selected for discussion (Robin, 1981; Robin & Weiss, 1980).

Each of these methods has advantages and disadvantages that depend in part on the purpose of collecting the sample of family interaction. In clinical use, the major purpose is to obtain a sample of behavior that mirrors the family's communication at home. Creating conditions that duplicate home circumstances, such as choosing an issue of current concern, enhances the chances that a representative sample of home behavior will occur.

When the communication sample is used for research, the issue is more complex. In a study comparing the communication of distressed and nondistressed families, hypothetical problems standardize the task across families, increasing the likelihood that differences between groups of families are primarily a function of the family's interactional patterns, not task characteristics such as the topic under discussion. For example, the most intense disagreement is likely to be more severe for distressed than for nondistressed families (Robin & Weiss, 1980). In an outcome study, real problems discussed at preassessment that have been resolved during treatment are unsuitable for discussion at postassessment.

The unresolved issues that remain may be more severe than preassessment topics, since they are still problems after treatment. On the other hand, some family members (especially teenagers) find it difficult to become involved in discussions of hypothetical problems, limiting the generalizability of the communication they display. Interactions around hypothetical problems may be generalizable for clinic families only to those problems in which participants do not have strong, well-established positions—not the kinds of problems that typically lead to clinic referrals.

Real-life problems have the advantages of maximizing the salience of the topic to the family, hopefully enhancing the involvement of all members, and increasing the external validity of the resulting behavior sample. As mentioned above, real problems do pose confounds due to differences in the intensity of the topics across families and changes in intensity of problems over time. Investigators might compensate for these problems statistically by using analyses of covariance with the intensity of the topic under discussion as the covariate. Alternatively, they can select real topics matched on intensity across families.

At the present time, there are few empirical guidelines for selecting topics. A few studies, however, have indirectly touched upon the problem. Henggeler, Borduin, Rodnick, and Tavormina (1979) compared nondistressed families' discussion of where to go on vacation to identification of their biggest family problems. Observer ratings of attempted interruptions and simultaneous speech were higher for the latter task; successful interruptions, talk time, and ratings of affect did not differ across topics. Zuckerman and Jacob (1979) compared nondistressed parents' and sons' communication when making up a story together, discussing family problems, and resolving differing opinions on a questionnaire. The last of these tasks was related to greater numbers of times each family member spoke, but not to successful or attempted interruptions.

Studies including distressed families are perhaps more relevant to the issue of task comparability. Gilbert, Christensen, and Margolin (1984) assessed family alliances with parents and children aged 5–13 in two different tasks: planning a hypothetical dinner menu and discussing a current family problem. Although alliances were weaker in clinic than in nonclinic families in both tasks, patterns of weaker marital alliance and more unequal parent–child alliances emerged only in discussions of family problems, supporting the use of discussion of problems to elicit more pronounced conflict.

Two other studies bear on the question of what kind of problems family members discuss. In an outcome evaluation of problem-solving communication training (Robin *et al.*, 1977), dyads discussed both hypothetical and real problems; treatment resulted in large gains in problem-solving behavior across both types of discussions. Robin and Weiss (1980) asked distressed and nondistressed mother–son dyads to discuss the topics with the highest intensity by frequency product scores on the mothers' and sons' IC. There were no differences in problem-solving behavior during discussion of parents' versus adolescents' topics, but topics selected for distressed dyads had significantly higher intensity scores than the topics selected for nondistressed dyads. However, the behavioral differences between the two dyads were robust, even when the intensity of the topic under discussion was covaried out. Taken together, the results of studies on task and topic variations indicate that these influence different behaviors in different ways. The consistency, loci, and impact of these effects await more systematic exploration.

Another concern lies in how generalizable audio- or videotaped discussions are to family interaction at home. Foster (1978) collected data on this issue. After participating in a taped discussion, mothers and adolescents answered the question "How much was this discussion like those you have at home?" (1 = exactly the same, 5 = very different). Half of the adolescents and 25% of the mothers said their discussions were either "somewhat" or "very" different. Only 11% of the adolescents and 25% of the mothers said the discussion was "exactly the same." Following audiotaped assessments with these kinds of questions can give an indication of family members' perceptions of generalizability of their discussions. Follow-up questions can sometimes yield information on the ways the family's communication resembled and differed from their usual patterns. In addition, family members' communication in session can be compared with their taped discussion in the search for consistent patterns of interaction.

Even reactive communication samples can be informative to the clinician. A conversation that goes well indicates to both family and therapist that, under certain circumstances, the family can resolve its problems through discussion. The therapist can then examine conditions that differentiate clinic from home discussions, such as lower levels of affect and fewer external interruptions, as possible variables related to the ineffective communication at home. Reactivity is a persistent problem, however, for the researcher or clinician who wishes to infer that the behavior sample s/he collects in a controlled environment duplicates behavior at home.

Coding an Interaction Sample

Approaches to coding a video- or audiotape of a parent–adolescent discussion vary in complexity and include informally reviewing the tape without using any standardized code, coding it with a global-inferential system, or coding it with a detailed, frequency-based coding system. Selection of an appropriate approach depends upon the time, resources, and purpose for which the data are collected. The clinician wishing to obtain a useful picture of the interactions of a family for treatment planning may wish to review the tape informally and/or rate it with a global-inferential coding system, since the resources and time necessary to use a detailed frequency-based code go beyond the practical capabilities of most practicing clinicians. Researchers who need an overall summary of the amount and valence of problem-solving communication behavior can also rely upon a global-inferential code. Frequency breakdowns of component behaviors or sequential patterning of interactions, however, require a detailed frequency-based coding system.

Three observation systems (the modified Marital Interaction Coding System, Interaction Behavior Code, and the Community Members Rating Scale) developed in our research will be reviewed in depth here. Table 5-5 lists these and other observational coding systems that have been developed or could be adapted for coding parent–adolescent interaction.

Modified Marital Interaction Coding System

The MICS was originally developed for coding videotaped samples of marital problem-solving communication behavior (Weiss, Hops, & Patterson, 1973; Weiss & Margolin, 1977). We adapted it for use with parents and adolescents. The modified MICS is a content-oriented coding system requiring extensive training designed to classify all verbal behavior emitted by parents and adolescents into 23 mutually exclusive categories (Robin & Fox, 1979; Robin & Weiss, 1980). Verbal behaviors are categorized within 30-second intervals; there is no artificial constraint on the number of verbal behaviors that could be coded

TABLE 5-5   Observational Coding Systems for Parent–Adolescent Interactions

Code	Target	Type	References
Community Members Rating Scale	Problem solving, communication	Global-inferential	Robin & Canter (1984)
Interaction Behavior Code (IBC)	Problem solving, communication	Global-inferential	Prinz & Kent (1978)
Modified Marital Interaction Coding System (MICS)	Problem solving, communication	Frequency	Robin & Weiss (1980)
Parent–Adolescent Interaction Coding System (PAICS)	Problem solving, communication	Frequency	Robin (1981)
Centripetal/Centrifugal Family Style Scales	Cohesion	Global-inferential	Kelsey-Smith & Beavers (1981)
Defensive/Supportive Behavior Code	Defensive and supportive behavior	Frequency	Alexander (1973)
Family Alliances Coding System	Dyadic alliance	Frequency	Gilbert, Christensen, & Margolin (1984)
Family Interaction Coding System	Positive and negative verbal and nonverbal behavior	Frequency	Loeber, Weissman, & Reid (1983); Reid (1978)
Family Interaction Scales	Communication, affective expression	Frequency and global-inferential	Riskin & Faunce (1970a, b)
Problem-Solving Code	Problem solving	Frequency	Robin, Kent, O'Leary, Foster, & Prinz (1977); Foster, Prinz & O'Leary (1983)

separately within each interval. A "verbal behavior" is defined as a statement by one family member that is both homogeneous in content and bounded by the statements of other family members. Each statement may be classified sequentially into one or more categories depending upon whether its meaning changes before the speaker concludes. The modified MICS categories include accept responsibility, agree, approval, assent, command, complain, compliance, compromise, deny responsibility, disagree, evaluation, humor, interrupt, laugh, negative solution, no response, noncompliance, positive solution, problem description, put-down, question, specification of the problem, and talk.

The modified MICS provides information on the frequency and temporal patterning of a variety of problem-solving communication behaviors. Category scores are expressed as proportions, obtained by dividing the total number of behaviors within the category by the total number of behaviors for the target speaker across all of the categories.

Robin and Weiss (1980) established the criterion-related validity of the modified MICS by showing that distressed mother–adolescent dyads exhibited more commands, put-downs, and no-response statements than did nondistressed dyads, and fewer accept-responsibility, agree, approval, assent, evaluation, humor, laugh, positive-solution, and specification-of-the-problem statements. Interobserver agreement (percent agreement) computed tape by tape (across categories) ranged from 58% to 68%, averaging 76%. When we recomputed interobserver agreement on a category-by-category basis, figures were less satisfactory, ranging from 0% to 100%, with 10 of the 23 categories (most very low frequency) having percent agreement below 70%.

Evidence for the construct validity of the modified MICS came from a study where MICS summary scores correlated in the .90 range with community members' global ratings of conflict, communication, and problem solving (Robin & Canter, 1984). The modified MICS has now been revised and is called the Parent–Adolescent Interaction Coding System (PAICS), which has been reduced to 15 categories. Treatment studies have demonstrated the sensitivity of the PAICS to changes produced by therapy (Robin, 1981). Further revisions have yielded a version of the PAICS that has six major categories, maintains frequency-based coding, is comparable to the more complicated versions psychometrically, but is easier to use (Adams, 1987).

Interaction Behavior Code

Partially in response to the time-intensive nature of sequential and interval coding systems, Prinz and Kent (1978) developed the global-inferential Interaction Behavior Code (IBC) for assessing parent–adolescent communication. The IBC relies upon the consensus of several raters who listen to and evaluate audiotapes of family interaction after approximately 2 hours of training with the rating criteria. The IBC consists of 32 categories such as negative exaggeration, yelling, making suggestions, and compromise, each of which is accompanied by a brief definition (see Appendix B). Twenty-two categories are rated "yes" (given a 1-point value) if they occurred at all during the discussion; otherwise, they are rated "no" (0 points). Eleven other categories are rated either "no" (0 points), "a little" (.5 point), or "a lot" (1 point). Points are totaled separately for positive and negative items, then divided by the total number of positive and negative items (respectively) to yield composite positive and negative interaction scores for each interactant. In addition, observers rate each family on 4-point Likert scales for degree of resolution, friendliness, insults, and general problem-solving effectiveness. The means of the raters' figures are used as dependent measures in analyses. The reliability of these scores is assessed using the Spearman–Brown formula, which uses correlations among all possible pairs of scores to estimate the reliability of the mean, which is more stable than the value of any single score (Hartmann, 1977; McNemar, 1969).

Three separate investigations using the IBC have reported consistently high reliability estimates, ranging from .83 to .97 (Foster *et al.*, 1983; Prinz & Kent, 1978; Robin & Koepke, 1985). These figures were based on means of four raters; agreement between any two raters would be much lower. Foster *et al.* found that only negative maternal behavior showed changes as a function of problem-solving communication training. Although it is possible that actual behavior changes did not occur, it should be noted that positive and negative summary categories reflect the *number* or *diversity* of behaviors displayed by mothers and adolescents, not frequencies of any of the component behaviors. For this reason, the code may not be sensitive to real changes in frequency of occurrence. Robin and Koepke also examined the relationship of global-impressionistic IBC ratings and frequency-based modified MICS coding of parent–adolescent interactions, finding correlations between the two codes ranging from .51 to .82. Based upon these findings, clinicians and researchers can select the coding scheme that meets their needs, taking into consideration factors such as degree of detail required and available resources.

Community Members Rating Scale

Robin and Canter (1984) developed the Community Members Rating Scale as an alternative to the complex modified MICS. Representative parents, teens, and/or mental health professionals from the community rate audiotapes on 7-point Likert scales on 21 of the 23 MICS categories and also provide global ratings of communication positiveness, problem-solving effectiveness, and conflict. Like the IBC, tapes are scored by several individuals and the mean of their ratings is used.

Interrater agreement scores based on 13 to 15 raters were excellent for the global ratings (all >.90), but more variable for individual categories, ranging from .00–.96. Mothers scored above .70 on 71% of the specific categories they rated; fathers did somewhat better (81%), while adolescents did somewhat worse (62%). Reliabilities for the group of professionals exceeded .70 for all but one category. However, we computed average pairwise agreement to be much lower, with all figures below 60%, indicating that reliable data can only be obtained with large numbers of raters.

Correlations of specific categories with their modified MICS counterparts were also generally below .60, although (as indicated previously) global ratings all correlated .81 or more with MICS global ratings. Thus, this rating scheme seems most useful when numerous raters are available and only global estimates of problem solving, positive communication, and conflict are needed.

Concluding Comments on Direct Observation

Direct observation has several clear assets, not the least of which is the opportunity to assess potential intervention targets directly. The objectivity and lack of susceptibility to some of the biasing factors that limit self-reports also justify its use. However, researchers and clinicians need to be aware of the methodological problems that beset direct observation, including reactivity to the observation situation, biases inflating reliability, expectation effects, and observer drift. Reviews by Hartmann and Wood (1982), Cone and Foster (1982), and Foster and Cone (1986) provide in-depth analyses of these difficulties.

The coding systems and interactional tasks we have presented tap problem-solving communication behavior but fail to assess directly family structure and the functions of behavior within systems. Two other observation systems assess structural dimensions of families, however, using categories and methods compatible with a behavioral assessment framework. Kelsey-Smith and Beavers (1981) describe a global-inferential rating system for assessing a continuum they term centripetal–centrifugal, very similar to the cohesion continuum described in Chapter 2. This was used to rate five family discussions (totaling 50 minutes per family). Unfortunately, interrater agreement was below 79% for all 13 rating scales included in the coding system.

Gilbert et al. (1984) provided more promising interobserver agreement data (above 97%) for a system used to assess alliances among family members. Gilbert et al.'s observation system requires that each speech act be coded in terms of to whom it was directed, its content, and its affective quality. Each content and affect code is then multiplied by a weighting based on average ratings provided earlier by graduate students evaluating how much the code represented a positive or negative alliance. The code discriminated weaker alliance rates in distressed than nondistressed families with preadolescent children, and it provides a promising method of assessing this aspect of family structure.

Unfortunately, neither Kelsey-Smith and Beavers nor Gilbert et al. presented data directly aimed at evaluating their particular codes as indices of cohesion and alliance. Given the molarity of such systems-oriented constructs, further attention to content and construct validity is particularly important.

In addition, coding systems have not yet been used to assess functional relationships among interactional behaviors. Data from the modified MICS or the PAICS, for example, could be analyzed sequentially for patterns of coercion or for common interaction chains, much as Patterson and his colleagues (e.g., Patterson, 1982) examined observational data from aggressive children and their parents, and Gottman (1979) derived common patterns in marital discussions. Examination of function over longer time frames may prove more challenging, since observations of brief discussions are inherently unsuitable for this analysis. Nonetheless, it may be possible to develop home-based assessment devices to yield a data base for these efforts, or to gather information via interview and then analyze it for sequential patterns.

Direct observation measures have to date relied on small samples of communication collected in laboratory or clinic settings, where the focus is on decision-making or problem-solving tasks. No one has to date explored the generalizability of these samples to the ways parents and adolescents discuss problem issues at home. Direct observational investigation of home communication patterns, while logistically difficult, is important both for establishing the external validity of laboratory-analogue measures and for establishing the accuracy of self-report measures of home behavior. Placing microphones in the home that transmit at randomly selected, unsignaled times to out-of-sight audiorecorders (Christensen, 1979) provides one way of doing this unobtrusively. This option, of course, requires fully informed consent by all participants for it to be implemented ethically.

Finally, all the systematic observation systems described here have been used to code communication samples, but never applied to observing family behavior during therapy sessions. Because behavior during sessions provides a rich source of information to the therapist, it would be especially useful to examine the extent to which behavior displayed in his/her presence is generalizable to home interaction. Other types of in-session observation codes may also be helpful for understanding the interview process (e.g., Chamberlain, Patterson, Reid, Kavanagh, & Forgatch, 1984).

NOTE

1. A recent study with black, impoverished 16–20-year-old youth found that scores for distressed and nondistressed adolescents were comparable to previous norms for white, middle-class youth (Schubiner & Robin, in press).

CHAPTER SIX

Conceptualizing and Integrating Assessment Data

The clinician who conducts an interview, administers the CBQ, the IC, the HR, and a marital questionnaire, and rates a taped discussion using the IBC will wind up with over 900 bits of data for a two-parent family. Collecting and scoring such data are only preliminary steps in the conceptual process that integrates assessment information into (1) themes regarding response patterns and (2) hypotheses about the interlocking contingency arrangements that maintain problematic family interaction patterns. Such themes and hypotheses are based on the content and process of the interview, questionnaire and home monitoring measures, and audiotapes of interaction samples.

Critical to this process is a functional analysis of interlocking contingency arrangements. First this involves describing the patterns common to important family interaction patterns, including behavioral, cognitive, and affective antecedents and consequences, thereby relating each member's interaction behavior to both internal and external events. The latter are comprised primarily (but not exclusively) of other interactants' behavior. Thus, the behaviors of each participant in an interaction serve as critical antecedents and consequences for the behaviors of the others. Each individual's behavior can be described as a behavior sequence in which many of the antecedent and consequent actions are provided by other participants. The *interlocking* nature of these sequences is a crucial parameter of descriptions of family interactions.

The next step involves hypothesizing what functions problem behaviors in the chain serve for different involved parties. The functions that the therapist examines include reinforcement, punishment, avoidance, reciprocity, and coercion. Structural configurations such as coalitions, triangulation, and cohesion, which are maintained by functional outcomes of family members' behavior, are also postulated as ways of describing cross-situational patterns of interaction. As hypotheses are generated, the clinician attempts to test them by asking pinpointing questions, administering additional self-report inventories, or informally introducing manipulations in the family system that should produce predictable changes in interaction consistent or inconsistent with the original hypotheses. In the pages that follow, we elaborate on these methods for generating and testing hypotheses concerning functional and structural interaction patterns.

Functional analysis is central to planning successful interventions, particularly with severely distressed families. Without an adequate understanding of the

99

antecedents and consequences of problematic family interaction patterns, the therapist may fail to take crucial functions of behavior into account, and change will either fail to occur or be short-lived. Intervention must be planned and sequenced considering family functional and structural patterns. The following example illustrates the results of failure to do this.

Example. Mrs. Jones and 13-year-old Andrew regularly argued over Andrew's failure to complete his homework. She checked on him repeatedly to determine whether he was working on his homework. Often he was not. Mrs. Jones was also depressed about her recent separation from Andrew's father and had become something of a social recluse since the separation. The therapist taught the dyad to problem-solve the homework issue. During three separate sessions, mutually acceptable solutions were negotiated and renegotiated. One or both family members, however, sabotaged the solutions at home. From talking individually with Mrs. Jones, the therapist learned the seriousness of her social isolation, her anxiety about reinitiating dating, and her depression. The therapist hypothesized that Mrs. Jones's intense preoccupation with Andrew's homework functioned to keep her in close contact with her son, to help her avoid anxiety-provoking dating situations, and to fill the void left by her separation from his father. Andrew contributed to the situation by working on his homework only intermittently. Given this analysis, problem solving would not be expected to be effective unless the "problem" was adequately defined in a broader context. Using cognitive restructuring, the therapist helped Mrs. Jones overcome her social isolation, decrease her anxiety about dating, and begin to see other men. Then she and her son were able to implement the agreed-upon solutions to the homework problem.

Commentary. In this case, parent–adolescent conflict was not solely the result of skill deficits. Arguing with Andrew fulfilled important functions for Mrs. Jones: It helped her to avoid interpersonal anxiety associated with dating and provided her with a source of interpersonal closeness (albeit negative) to replace her lost husband. Only when the therapist recognized the functions of the arguing and helped Mrs. Jones to overcome her anxiety and to achieve other sources of interpersonal closeness was problem solving effective with the presenting problem—homework.

THE PROCESS OF INTEGRATING INFORMATION

The process of thematic data integration and functional analysis, while crucial to planning a coordinated treatment strategy, only begins during the assessment phase, and continues throughout treatment. Themes and treatment plans are refined as the therapist observes family interaction during problem-solving sessions, notes members' responses to therapeutic interventions, and listens for new information. Thus, synthesis of assessment information leads to preliminary hypotheses about crucial family patterns and their determinants. These hypotheses are supported by data but subject to change should new information disconfirm them.

Pinpointing Questions

Interview questions asking the family to pinpoint conditions in which problematic interactions occur or are absent can be used to postulate events that consistently correlate and may be functionally related. In the following example, pinpointing questions are used to elicit descriptions of sequences of family interaction that form the essential raw material for clinical hypotheses.

Example.

THERAPIST: Tell me exactly what happens when you have a disagreement about curfew.

MRS. SMITH: I tell John to come home at 11:30, but he gets in at 1:00 a.m.

MR. SMITH: Without even calling us!

JOHN: Well, they just *tell* me, they don't care what I want.

THERAPIST: So, John, Mom tells you when to come home. Then you come home late without calling. What happens when you come in the door?

JOHN: They jump all over me.

THERAPIST: Who says what?

JOHN: She starts yelling and threatening to ground me.

MR. SMITH: His mother is really worried that he might have gotten hurt, like in a car accident.

THERAPIST: What about you, Mr. Smith? What do you do when John comes in the door at 1:00 a.m.?

MRS. SMITH: He never does anything. He's usually in bed. Seems like I have to do all the dirty work in this family. . . .

MR. SMITH: *(Interrupting)* That's not true! How many times have I tried to reason with the boy. . . .

THERAPIST: *(Interrupting)* Wait a minute! Sounds like the two of you disagree about this, and Mom feels like she is the heavy.

JOHN: She is!

THERAPIST: Hold on! Let me see if I have this straight. Mom first takes charge of talking to John when he comes in late. And Mom comes on loud and clear, with threats of grounding. Then, Mom tries to bring Dad into the act. Dad would rather use reasoning while Mom would rather use punishment. Right?

MRS. SMITH: Yes.

MR. SMITH: I guess so.

THERAPIST: So how does this end?

JOHN: They ground me for 2 weeks.

MRS. SMITH: And my husband sometimes feels sorry for him and lets him off early.

MR. SMITH: You can't keep the boy in the house forever.

THERAPIST: *(To the parents)* And what happens to the disagreement between you two?

MRS. SMITH: We usually wind up in a fight after John goes to bed.

MR. SMITH: We end up angry with each other for several days, too.

MRS. SMITH: All I want is some support in disciplining John.

THERAPIST: I understand how you must feel, Mrs. Smith. John, it appears that this kind of argument between you and your parents ends up in a fight between your parents. Dad is laid-back until Mom forces the issue and pulls him in. Then, you get punished, but Dad sometimes undoes Mom's punishment. This all must be very hard on everyone.

Commentary. The therapist uses pinpointing questions about a representative interaction pattern. As the family supplies information that suggests patterns and hypotheses about the functions of each person's behavior, the therapist reflects back coherent statements of the patterns s/he sees. John and his mother appear to be engaged in a reciprocal cycle of punishing behavior concerning curfew. In this incident, when Mrs. Smith established her son's curfew without consulting John, he "paid her back" by coming home late (a behavior that could be maintained by negative attention from both parents, temporary avoidance of negative interactions at home, and/or positive reinforcement from peers). Mrs. Smith attempted to provide a consequence for John's tardiness, and an argument ensued. Mr. and Mrs. Smith were also engaged in a reciprocally negative cycle, elicited either by their disagreement about how to discipline John, or as a function of cognitive variables not yet assessed. Mr. Smith encouraged John's defiance of his wife's curfew by undoing the punishment she administered, thereby punishing her efforts to discipline John. He also avoided negative interactions with his son by leaving the discipline to his wife, and fostered positive interactions with his son by easing John's punishments. Mrs. Smith's arguing with her son, while serving as an ineffective punishment for his coming home late, functioned successfully to coerce her distant husband to participate more actively in the disciplinary process; without her prodding, he remained aloof and unsupportive.

Of course, this analysis is based upon a single retrospective sample of family interaction. The therapist should attempt to verify these hypotheses by collecting additional information (e.g., by observing the interview process while attending to the content of family members' statements).

Using Observational Data to Formulate Hypotheses

Audio- or videotapes of parent–adolescent interactions also provide sources for generating hypotheses concerning interlocking contingency patterns. Observations of family interaction during the interview often supply another rich source of data. Even without the use of formal coding systems, the astute clinician can infer the presence of patterns of reciprocity, avoidance, and coalitions from informal reviews of taped discussions or therapy sessions. Strong reciprocity of negative affect and behavior, for example, might be inferred if parents and adolescents repeatedly enter into accusatory–defensive interchanges, where one rebuts the other's blaming statements in a defensive manner. Avoidance might be inferred if a mother repeatedly changes the topic when a father and son begin to have a heated, accusatory interchange. A father who "softens" his wife's demands on their son when the son complains, by making comments such as "Leave the boy alone" or "Go easy on him," might recurrently form coalitions with his son against his wife, reinforcing the boy's complaints. The key to making reasonable hypotheses is listening for *recurring* sequences of interaction, not single instances of behaviors. Sequential analyses of coded interaction data using formal coding systems such as the modified MICS data (see Chapter 5) can also form the basis for inferring functional interaction patterns, if such data are available.

Informal Manipulations of Interaction Patterns

One way to test hypotheses about the antecedents and consequences of interaction patterns involves introducing interventions designed to alter the family's interaction patterns and observing their responses. This technique is based upon the ABAB reversal design derived from applied behavior analysis (Baer, Wolf, & Risley, 1968). In applied behavior analysis, cause–effect relationships are established by altering or removing the hypothesized causal variable *(B)* following collection of baseline data *(A)* and examining the ensuing effect of this manipulation on repeated measurements of a dependent variable. While therapists cannot usually conduct full controlled experiments during the course of treatment, informal ABAB probes can be constructed by using therapists' instructions and feedback to alter temporarily one or more aspects of family members' interactive behavior and to observe the impact on their relations during the session.

Example.   Lani Phillips was a 13-year-old whose weight had dropped from 95 to 60 pounds over a 4-month period, prompting a great deal of conflict between Lani and her parents, mostly about eating. The following excerpt is from a family assessment session conducted while Lani was hospitalized on a pediatric ward for anorexia nervosa. Lani, her mother, her father, and the therapist were present.

THERAPIST: Tell me exactly what happened at home at the dinner table during the last few days before Lani came into the hospital.

MR. PHILLIPS: She wouldn't eat, and I'd have to yell at her to get her . . .

LANI: *(Interrupting)* You didn't have to yell that much. . . .

MRS. PHILLIPS: Doctor, I don't want you to get the idea that we fight a lot. It really isn't . . .

LANI: *(Interrupting)* . . . that bad.

THERAPIST: Hold on! One at a time. Lani, what did you do when your dad tried to get you to eat?

LANI: I ate. I was getting better. Then . . .

MRS. PHILLIPS: *(Interrupting)* She really was . . .

MR. PHILLIPS: *(Interrupting)* But not enough. She was real fussy about what she would eat. . . .

LANI: *(Interrupting)* That's why I went shopping with Mom. To make sure she got what I like.

MRS. PHILLIPS: She is a real help. But recently she started dictating what I could buy.

THERAPIST: Tell me more about this.

MR. PHILLIPS: She was only trying to keep her mother from eating fattening foods. Mom really should . . .

LANI: *(Interrupting)* Dad! Mom doesn't eat junk. I love junk foods, especially potato chips.

MR. PHILLIPS: That was our real problem. All she would eat was junk foods. Doctor, what should we do?

THERAPIST: I'm getting dizzy listening to this discussion. Every time one of you begins to say something, another interrupts.

MRS. PHILLIPS: We're a close family.

LANI: I can read Mom's mind.

THERAPIST: You're right. You are a close family. You help each other quite a bit. Whenever someone disagrees with another, the third person interrupts to play it down. But, Mr. Phillips, you raised an important question. To answer it, I need to hear everything each of you wants to say. Therefore, whenever anyone interrupts another, I'm going to stop it. Now, let's come back to what happens at the dinner table.

MR. PHILLIPS: I yell, but I can't understand why Lani doesn't eat. It's like she wants to get us upset. . . .

LANI: *(Interrupting)* I . . .

THERAPIST: *(Interrupting)* No interrupting. Now, Mr. Phillips.

MR. PHILLIPS: I think she wants to get us upset at her.

LANI: I'm not trying to get you upset. You're getting yourself upset. . . .

MRS. PHILLIPS: *(Interrupting)* Dad's not . . .

THERAPIST: *(Interrupting)* Remember . . .

MR. PHILLIPS: I'm upset. I have enough to worry about at work without this thing with Lani's not eating. . . .

LANI: *(Interrupting)* I do . . .

THERAPIST: *(Interrupting)* You will have a chance. Mrs. Phillips, you look upset.

MRS. PHILLIPS: I'm upset about a lot of things. And not only Lani's eating. . . .

MR. PHILLIPS: *(Interrupting)* I thought we . . .

THERAPIST: *(Interrupting)* Remember, one at a time.

MRS. PHILLIPS: Doctor, we may as well be honest. That's what we are here for. It's his drinking. He drinks too much.

LANI: When will this meeting be done?

THERAPIST: We are just getting started. . . .

Commentary. The therapist uses instructions and feedback to alter one aspect of the family's interaction and conduct a functional analysis. At first, the therapist noted a great deal of interrupting and evasive conversation. In particular, when one family member disagreed with another or hinted at an area of conflict, a third immediately interrupted. The interruptions served either to change the topic or to play down the area of disagreement. The therapist hypothesized that open conflict was extremely aversive for the family and that interrupting functioned as avoidance or escape behavior. Interruptions that successfully sidetracked the discussion were negatively reinforced by reducing open conflict. (Minuchin *et al.*, 1978, noted similar "protective" interactions in the families of many anorectic teenagers.)

To test this hypothesis, the therapist intervened to short-circuit interruptions and prevent avoidance of the aversive stimulus. Notice how the therapist avoided answering Mr. Phillips's direct question but instead used the question to construct a rationale for targeting interruptions as changeworthy. If the hypothesis were correct, one would expect increased evidence of conflict when interruptions were stopped. In fact, a serious disagreement between Lani's parents over her father's drinking emerged. The hypothesis about the avoidance function of interrupting comments was tentatively confirmed, further suggesting that family members were avoiding discussion of marital conflicts. Further assessment revealed that patterns of avoidance behavior permeated all of this family's interactions.

GROUPING INFORMATION THEMATICALLY

Functional analysis of every bit of interactive behavior sampled by an assessment battery is obviously not feasible. To make this process less cumbersome, information can be grouped or "chunked" into broader categories, based on thematic content. This grouping process facilitates hypothesis generation and helps in planning interventions that simultaneously target multiple problems with a common theme.

The IC provides a good starting place for this process. The most intense conflicts are usually those with anger-intensity ratings of 4 and 5. Often these are the initial presenting problems and are likely to be the products of central functional patterns within the family. These can serve as springboards for further analyses and grouping.

Grouping of issues is accomplished by assessing the situational factors surrounding specific disputes. Disputes that share common situational antecedents and consequences can be grouped together, and reasonable inferences can be made concerning the interactional patterns that they exemplify.

Example.   Mr. and Mrs. Jones and 14-year-old Betsy assigned curfew, dating, going places without parents, and homework anger-intensity ratings of 5 on the IC. Interview information revealed that when Betsy's parents established specific limits on her weekend curfew, whom she could date, and where she could go with her dates, Betsy disobeyed. Loud arguments would ensue, during which Betsy's parents would say that they needed to protect her from "being hurt by boys." Betsy maintained she was capable of handling herself with boys. Arguments culminated in Betsy's begrudgingly agreeing to parental restrictions which she had no intention of honoring. In contrast, disputes over homework revolved around the sloppy, impulsive manner in which Betsy completed her assignments. The disputes were prompted by notes from the teacher and resulted in parental withdrawal of selected privileges, losses that Betsy did not contest. The therapist grouped curfew, dating, and going places without parents as examples of the theme of parental attempts to avoid perceived catastrophic consequences by limiting Betsy's contacts with boys. Since disputes over homework were elicited by different situational factors, they were considered separately.

Summary scores on the IC and CBQ can also be useful for generating hypotheses about structural interaction patterns. In the case of triads, the therapist can examine the relative levels of conflict in the mother–adolescent, father–adolescent, and even mother–father dyads when marital questionnaires have been administered. If, for example, there is more conflict in the mother–adolescent than in the father–adolescent dyad, the therapist might explore the following hypotheses: (1) the mother is overly involved in disciplinary actions while the father either avoids or is excluded from the process; (2) the mother is overly protective and the father is not; and (3) the father and adolescent support each other's view, forming a coalition and undermining the mother's parenting attempts. When high conflict is reported in both parent–adolescent dyads, but the parents report minimal marital conflict, the therapist might hypothesize that the parent–teen conflict is relatively independent of marital functioning. When spouse conflict is high and parent–teen conflict is low, it is reasonable to suspect that the teenager's problematic behavior may have some functional relationship to the parents' relationship disturbances.

Observations of the family during the interview and in taped discussions can also assist the therapist in isolating problematic structural patterns. The key to identifying coalitions, triangulation, and shifting hierarchies lies in identifying molar-level patterns of interaction that are repeated across problem areas. Chapters 2 and 10 present some of the structural patterns associated with excessive parent–adolescent conflict, and Chapter 10 describes how treatment plans can be adapted to address these patterns.

PROBLEMS IN HYPOTHESIZING FUNCTIONAL PATTERNS

Elaborating the interlocking nature of sequences of behavior within the family system is made difficult by the fact that, unlike linear analysis of an individual's behavior, it is difficult to decide where in time to punctuate the beginnings and endings of sequences. When focusing on an individual, environmental antecedents and consequences can be specified by observing what happens before and after the target behavior. However, when the focus is on the interactions of an adolescent and two parents, the unit of analysis is more ambiguous. Through observation, circular processes emerge, with each person's behavior serving as both antecedent and consequence for others' behavior. The selection of "beginning" and "ending" points often becomes arbitrary with such circular patterns of interaction. Similarly, the level of analysis at which to process interaction is open to debate: Should molecular behaviors (e.g., accusatory statements) be the primary focus of analysis, or should the analysis consider larger groupings of behavior (e.g., an argument)?

Under these circumstances, the model of human behavior used by the therapist to view interaction patterns may become a more important determinant of how "raw interaction data" is punctuated and categorized than the reality of the behavior itself. Proponents of social-learning theory, who apply concepts such as reinforcement, reciprocity and coercion, are likely to slice behavior in terms of sequences of molecular dyadic interaction. Proponents of family systems theory, using concepts such as triangulation, are more likely to group behaviors into molar-level descriptions of triadic interaction. Ideally, a behavior analysis (Goldfried & D'Zurilla, 1969) of family interactions should be conducted to derive an empirically based taxonomy of important functional patterns seen at molecular and molar levels of analysis. But until such an analysis has been completed, the therapist must rely on a "trial and error" approach.

Roadblocks sometimes occur in formulating reasonable functional analyses. When the therapist encounters difficulties formulating interlocking positive and negative reinforcement patterns that make sense and seem to explain an interaction pattern fully, s/he should reconsider whether (1) avoidance patterns are operative, (2) private events are critical either as antecedents or in determining the valence of a consequence, or (3) the level of analysis employed is too molecular.

Avoidance is most often seen in family interactions in which historically one family member's behavior has either been punished or served only to terminate a negative interaction with no resolution of the original problem. For instance, Lani and her parents avoided arguments via interruptions, in an earlier example in this chapter. Avoidance patterns are sometimes illuminated by blocking the avoidance response (as with Lani and her parents). Alternatively, the therapist can ask family members to anticipate what would occur if the "avoider" engaged in a more active response. The predicted outcomes of alternative responses can reveal real or imaginary negative consequences, further revealing factors that maintain the interaction. Parents and teenagers who fail to bring up pressing issues at home with each other, for example, frequently say that they avoid this because "it wouldn't do any good anyway." When pressed for imagined scenarios, parents may describe scenes of angry yelling, stony silence, or unkept agreements on the part of the teenager. Teens may anticipate moralizing or unreasonable demands from their parents. Prompting the family to specify further the experiences and behaviors that have led to these predictions may bring out potential targets for intervention, such as voicing negative statements in a nonaccusatory fashion, suggesting reasonable compromises, and/or evaluating the probable outcomes of behavior changes more realistically.

Other nonobvious functions of behavior may derive from unobservable cognitive, affective, and physiological states. Reduction of unpleasant experiences of guilt, anxiety, or tension can negatively reinforce interactive behavior. In addition, affective and cognitive events sometimes reveal the valence of behavioral consequences: Chatty conversations with parents may be enjoyable to some adolescents and aversive to others. The affect, cognitions, and evaluative self-statements that accompany interactions often provide clues to the valence of consequences as well as supplementing behavioral aspects of interaction chains, as the following example illustrates.

Example. Mr. and Mrs. Edwards complained of difficulties setting limits for their daughter, Marilyn. Mr. Edwards set very strict curfews and deadlines when he was at home. When he was away (about 2 days per week), Mrs. Edwards failed to enforce these rules and initiated extra activities with her daughter. When Mr. Edwards came home, he often became angry with his wife, stating that "she knew Marilyn needed a firm hand." Mrs. Edwards felt that Marilyn "needed freedom to grow." Both parents ascribed their discipline conflict to a fundamental difference in values.

Upon further probing, the therapist discovered that when Mr. Edwards imposed strict limits, he evaluated himself positively as a father and avoided his fear that Marilyn would get involved with drugs and a "bad" crowd. Mrs.

Edwards reported feeling guilty about her husband's contingencies, which she judged to be unfair. She told herself that by relaxing the rules, she was compensating for his unfairness. In so doing, her guilt was appeased.

Commentary. The above sequence of interactions could not be completely analyzed without attention to private events, that is, cognitive and affective components. Mr. Edwards's strict discipline would best be seen as supported both by avoidance of fear and of negative self-evaluation, and by positive reinforcement via self-commendation after setting strict limits. Mrs. Edwards relaxed the regulations under two conditions: (1) when her husband was away, and (2) following thoughts about the rigidity of his rules and feelings of guilt. Her behavior appeared to be negatively reinforced by guilt reduction. Initiation of extra activities might also be negatively reinforced; alternatively, positive reinforcement in the form of pleasant interactions with her daughter might be operative. Notice that in this situation, the short-term consequences of Mrs. Edwards's guilt reduction outweigh the long-term consequence of her husband's anger. Note, too, that the parents' attribution of the problem to incompatible values, while representing an accurate description of differences in their *cognitions,* does not accurately describe the immediate factors that maintain the Edwardses' interaction patterns.

Up to this point, we have used the concepts of positive and negative reinforcement, avoidance, punishment, and private events to illustrate relatively molecular analyses of family interaction sequences. At times, the clinician may have difficulty inducing useful functional patterns from such point-by-point description. More molar focus can be achieved by broadening either the time frame and/or the level of analysis used to describe target behavior sequences and their functions.

Broadening the time frame means examining longer term antecedents and consequences of interaction patterns. An adolescent who smokes marijuana in his bedroom may gain considerable peer esteem a day or two later when he recounts his challenge of parental authority to his pals. An argument between mother and daughter may lead to intimate sharing between the parents hours after the teenager has gone to bed. Exploring longer term components of behavior sequences can sometimes lead to hypotheses about functional relationships that would go unnoticed if the therapist focused only on immediate antecedents and consequences.

Broadening the level of analysis implies shifting the punctuation of behavior and behavior sequences to yield different descriptive constructs that summarize behavior. In analyzing an argument, for example, a clinician can ask on a molecular level, "What is the function of the mother's accusatory comments?" Broadening the level of analysis to include a larger chunk of interaction, the question becomes, "What is the function of the mother's repeated accusations followed by her daughter's counteraccusations?" And at a still broader level, "What function do these arguments play in the family?"

The use of broader constructs can be applied to descriptions of antecedents and consequences as well as target behaviors. Experimental work examining the role of positive reinforcement in maintaining patterns of choice behavior in the animal laboratory illustrates this nicely. These efforts have in fact channeled little attention into examining single response–consequence segments. Instead, analyses based on relative rates of responding and reinforcement have yielded conclusions with greater predictive power. Among these conclusions is the idea that one factor that can maintain behavior is access to particular situations. Based on animal work with concurrent chain schedules in controlled laboratory settings, it appears that an organism will respond to place itself in a situation based on the reinforcement within that situation, relative to reinforcement obtainable in simultaneously available situations (Herrnstein, 1970, 1979; McDowell, 1982). Applying this to families, teenagers who increasingly choose to spend time away from their parents or to lie about their companions or activities may be responding in ways that allow them access to situations providing major sources of reinforcement—time with their friends. The weaker the reinforcement value of alternative situations, such as family activities, the greater the relative amounts of time that the adolescent will allocate to peers. In this case, the molar concept of situational access as a maintaining variable may prove more fruitful than simple stimulus–response chains.

Alexander and his colleagues utilize other molar conceptualizations of the consequences of family interaction as the basis for their "functional family therapy" (Alexander & Parsons, 1982; Barton & Alexander, 1981). They theorize that the functional outcomes of most interactive processes in families can be described by one of three relationship outcomes: distance, intimacy, or regulation. Distancing behaviors produce privacy and reduce interpersonal contact; examples might include reading a newspaper, a parent working two jobs, a teen spending excessive time with peers, or the parents devoting so much time to the teen that they have no time together. Intimacy-producing behaviors promote closeness and interpersonal contact, and include communicating feelings, sexual intercourse, discussing problems, or asking for help. Regulation, an intermediary process, blends intimacy and distance. Regulation is exemplified by actions such as being polite but reserved, double-dating, taking someone to a movie, or fighting between siblings. Within this framework, the therapist assesses the relative frequency of behaviors in each class for each family member as a means of determining functional payoffs for problematic behavior sequences. Barton and Alexander note that since the developmental tasks of adolescence include becoming autonomous or "distant" from parents, many parent–teen conflicts involve teenagers struggling to increase interpersonal distance while parents attempt to maintain contact and closeness.

While we have trouble accepting the assumption that all family interactions can be reduced to attempts to produce intimacy, distance, or regulation, we have found the framework useful for analyzing some functional interaction patterns. From a social-learning perspective, intimacy and distance can be translated into scheduling phenomena related to social reinforcement. Intimacy can be viewed as a preference for high density, low ratio, and short interval schedules of social reinforcement, while distance can be conceptualized either as a preference for a low density, high ratio, and long interval social reinforcement schedules, or as an avoidance of particular types of interaction. Family members differ in their preferences for rich or lean schedules of social reinforcement, probably as a function of both constitutional predispositions and earlier reinforcement histories. According to Alexander and Parsons (1982), each family member attempts to obtain an optimal schedule of social reinforcement from the family; in doing so, problematic interaction patterns can result, especially if one member prefers a richer schedule than another.[1]

The utility of Alexander's framework is illustrated in the following example. This case also demonstrates the use of molar punctuation of interaction sequences over a broad time frame.

Example. Mr. Jones worked 16 hours a day at two jobs. Mrs. Jones was a housewife who had few friends and whose life had focused on her three children, ages 14, 10, and 8, for many years. As the eldest reached adolescence, he began to spend less time at home and more time with his peers. Adolescent conflicts around independence issues began, and Mrs. Jones cracked down in a very domineering way on her son. He reacted by becoming depressed and starting to fail in school. Mr. Jones blamed his son's problems on his wife, feeling that she should be able to take care of the kids since she "had nothing else to do." Mrs. Jones attempted to enlist her husband to help with their son, but he refused. A pattern emerged where Mr. Jones would come home from work to be greeted at the door by his wife, extremely upset about their 14-year-old's latest exploits. The parents would argue, and Mr. Jones would finally talk to his son, who would act receptive but later ignore his father's demands for change. Mr. Jones then withdrew until his wife coerced his attention with another crisis involving their son.

Commentary. Using Alexander and Parsons's framework, we can see Mrs. Jones as preferring intimacy in family affairs while Mr. Jones appears to prefer distance. Since her husband did not provide her with a rich schedule of social reinforcement, Mrs. Jones came to rely on her children for support. As the eldest approached adolescence, he began to distance himself from his parents, a withdrawal that had little impact on his father but represented a loss of an important source of attention for his mother. She attempted to stop his distancing, and he reacted by rebelling and becoming depressed, reestablishing at least some distance. When he misbehaved severely, his mother was able, at least temporarily, to coerce her husband into interacting more with her, replacing some of the lost contact. A self-perpetuating cycle evolved in which the son's rebellious behavior permitted him to achieve distance from his parents while his mother obtained more contact from his father. If the therapist attempted to teach

Mrs. Jones to solve her differences with her son without arranging alternative sources of social support for her, the solutions might well be unsuccessful. The analysis of the process in terms of intimacy and distance as functional payoffs can help the therapist to recognize how to deploy skills and other intervention techniques to optimize long-term change within the system.

CONCLUDING COMMENTS ON ASSESSMENT

In the past three chapters, we have tried to convey a picture of many options for both gathering and conceptualizing information that are available to the clinician or researcher assessing parent–adolescent conflict within a behavioral–family systems perspective. Various standardized assessment instruments and methods can be supplemented by other data sources, such as direct observation of family process during the interview, that as yet have not been evaluated systematically but are still potentially useful. The level of analysis used in assessment may vary from molecular to molar, depending upon target problems and family interaction style. It is clear that multidimensional problems require multidimensional assessment tools. In future years, we hope that investigators will improve the quality and variety of tools that are available, as well as expand our knowledge of how best to conceptualize, integrate, and utilize the information yielded by these tools.

NOTE

1. We recognize that in reframing Alexander's concepts of intimacy, distance, and regulation in terms of reinforcement phenomena, we may be engaging in semantic reductionism. The ultimate test of which vocabulary to adopt will eventually lie in which concepts direct the therapist toward the most effective intervention strategies.

CHAPTER SEVEN

Treatment—Overview and Problem-Solving Training

The next six chapters describe our intervention program for parent–adolescent conflict. This program is based upon the behavioral–family systems analysis of parent–adolescent relations outlined in Chapter 2. To teach family members to resolve conflicts effectively, the therapist must employ a comprehensive approach that addresses the major factors believed to underlie adult–teenage relational problems: skill deficits, distorted cognitions, structural problems, and functional interaction problems. Components of the intervention address each factor; which components are emphasized depends on the families' specific problems. In the problem-solving communication training component, families learn a democratic approach to problem solving as a strategy for discussing specific issues about which they disagree. During problem-solving training, negative communication habits that interfere with productive verbal interchanges are targeted for change. When irrational thoughts are linked to conflict, cognitive restructuring and social–psychologically based attributional techniques are employed to transform rigid, extremist attitudes into more flexible, solution-oriented cognitive sets. With families displaying problematic functional/structural patterns, selected techniques incorporated from family systems therapy are used to change these problems. Through the judicious selection of issues to problem solve, communication targets to modify, and attitudinal targets to alter, the therapist develops a behaviorally based strategy for modifying the family system, culminating in increased reciprocity of positive behavior and decreased reciprocity of negative behavior.

Environmental contingencies must also be arranged to maximize the chances that newly acquired interactional sequences will generalize across time and settings. Intervention consequently includes explicit techniques for programming these forms of generalization.

Chapters 7 through 10 present procedures for implementing the problem solving, communication training, cognitive restructuring, and functional/structural components of intervention. In our experience, most families need some training in problem-solving and communication skills. Cognitive restructuring is important for some but not all of these. Structural and functional treatment components may require little attention in families where parent–adolescent conflict is relatively circumscribed and parents work together as a team, but assume major importance in building a comprehensive treatment for multiproblem, severely distressed families. Thus, these components are best thought of as treatment modules, not all of which will be applicable in every case.

Sequencing components of intervention and programming generalization are considered in Chapter 11. Chapter 12 examines resistance and implementation problems, and suggests solutions.

Before beginning this description, however, one caveat: Most of our work has involved lower to upper middle–class Anglo-American families. Certainly aspects of the procedures, philosophy, and targets of intervention will require modification for this approach to be used with recent immigrants, inner-city poor, and Hispanic, Asian, and other subcultures with strong ethnic norms. Our limited experience with these populations does not equip us to provide specific guidelines for these modifications, which will require sensitivity both to the goals of treatment and to strong cultural contingencies and norms.

OVERVIEW OF TREATMENT

Problem-solving communication training has four phases: engagement, skill building, resolution of intense problems, and disengagement. While intervention can vary from 7 to 20 sessions depending upon the severity of the family's distress, the therapist always establishes a time-limited contract for a pre-specified number of meetings, with an option to renew the contract if necessary (see contract points in Chapter 4).

A typical family progresses through four phases of intervention. During the engagement phase (typically two to four sessions), the therapist "joins" the family by establishing rapport, conducting the type of thorough behavioral assessment discussed in Chapters 4 through 6, fostering change-oriented attitudes, and specifying therapeutic goals. The engagement stage is crucial since families are unlikely to follow the therapist's later instructions unless they have formed a trusting relationship and they clearly understand the rationale for a family-oriented, skill-training intervention. The therapist introduces the family to problem solving during this phase of treatment and uses instructions, modeling, behavior rehearsal, and corrective feedback to guide the family through the stages of problem solving for a mild disagreement. Afterwards the family is sent home to implement the solution. The experience of successfully resolving a dispute early in treatment is designed to build trust in the therapist and the procedures.

Skill building typically begins with the third or fourth session and continues for two to four sessions. During this phase of treatment the therapist emphasizes acquisition of new problem-solving and communication skills. Sessions are organized primarily around specific conflictual issues. At each session, the family problem-solves a new topic, renegotiates a failed solution, or completes an unfinished discussion. Negative communication habits are targeted for change. When an inappropriate response occurs, the therapist interrupts the discussion, gives feedback concerning the negative interaction sequence, models incompatible responses, and requires the family to rehearse the positive interaction sequence. Families learn reflective listening and nonaccusatory expression of feelings and opinions, particularly negative affect. The role of unreasonable cognitions in impeding effective conflict resolution may be explained, and cognitive restructuring techniques are introduced if needed. Strategic decisions regarding which topics to problem-solve, communication targets to correct, and beliefs to challenge are made with an eye towards the main purpose of this stage—teaching skills.

The skill-building phase of therapy blends naturally into the resolution-of-intense-conflicts phase, when the therapist and family tackle the intense, knotty issues that are usually the major presenting problems. Entrenched, unreasonable beliefs are addressed, using cognitive restructuring or reframing techniques. The therapist uses the information collected throughout earlier sessions to formulate hypotheses and change problematic functional/structural patterns. In-session and home tasks are integrated into intervention as needed to change functional/structural interaction patterns. Decisions concerning problems to solve, communication targets to correct, and beliefs to challenge are based on a coordinated strategy to move the family system in targeted directions. Teaching the family to de-escalate intense affect when target problems arise at home may be important during these sessions. Intense conflict resolution continues for as many sessions as are needed in clinical practice or for two to three sessions in research applications.

During the final phase, disengagement, the therapist prepares the family for termination. The therapist fades his/her prompts during sessions, encourages the family to progress naturally from step to step of problem solving, recognizing when they are getting bogged down and moving forward. The therapist and family develop strategies for continued self-initiated use of problem-solving communication skills and plans for fitting their newly acquired skills into their daily routines. The therapist frames this endeavor so that families perceive their gains to be a function of their own, rather than the therapist's efforts. By termination, a successfully treated family will have resolved many of their presenting conflicts and learned skills and attitudes that will permit continued resolution of new disagreements in the future.

As mentioned previously, whether and how each component of intervention is incorporated into treatment varies from case to case, depending upon the therapist's initial assessment of the family and their response to treatment. The following questions should help guide the practitioner in deciding which components to emphasize.

1. Does the family exhibit significant skill deficits in resolving disagreements or communicating? If so, emphasize problem-solving communication skill training.

2. Does the family have skills in their repertoire but fail to use them? If so, emphasize cognitive restructuring and functional/structural interventions.
3. Does the family adhere to unrealistic beliefs and expectations about parent–adolescent relations? If so, incorporate cognitive restructuring; if not, emphasize other elements of treatment.
4. Are there overt functional/structural problems in the family, or is there a history of resistance to family therapy? If so, emphasize functional/ structural interventions. If not, pursue straightforward problem-solving communication training.
5. Do members of the family have other problems such as marital conflict, depression, the Attention Deficit Disorder, alcoholism, or drug abuse? If so, add interventions beyond those described in this volume, to produce comprehensive change.

Problem-solving communication training is a highly structured intervention typically carried out by a directive therapist. Our presentation of the therapy emphasizes its structure. However, to be successful, each therapist must find an appropriate blend of structured behavioral training procedures and clinical flexibility. Structure is important to move in a goal-oriented direction within a time-limited framework; however, flexibility is equally important to respond to the idiographic exigencies inherent in the clinical picture presented by each family. The astute therapist enters each session with an agenda but knows when to modify or discard the agenda because of current crises or needs.

In order to make a clear-cut presentation of basic components of our intervention, we occasionally use what may appear to be simplified examples of clinical problems. For example, curfew, chores, backtalk, and homework are conflictual issues used to illustrate concretely our points about intervention. We do not mean to give the impression that these are the only or even the most important issues in parent–teen relations. In clinical practice we apply our intervention to a variety of issues and problems, some relatively circumscribed and some complex, as examples in later chapters should make clearer.

PROBLEM-SOLVING SKILL TRAINING

Problem-solving skill training is a central component of the intervention program. Because a major developmental task of adolescence is becoming independent from the nuclear family, it is important for the therapist to provide family members with independence-related skills. When we first began to work with parents and adolescents, we considered training parents to use contingency management skills to modify the "disruptive" behavior of their adolescents. However, as nonbehavioral clinicians have noted, the effective use of contingency management presumes that parents control the major reinforcers in their adolescents' lives (T. Gordon, 1970). Such an assumption is at best tenuous. In fact, as young adolescents' behavior comes increasingly under the control of antecedents and consequences provided by peers and other agents outside of the home, parents inevitably run out of power. Parents' attempts to use disciplinary contingencies that rely primarily upon their personal authority may be successful in the short run, but be doomed to eventual, costly failure, eliciting negative emotional reactions from the adolescent. More important, through the imposition of primarily aversive control contingencies, parents undermine the developmental task of achieving independence and fail to provide appropriate role models for responsible exercising of adult decision-making skills. After all, independent adults resolve conflicts through a process of mutual accommodation. One adult does not establish a contingency management program for another adult, except in special circumstances (such as therapy). If the family is viewed as the "laboratory" where a child learns repertoires of behavior useful in later life, then the adolescent years should be viewed as the time to teach conflict-resolution behavior which will be useful to the teenager during adulthood.

D'Zurilla and Goldfried's (1971) conceptualization of problem solving as a heuristic framework for individuals to follow when faced with interpersonal conflicts has guided the development of our intervention. In discussing our model, it is important to remember that a heuristic teaching technique is defined as one that encourages the student to discover for himself/herself. In our case, it is a way of helping families to find their own specific solutions to disputes, not a way for the therapist to impose his/her favorite solutions upon the family. Problem solving is considered to be a means to the end of resolving specific disputes, not an end by itself.

The problem-solving model, adapted for use with families, consists of four basic steps: (1) problem definition, (2) generation of alternative solutions, (3) decision making, and (4) planning solution implementation. A fifth step, renegotiation, is invoked when the family is unsuccessful in resolving the dispute through the implementation of the initial solution. Families are taught to use the five steps of problem solving when a dispute arises concerning a specific issue such as curfew, dating, smoking, or household chores. These five steps codify in a systematic manner the generic skills in any verbal negotiation process.

In the following discussion, much of the material is geared toward the initiation of problem-solving training; it should be noted that the basic steps, without the rationales, are repeated during all of the subsequent attempts at problem solving.

Problem Definition Phase

Goals

The problem definition phase of the discussion has three goals: (1) for each family member to express clearly to the others his/her perspective concerning the topic under consideration; (2) for each family member to understand the others' perspectives; and (3) to limit the topic under consideration. In order to accomplish this, the family members must be able to approach disagreements with the cognitive set that differences of opinion concerning a topic are a normal, healthy sign of independent adult cognitive functioning, not an indicator of pathology, rebellion, disloyalty to the family, or any other catastrophic processes they may care to invoke.

Critical Attributes

Family members take turns defining the problem as they perceive it. As each family member expresses his/her viewpoint, the listeners verify their understanding of the statement by reflecting it back to the speaker. If the reflection does not match the initial statement of the problem, the speaker clarifies his/her position. An adequate definition describes explicitly what the other person is doing or saying that creates a problem for the speaker. It pinpoints why the other person's behavior is problematic to the speaker. It is nonaccusatory and concise, yet it is an accurate reflection of the affect experienced by the speaker concerning the topic. It addresses behaviors, feelings, and situations, not personality characteristics of individuals. It typically begins with an "I," not a "you."

An adequate reflection of a problem definition statement restates clearly and without the addition of new material the listener's perception of the speaker's definition of the problem. It is also nonaccusatory and concise, and addresses behaviors, feelings, and situations, not personality characteristics of individuals. The critical attributes of problem definition and problem definition reflection statements are illustrated in the following vignettes.

Example 1 (Curfew).
SALLY: My problem is that I want to stay out until midnight on weekends to party with my friends, but my curfew is 11:00 p.m. This bugs me because I miss out on the fun by having to leave parties early.
MRS. JONES: So you are saying that it bothers you to have an 11:00 p.m. curfew on weekends because you have to leave parties early. And then you miss out on having a good time with your friends.
SALLY: Yes, that's it.

Commentary. This was an adequate problem definition and an adequate reflection. The adolescent began with an "I," pinpointed the situation that was a problem, and indicated why the situation bothered her. She was concise and nonaccusatory. Her mother paraphrased accurately her daughter's perspective concerning curfew without distorting or adding to it.

Example 2 (Marijuana Smoking).
MRS. SMITH: My problem is that you are smoking pot and on the way to becoming a good-for-nothing bum.

JOHN: There's nothing wrong with pot. You and Dad drink, so why can't I smoke pot?

Commentary. This was an inadequate problem definition, followed by an inadequate response. Mrs. Smith began with a "you" and made a demeaning, accusatory statement. She addressed herself to a personality characteristic of an individual (bum) rather than a situation (smoking marijuana). She failed to pinpoint what she meant by a "bum." Not surprisingly, her son reciprocated her negative comment with a defensive, blaming statement.

Example 3 (Cleaning Up the Adolescent's Room).
MR. JONES: Billy, I'm very angry about the dust on the floor, the clothes on the bed, and the messy papers on the desk in your room because it really embarrasses me when Mom and I have friends over to visit.
BILLY: So you're saying that you want me to clean up my room just so you won't be uptight when your friends come to visit.
MR. JONES: Yes and no. Yes, I am saying I'm angry about the mess in your room. It does embarrass me. No, I'm not saying that I want you to clean it up because I'm uptight. I feel that the family needs to share the responsibility for the cleanliness of the house, and when your room is dirty, I feel like Mom and I are doing our part of the cleaning but you are not.

Commentary. Mr. Jones's initial definition of the problem started with an "I," pinpointed the behavior of his son that troubled him, and specified why the behavior troubled him. In addition, the intensity of his statements matched his level of anger concerning the problem. As is common when parents first begin to employ problem solving, his son responded in a sarcastic, accusing tone. Perhaps Billy was responding to the somewhat dubious rationale his father gave for his dissatisfaction with the room. Fortunately, Mr. Jones was able to remain cool and clarify his reason for being as angry as he was. Billy might have understood better the intensity of his father's anger and responded differently if Mr. Jones had initially shared his concern about family responsibility.

Example 4 (Sexual Behavior).
MRS. MARTIN: My problem is that I am really bothered by the fact that you are a promiscuous teenager.
BETTY: What you are saying is that you are upset that I mess around with guys, have sexual intercourse, and might get pregnant the way you did when you were my age.

Commentary. This was an inadequate problem definition. Mrs. Martin's statement is an excellent example of a disguised put-down. Although she begins well with an "I" statement of her feelings, the phrase "promiscuous teenager" is accusatory as well as vague. Betty, in turn, reciprocates with a not-so-veiled counterattack.

Teaching Problem Definition Skills

As the previous examples may have suggested, it can be tricky to teach family members to say what is on their minds precisely, concisely, and without accusations. After the family selects a topic for discussion, the therapist briefly describes the rationale and attributes of an adequate problem definition statement, and asks one of the parents to begin the statement. A parent is usually asked to define the problem first for several reasons. Parents are ordinarily more likely to be cooperative and less likely to be threatened by the therapist's corrections in the early stage of the discussion than are adolescents. By listening to their parents speak, adolescents can be exposed to several models of problem definition statements before being required to respond. In addition, parents are initially more likely to have explicitly formulated complaints than adolescents. The therapist might begin as follows:

Now that we have agreed to talk about curfew, I'd like you, Mr. Jones, to tell Sally exactly what she does and says that makes curfew a problem for you, without blaming her or putting her down. For instance, if I were you, I might say, "Sally, my problem is that I'm upset when you come home at midnight on weekends after I thought we had agreed to an 11:00 p.m. curfew. I'm upset because I worry that you might be hurt or in trouble." Now, tell her your problem while I listen.

After the parent has made an initial statement of the problem, the therapist gives the parent feedback. If the problem was clearly defined without accusations, the therapist provides positive feedback to the parent. Otherwise, the therapist pinpoints the deficiency in the parent's statement, models an improved version, and asks the parent to "replay the scene."

Example.

MOTHER: The problem with Danny is that he is irresponsible now and will grow up to be an irresponsible adult.

THERAPIST: That's a start, but please be more specific. You might want to say, "Danny, when you come home 2 hours late, fail to do your homework 5 out of 7 days, and fail to do your chores daily, I feel you are acting irresponsibly. I worry that if you keep this up you will act this way as an adult." Now, Mrs. Jones, tell Danny your problem again.

After the parent has defined the problem adequately, the therapist gives a rationale for and models a paraphrase of the definition and asks the adolescent to "say back to your parent exactly what s/he told you was the problem and no more." Following the paraphrase, the parent is given the opportunity to verify the accuracy of the reflection or correct any misunderstandings.

As the discussion progresses, the therapist gives each family member a turn to define the problem, followed by paraphrases and verification. The therapist takes the opportunity to point out how different family members quite naturally have different opinions about issues, and that it is unnecessary for each member to persuade the others of his/her opinions in order to talk about the issues. It is important for the therapist to control the flow of the discussion in a directive manner, interrupting digressions, put-downs, or other inappropriate comments.

Family members vary considerably in their ability to define problems appropriately. Some will give specific, nonaccusatory definitions on the first trial while others will require four or five corrections before producing reasonable approximations to correct definitions. During each problem-solving discussion the therapist must decide how much time to devote to correcting deficient definitions and stick to that decision. In the first session, where the primary goal is to get the family through the steps of the model in order to permit them to experience immediate success resolving a dispute, it is wise to limit refinement of problem definitions, accepting less-than-optimal performances and moving forward. In later sessions, where a primary goal is skill building, the therapist may allocate up to 30 minutes for refinement of problem definition statements.

Generation of Alternative Solutions

Goal

The goal of the generation-of-alternatives phase of the discussion is for the family members to list a variety of suggestions for ways to resolve the specific dispute.

Critical Attributes

Adherence to three rules of brainstorming derived from the educational–industrial creativity training literature (Osborn, 1963) is the key feature of the generation-of-alternatives phase of problem solving.

1. List as many ideas as possible.
2. Defer evaluation of the ideas until later in the discussion.
3. Suggest creative and outrageous ideas: anything goes.

These rules are designed to help family members move beyond the "rut" in which they are often stuck at the beginning of the discussion. By deferring the evaluation of ideas, the family members are able to suggest the unthinkable without fear of retaliation or without the implication that they are later committed to supporting a particular suggestion. By listing a variety of ideas, the members increase their flexibility, and maximize the chances of arriving at a high-quality, novel alternative. By encouraging the family to generate creative, outrageous ideas, the therapist helps to lighten the overall mood of the session and maintain a high level of involvement.

Teaching Generation of Alternative Solutions

The therapist introduces the generation-of-alternatives phase of problem solving with a comment such as

Now we are going to take turns listing as many ideas as possible to solve this problem. The goal of this is to make a list of lots of ideas, so that there are good ones to choose later on. I want you to think of the most creative, crazy ideas you can. Anything goes. And it's important now not to say whether we like the ideas or not; that comes later. If we do it now, it will discourage people. So let's just come up with as many ideas as we can.

Family members are asked to take turns suggesting ideas. One family member is assigned the task of writing down the ideas on a problem worksheet (see Figure 7–1). In the early sessions of therapy, we typically assign secretarial chores to the adolescent because the necessity for recording ideas helps maintain the interest and attention of most adolescents.

The therapist's role during the generation of alternatives phase is to keep the conversation on task, enforce adherence to the rules of brainstorming, and insure balanced participation by all family members. It is not the therapist's responsibility to generate the actual solutions, although under certain circumstances the therapist may choose to interject an idea. At first, family members are likely to suggest ideas that reflect their initial positions on the issue. As they become accustomed to the nonevaluative atmosphere of the discussion, they begin to suggest more creative alternatives. Inevitably, someone begins to evaluate an idea prematurely; the therapist should immediately interrupt to remind the family to defer judgment of the idea until a later time.

An excerpt from the Joneses' discussion of curfew illustrates the ebb and flow of this phase of problem solving.

Solutions	Evaluations (+ or −)		
	Mom	Dad	Teen
1.			
2.			
3.			
4.			
5.			
6.			
7.			

Agreed-upon solution:

FIGURE 7-1 Problem-solving worksheet.

Example.

THERAPIST: Now, I want you to take turns listing as many ideas as possible to solve the curfew problem. Be creative but don't say whether the ideas are good or bad. Just say whatever comes to mind. Bill, I want you to write down the ideas on this worksheet. Mr. Jones, why don't you begin?

MR. JONES: OK. Bill could come home when we tell him.

THERAPIST: I want you to talk to each other, not me. Bill, your turn.

BILL: I could come home whenever I want to. . . .

MRS. JONES: *(Interrupting)* That's what you do now.

THERAPIST: You're evaluating, Mrs. Jones. All I want you to do is suggest ideas, not evaluate. What would you like to suggest?

MRS. JONES: We could ground Bill for a week every time he comes home late.

BILL: That's not fair.

THERAPIST: Bill, now you're evaluating. Would you care to suggest another idea?

BILL: They could stop bugging me about coming home late.

THERAPIST: Remember, talk to each other. I have an idea. Bill, your parents could come home by nine on weekends and they could pay you a dollar for each minute they are late.

MRS. JONES: You're kidding.

THERAPIST: No, I'm not. Please don't evaluate. We can be as crazy as we like now. We'll pick the best idea later. Mr. Jones, your turn.

MR. JONES: We could let him stay out till midnight on special occasions, and if he is late he could pay a dollar fine from his allowance for each half-hour.

BILL: Or you could let me stay out until midnight on weekends if I come in by nine on weeknights.

MRS. JONES: He might stay out until midnight on Saturdays if he comes home by 10 on Fridays.

BILL: But what if there's a good party on Friday?

THERAPIST: Bill, you're evaluating again. Suggest another idea instead.

BILL: OK. How about I stay out till midnight one night each weekend, and I get to decide each week.

MR. JONES: If you weren't so irresponsible about not calling us if you are going to be home late, we might let you stay out until midnight both weekend nights.

THERAPIST: Mr. Jones, that's an evaluation again. Usually an evaluation comes up when people don't like a solution. It will work better if you turn your criticism into a positive solution.

MR. JONES: Well . . . you could call us if you are going to be late.

Commentary. At first, Mr. Jones suggested his previously ineffective authoritarian solution. Bill reciprocated with his previously ineffective, permissive alternative. When Mrs. Jones tried to make an accusing, evaluative comment, the therapist interrupted her. Instead, she gave a harsh negative idea followed by Bill's evaluation, which the therapist also interrupted. In essence, the family members were using the solution-listing format to make veiled, punishing remarks to each other. Such hidden agendas are common with distressed families.

To clear the air and reduce the high level of anger, the therapist suggested an outlandish alternative. Mr. Jones apparently began to get the message that the therapist was serious about finding a reasonable solution. He then proposed a late curfew on special occasions. At this point, the tone of the discussion mellowed. Afterwards, a series of increasingly flexible suggestions were given, despite occasional interference from accusations. From this interchange the therapist might also hypothesize that in the Jones family the father's movement towards a compromise may be a prerequisite for serious negotiation. In future problem-solving discussions with the Jones family, the therapist might develop strategies designed to have the father sanction flexible solutions earlier in the discussion. The excerpt illustrates not only how a family shifts gears during a discussion but also how the therapist can gain valuable information about functional interaction patterns by attending to the process of family interaction.

Occasionally, particularly rigid, angry families "run dry" after listing several clearly unacceptable alternatives. The therapist may use humor, as in the case of the Jones family, to defuse the tension and to prompt new, more creative ideas. Humor is a particularly potent weapon during all phases of problem solving and family therapy in general. By "innocently" suggesting an outlandish idea that may be constructed as a parody of a previously suggested rigid solution, the therapist metacommunicates to the members that they are being unreasonable, and that it is time to get on with the process of reaching a compromise.

Alternatively, one or more of the following guidelines can be given as prompts for constructing additional solutions.

1. What is the basic conflict concerning this issue? Can solutions address that conflict?
2. Is a trade possible?
3. Can the physical environment be rearranged to solve the problem?
4. Can cues be provided to help each family member remember to act differently?
5. Can the problem be solved by changing the way one or more family members think about the problematic situation?
6. Can one family member suggest a solution that explicitly addresses the problem as defined by another family member?

Generation of alternatives continues until the therapist judges that the family has a workable set of solutions. There are no general guidelines for making this judgment. Typically, 8 to 10 solutions are the minimum required before the family is ready to proceed to decision making, although fewer may suffice in the later stages of therapy if the problem is of mild or moderate severity. It is important that the list contain at least three or four ideas that go beyond the initial positions embodied in the family's definition of the problem and can meet at least some of the objectives set forth by each family member in defining the problem. Lightening of the tone of the discussion, as was evident in the second portion of the Joneses' excerpt, is also an indicator that family members are prepared to compromise. When the therapist's criteria for workable solutions have been satisfied, the family continues to the decision-making phase of problem solving.

Decision Making

Goals

The goals of the decision-making phase of the problem-solving discussion are for the parents and adolescent (1) to evaluate each idea by projecting its positive and negative consequences, (2) to rate independently each idea as positive or negative for them, and (3) to negotiate an agreement to implement one or more solutions that maximize the positive and minimize the negative consequences for each family member.

Critical Attributes

In order to achieve these three goals, family members must become proficient at the cognitive-interpersonal problem-solving skills of consequential thinking and taking another's perspective (Spivack *et al.,* 1976) as well as the verbal-interactional skills of negotiation. The family members take turns evaluating each idea on their list of solutions. Each member makes a clear statement to the others projecting the consequences of the solution for himself/herself and for the remainder of the family, culminating in the assigning of a rating of plus or minus to the solution. The ratings are recorded next to the written solution in separate columns of the problem worksheet for the mother, the father, and the adolescent. When all of the solutions on the worksheet have been evaluated by each of the family members, they review their ratings to determine if any ideas were rated plus by everyone. If they have reached consensus on one or more ideas, then they decide to select one or combine several ideas. If they did not reach a consensus, then they begin to negotiate a compromise.

It is important to specify the critical attributes of a clear statement projecting the consequences of a solution, because parents and adolescents tend to limit their evaluatory comments to brief remarks such as "I like that" or "That won't work" unless prompted to elaborate by the therapist. An appropriate evaluatory statement expresses an opinion about the solution and answers one or more of the following questions: (1) What will the effects of this solution be on the problem as I defined it? (2) What will the effect of this solution be on the problem as others defined it? (3) What will be both the short-term and the long-term effects of this solution? and (4) What, if any, additional problems will be created by implementing this solution? Several illustrations of correct and incorrect evaluatory statements follow.

Example 1.

PROBLEM: Drinking alcoholic beverages

SOLUTIONS: The adolescent will be permitted to drink beer only under parental supervision.

MOTHER'S EVALUATION: I like that idea because then I won't have to worry that he is out driving and drinking with his friends.

Commentary. The mother's evaluation clearly projected a positive consequence of the solution for her, and would be acceptable in early sessions. However, she failed to consider any of the consequences of the solution for her son. What if his friends offer him a drink and tease him for refusing, for example? What if he feels rejected by them? These consequences can be elicited by prompting her or her son to voice them.

Example 2.

PROBLEM: Invading teenager's privacy

SOLUTION: Ask permission before searching teen's room.

MOTHER'S EVALUATION: That's a good idea because then my son won't feel I've invaded his territory. But he might have time to hide what I'm after. Overall, I'd give it a minus.

Commentary. This was a well-executed evaluation. The mother weighed both the positive and the negative consequences of the solution and then gave it an evaluation.

Example 3.

PROBLEM: Smoking marijuana

SOLUTION: The adolescent will stop smoking marijuana.

ADOLESCENT EVALUATION: I hate that idea because then you get what you want and I don't get anything.

Commentary. The solution may indeed be one-sided, but the adolescent has nonetheless failed to project its consequences. A better evaluation would have been "I don't like that idea because then I'll be laughed at by my friends at parties where I turn down a joint; it's not realistic to expect me to stop smoking at parties if all my friends smoke."

Teaching Decision-Making Skills

The therapist begins the decision-making phase of the first problem-solving discussion with a brief rationale.

Next, we are going to decide upon the best idea. I'm going to ask each of you to say whether each idea is good or bad and why. Consider whether the idea will solve your problem and the others' problem, as well as whether you could really carry it out. If you like an idea, we will record a plus for you on the worksheet. If you dislike an idea, we will record a minus.

The therapist models a hypothetical evaluative statement using the first idea on the problem worksheet. Afterwards, family members are prompted to take turns evaluating the first idea. The remaining ideas on the worksheet are evaluated in a similar vein. Whenever a family member truncates an evaluation, the therapist requires the member to project the consequences of the solution. The therapist interrupts digressions, redirecting the family to remain on task, but does not offer personal evaluations of any of the solutions. Novel solutions that emerge during the decision-making stage are added to the problem worksheet.

Most families readily catch on to the format for evaluating solutions. The more difficult task for the family is learning to negotiate a compromise when no solution is rated positively by everyone. During negotiations the therapist plays an extremely directive role. The starting point is usually a solution evaluated positively by at least one parent and the adolescent.[1] The members are asked to restate succinctly their evaluation of this solution, noting the areas of disagreement between them. Then, the person for whom a compromise would represent the largest concession is asked to propose a variation on the solution under consideration that might be potentially acceptable to the others. As a proposal is made, the remaining members are asked to evaluate it. The therapist mediates closely by (1) directing every comment toward the goal of achieving a compromise, (2) supporting strongly any emerging compromises, (3) suggesting novel compromises, and (4) lavishly praising family members who take a flexible stance on the issues. In essence, the therapist repeatedly enters and exits brief alliances with the parents and the adolescent in an attempt to represent convincingly and empathetically the interests of each family member while maintaining an overall neutral stance. If either the parents or the adolescent perceive the therapist as consistently aligned with the other, the therapist will be unable to use his/her power to push the family toward a compromise. Since the family may perceive a compromise as a "loss of face" or "giving in," it is important for the therapist to reframe a compromise as a protective ploy that helps to maintain family harmony and togetherness.

Example. The disagreement between Mrs. Bradley and her 12-year-old son Jim illustrates a problem requiring negotiation training. Mrs. Bradley defined the problem of putting away clothing in terms of her dissatisfaction with the appearance of Jim's room when he left clean laundry all over the bed, dressers, and chairs. Jim defined the problem in terms of dissatisfaction with his mother's frequent, accusatory reminders to put his clothing away. The dyad generated a list of solutions but did not reach a consensus regarding any of the solutions. Jim was willing to fold the clothes neatly but refused to put them in his dresser. The therapist directed them to consider a variety of compromises such as building a chute from the bed to the dresser, or putting half of the clothing in the dresser and leaving the other half on the chair. The laborious discussion of this seemingly trivial point continued for 25 minutes until they finally agreed that on Monday, Wednesday, Friday, and Saturday, Jim would put the clothing in the dresser, but that on Tuesday, Thursday, and Sunday, he would be permitted to leave the clothing on the bed. The underlying issue was really not where the clothes would remain, but who would "win" the "power struggle." In more behavioral terms, a suggestion by one party was regularly vetoed by the other, regardless of the content. However, direct discussion of the "power struggle" is ordinarily much less productive than a new experience that breaks repetitive, coercive interchanges. In this case, the therapist guided the dyad toward a solution that permitted both the mother and her son to "save face" by appearing to "win."

Such stalemates during negotiations provide the therapist with valuable information concerning functional interaction patterns between parents and adolescents. As a postscript, after 1 week, Jim "spontaneously" decided that it was easier to put his clothing in his dresser every day. By permitting young, rebellious adolescents to "win" such "debates," parents model flexible decision making and often end up achieving their original goals.

When negotiations get bogged down, the therapist can frequently help resolve the dispute by suggesting the "try it for a week" strategy. This can work well if the solution suggested by the teenager is chosen. Teens are often willing to assume extra responsibility in implementing the solution in exchange for choosing their ideas. Furthermore, by adequately fulfilling their agreements, adolescents avoid a renegotiation of the problem. On the other hand, parents are often willing to try the adolescent's solution if they know they can renegotiate the issue in therapy if the teen fails to follow through.

In some cases, despite the previous strategies, family members rigidly refuse to consider each others' perspectives concerning intensely contested issues. Social–psychological techniques derived from research on international conflict have proven useful with this problem (Robin, 1981). Two particularly helpful strategies are fractionation of the conflict and appeal to a higher authority figure, followed by graduated reciprocal initiatives in tension reduction.

Fractionation of the conflict (Fogg, 1972) entails breaking a dispute into several elements that might each be settled separately. The more easily managed elements are dealt with first to build up a reciprocity of positive interactions. If such reciprocity is not forthcoming, a partial solution may at least be salvaged.

Example.   Mrs. Janis found several marijuana cigarettes in her son Tom's dresser. She had suspected that Tom was smoking marijuana and had surreptitiously searched his room. Tom was incensed by his mother's invasion of his privacy and refused to give up smoking marijuana. His mother was unalterably opposed to Tom's use of marijuana, at home or outside the home, and had responded to her discovery by grounding him indefinitely. They were unable to resolve this dispute.

The therapist fractionated the issue into three elements and addressed each individually: (1) Tom's use of marijuana outside the home, (2) Tom's use of marijuana at home, and (3) Mrs. Janis's invasion of Tom's privacy. Even though Mrs. Janis could not condone any form of marijuana smoking, she did recognize that it would be difficult to prevent her son from smoking outside the home. After an extended discussion, she "agreed to disagree," that is, to cease making an issue of marijuana smoking outside the home although she made clear her continued opposition to his smoking. Tom was able to provide convincing evidence that he was discreet in selecting the locations where he smoked. Given the positive climate created by his mother's compromise, Tom agreed to refrain from smoking and storing marijuana in the home. The resolution of the first two issues set the stage for a discussion of Mrs. Janis's invasion of Tom's privacy. Mother and son agreed to communicate future suspicions directly rather than obtain information surreptitiously.

Appeal to a higher authority entails locating a higher authority whom the parents, the adolescent, or both respect, and arranging for the authority to sanction a compromise by one or more family members. Such authorities include friends of the family, clergymen, physicians, and political or media personalities. The therapist prepares one family member to announce a "spontaneous" de-escalation of the conflict, taking the others by surprise. As a consequence, the other family members feel obligated to follow suit with a second de-escalation step, reciprocated by further compromises, and the conflict is rapidly resolved.

Example. This strategy was inadvertently used in the case of a disagreement concerning religion. Sixteen-year-old Joey Hayne was a passive adolescent who was unable to verbalize his opinions and feelings to his parents; instead, he would "save up" his affect until he exploded in a rage. During the first two therapy sessions, the therapist taught Joey to define problems assertively to his parents, and the family appeared to be benefiting from treatment. Then a discussion of church attendance was held. Displaying his newly acquired assertive repertoire, Joey stated for the first time that he was agnostic and therefore considered it hypocritical to continue attending church services. Mr. Hayne became livid; Mrs. Hayne began sobbing uncontrollably, while her husband stated that his son would be damned for the remainder of his life if he ceased to attend Mass every week. Enraged, Joey threatened to run away if his parents forced him to continue attending Mass. Because the intensity of all family members' affect implied that no solution would be reached during that session, the therapist adjourned the session after instructing each family member to consider the issue very carefully during the week but not to discuss it without the therapist's help.

Serendipitously, Mr. and Mrs. Hayne consulted their priest, who advised them that a flexible attitude was appropriate with teenagers who were going through the stage of doubting religious beliefs. With permission from the priest, a credible higher authority figure, Mr. and Mrs. Hayne were willing to announce a de-escalation of the conflict at the beginning of the next session: they suggested that Joey attend church twice a month and read a passage from the Bible on the weeks when he did not attend Mass. Aware of his parents' orthodox religious beliefs, Joey was genuinely surprised that they would even consider a compromise. He indicated that since he recognized how much religion meant to them and what a great sacrifice they were making, the least he could do was attend church twice a month "to please them," even though he would continue to maintain his agnosticism.

In cases of conflicts revolving around medically related issues, the therapist might enlist the assistance of a physician as a higher authority figure who sanctions a compromise.

Example. Mrs. Smith and her daughter Wanda were fighting over Wanda's sexual activities. Mrs. Smith was afraid that Wanda would "sleep around" and become pregnant, as had many of her peers, yet she refused to permit Wanda to use birth control. Wanda insisted that she was highly discriminating in her decision to make love with boys and had no desire to become pregnant; she wished to obtain birth control information. The dyad was referred for treatment by Wanda's pediatrician.

The pediatrician was asked to attend a session together with the therapist and Mrs. Smith. The pediatrician indicated that many of the teenagers she treated held beliefs similar to Wanda's concerning sexual intercourse, and that they would find a way to engage in intercourse whether or not their parents approved; therefore, the benefits of providing access to contraception outweighed the risks of teenage pregnancy. These risks were described in detail. Hearing this opinion expressed by a trusted physician, Mrs. Smith was more willing to compromise with her daughter.

Planning Implementation

Goal

The goals of the planning-the-implementation phase of problem solving are for the parents and the adolescent to (1) specify the details that are necessary to put an agreed-upon solution into operation, and (2) anticipate difficulties that may arise during the implementation of the solution.

Critical Attributes

A thorough plan for implementing a solution includes operationalizing which behaviors constitute compliance with the terms of the solution, delegating behavioral tasks to particular family members, formulating record-keeping systems for monitoring compliance with the terms of the solution, and planning for coping with noncompliance.

Example. Consider the previously mentioned case of the agreement between Joey Hayne and his parents. Joey agreed to attend church twice a month and read a passage from the Bible on the weeks when he did not attend Mass, if his parents agreed to refrain from nagging him about religion. Three behaviors needed to be specified: attending church twice a month, reading a passage from the Bible, and not nagging Joey about religion. "Attending church twice a month" was defined as Joey's going to church with his parents and remaining in church until his parents left, on the first and third Sundays of each month. "Reading a passage from the Bible" was defined as taking the family Bible from the living room and sitting anywhere in the house and reading any portion of the Bible for 15 minutes on Sunday morning of the weeks when Joey did not attend church; the TV and radio were to be turned off during this time. "Not nagging Joey about religion" was defined as Mr. and Mrs. Hayne's refraining from making comments or asking questions about Joey's personal religious beliefs; they were permitted to continue to discuss their reactions to shared church attendance experiences. The first two behaviors were assigned to Joey; the third to his parents. In this case, the family agreed that it was unnecessary to keep a written record of compliance with the solution; Joey's presence at church would be self-evident, as would be his parents comments to him concerning his religious beliefs. However, his parents needed a system for monitoring Joey's reading of the Bible. He suggested and they agreed that he would show them the passage that he had read and discuss it with them.

The importance of attending to details when planning the implementation of a solution can not be overemphasized. Questions such as who will do what, when, how, and in what way need to be answered, especially since many solutions are stated in general terms. The therapist should not assume that the parents and adolescent agree concerning the meaning of terms such as "a clean room," "no talking back," or "completion of chores on time." The therapist should help the family to operationalize the solution to clear, behavioral terms. In many cases compromises in the specifics of the agreement may require the therapist to recycle informally through the decision-making phase of problem solving.

Either a written plan or an oral strategy should be designed to monitor compliance with the solution. If a written plan is selected, a chart, graph, or table can be constructed that specifies the tasks to be completed and the occasions when the tasks are scheduled to be completed. The chart should include both the parents' and the adolescent's tasks. In order to insure balance and involve the entire family in the monitoring process, each member should be instructed to observe and record the others' behavior. For instance, when the Levin family agreed to resolve a dispute concerning Tammy's curfew, the chart in Figure 7–2 was constructed. Tammy monitored her parents' nagging while her parents monitored her compliance with the curfew.

If an oral strategy for monitoring compliance with the solution is utilized, the therapist should clearly indicate who will be responsible for reporting what information at the next session. Again, the task of monitoring solution compliance should be shared by all of the members. With most parents and teenagers, for whom *perceptions* of interactional processes are important determinants of family accord, it is usually sufficient to obtain an oral report of the outcome of solution implementation. Because of the difficulty most parents and adolescents experience keeping written records of behavior that occurs across multiple settings, we do not typically assign written monitoring tasks. The exception to this rule occurs in the case of severely distressed families where, in our experience, the members are likely to provide distorted reports of solution implementation. For such families, we routinely summarize agreements in the form of written contracts with written monitoring schemes.

Renegotiation

At the beginning of the next session, the family is asked to report the outcome of their implementation of the previously negotiated solution. If the solution was perceived as effective, the therapist praises the family for its effort, asks them to continue their implementation, and moves ahead to problem-solve a new issue. If the solution was perceived as ineffective, the therapist requests a detailed, step-by-step report of attempts at implementation. The failure of the implementation is placed within a constructive, problem-solving framework rather than a

Behavior	M	T	W	Th	F	Sat	Sun
Tammy comes home by 9:00 p.m. weekdays, 11:00 p.m. weekends							
Parents nag Tammy about curfew							

Agreement
1. Tammy agrees to come home by 9:00 p.m. Sunday through Thursday and by 11:00 p.m. Friday and Saturday.
2. Mr. and Mrs. Levin agree not to nag Tammy about curfew by reminding her to come home on time throughout the week.
3. Tammy will record her parents' nagging by checking each day on which they nagged one or more times.
4. Mr. and Mrs. Levin will check each day on which Tammy came home by the agreed-upon curfew.

FIGURE 7-2 Levin family curfew chart.

defensive, mutually accusatory framework. In other words, the therapist attributes the unsuccessful implementation to difficulties in defining the problem, projecting the consequences of the adopted solution, and planning the details of implementation, and so forth. The metaphor of learning a new skill, with the difficulties involved in its initial performance and the necessity for continued practice, is used to explain the failure of the solution. Afterwards, the family recycles through the problem-solving process to renegotiate an alternative solution to the disagreement. An analysis of case records from one of our outcome studies revealed that 21.2% of the solutions needed to be renegotiated (Foster, 1978).

NOTE

1. The exception to this occurs when the teen and one parent form a strong coalition against the other. In this case, the parents would be encouraged to find mutually agreeable solutions, and the therapist would avoid reinforcing coalitional behavior.

CHAPTER EIGHT

Communication Training

When we originated our treatment program in 1975, we intended to rely primarily upon the use of problem-solving skill training to teach parents and adolescents to resolve disagreements effectively. We quickly learned how naive it was to assume that parents and teenagers would behave in a reasonable, logically consistent fashion and unemotionally follow our step-by-step outline. There were multiple interferences with effective verbal problem-solving behavior during problem-solving discussions. These "interfering events" often took the form of biting, accusatory, sarcastic comments, distracting nonverbal gestures, and other negative expressive and receptive communication behaviors. Negative communication behaviors sidetracked the problem-solving discussion, elicited angry, reciprocally defensive interchanges between family members, and made it difficult for parents and adolescents to negotiate mutually acceptable solutions to their disagreements. In fact, our clinical experiences suggest that the frequency and intensity of negative communication behaviors exhibited by a family during a problem-solving discussion are directly proportional to the overall level of clinical distress, although we have not yet substantiated this hypothesis empirically. Communication skill training currently forms a major part of our treatment program.

Communication training is germane to a variety of relationship problems, and behavior therapists have no monopoly on communication training. There are humanistic (T. Gordon, 1970), eclectic–empirical (Gottman, Notarius, Gonso, & Markman, 1976), combined behavioral–humanistic (Guerney, 1977), as well as behavioral (Jacobson & Margolin, 1979; Piaget, 1972) approaches to communication training. Behavioral communication training can be distinguished from other approaches, however, by its emphasis on both specificity in defining targets for modification and systematic programming of skill acquisition.

Communication training takes place during the problem-solving discussions. Unlike the five-step model of problem solving, which is a standardized procedure used with all families whom we treat, communication skill training is a more informal procedure tailored to the idiosyncratic needs of each family. During the initial assessment, particular deficits and excesses in positive and negative communication skills are analyzed for each family (see Chapter 4). Based on this assessment, the therapist develops a list of problematic communication patterns, which assists in selecting one or two targets for change during each problem-solving discussion. These can be discussed at the beginning of the session, or brought up as they occur. In either case, the therapist describes the communication target, then provides instructions and models of the inappropriate versus the appropriate behavior. Whenever the inappropriate behavior occurs, the therapist interrupts the discussion, labels the behavior, prompts and/or models a more appropriate response, and requires the family to "replay the scene." The four-step procedure of feedback, instructions, modeling, and behavior rehearsal, used repeatedly, is a hallmark of behavioral communication training. Slowly, over a number of sessions, a variety of negative communication patterns can be modified.

COMMUNICATION TARGETS AND INTERVENTION METHODS

Table 8-1 summarizes 20 common negative communication targets, along with suggested alternative responses. The problematic behaviors range from verbal responses such as accusing, lecturing, mind reading, and interrupting to nonverbal responses such as failing to maintain eye contact and fidgeting. As mentioned above, communication training proceeds on a "catch it–correct it" basis. Ultimately, family members are taught to self-monitor and correct inappropriate communication patterns without external feedback.

TABLE 8-1 Dictionary of Communication Targets

Problematic behavior	Possible alternatives
1. Talking through a third person	Talking directly to another person
2. Accusing, blaming, defensive statements	Making I-statements (I feel _____ when _____ happens)
3. Putting down, zapping, shaming	Accepting responsibility, I-statements
4. Interrupting	Listening; raising hand or gesturing when wanting to talk; encouraging speakers to use brief statements
5. Overgeneralizing, catastrophizing, making extremist, rigid statements	Qualifying, making tentative statements (sometimes, maybe, etc.); accurate quantitative statements
6. Lecturing, preaching, moralizing	Making brief, explicit problem statements (I would like _____)
7. Talking in a sarcastic tone of voice	Talking in a neutral tone of voice
8. Failing to make eye contact	Looking at the person with whom you are talking
9. Fidgeting, moving restlessly, or gesturing while being spoken to	Sitting in a relaxed fashion; excusing self for being restless
10. Mind reading	Reflecting, paraphrasing, validating
11. Getting off the topic	Catching self and returning to the problem as defined

(*continued*)

TABLE 8-1 (*continued*)

Problematic behavior	Possible alternatives
12. Commanding, ordering	Suggesting alternative solutions
13. Dwelling on the past	Sticking to the present and future; suggesting changes to correct past problems
14. Monopolizing the conversation	Taking turns making brief statements
15. Intellectualizing, pendanticizing	Speaking in simple, clear language that a teenager can understand
16. Threatening	Suggesting alternative solutions
17. Humoring, discounting	Reflecting, validating
18. Incongruence between verbal and nonverbal behavior	Matching verbal affect and nonverbal posture
19. "Psychologizing"	Inquiring about maintaining variables for another's behavior
20. Remaining silent, not responding	Reflecting, validating, expressing negative affect

Note. From Robin and Foster in *Adolescent behavior disorders: Foundations and contemporary concerns,* by P. A. Karoly and J. J. Steffen (Eds.), 1984, Lexington, MA, D. C. Heath. Copyright 1984 by D. C. Heath. Reprinted by permission of the publisher.

Feedback

The first portion of the correction procedure consists of giving the family feedback concerning the emission of an inappropriate behavior. From a behavioral perspective feedback consists of specific, descriptive information concerning the nature of the behavior in question. Additional information can be added as to the specific negative impact of the problematic response. In doing this, it is best to avoid vague, interpretive, or metaphorical feedback, which can pull the topic away from the issue at hand.

   Example.
MOTHER: I think that the best solution is for you to cut out your irresponsible behavior. . . .
EXPLICIT FEEDBACK: Wait a minute, Mrs. Jones. The phrase "your irresponsible behavior" and your tone of voice sounded to me like you were accusing or threatening John. Perhaps, instead, you could suggest a specific idea for change.
VAGUE FEEDBACK: Wait a minute. Sounds like you're projecting your own anger onto John by accusing him of being irresponsible.

Commentary. In the first case the therapist stuck to a descriptive statement with a relatively low level of inference. In the second case the therapist made an interpretive statement, which requires inferential leaps.

Feedback may vary in terms of its directness. At one extreme, the therapist may clearly indicate which statement or behavior was inappropriate and why. At the other extreme the therapist may engage the family in a Socratic discussion designed to have them "discover" which statement or behavior was inappropriate and why. Intermediate degrees of directness may also be used to give feedback. Direct feedback has the advantage of being concise, precise, and quick to administer without diverting the family's attention from the problem to be solved; however, the therapist may occasionally face a confrontation with one or more family members.

Indirect feedback has the twin advantages of actively involving the client in the feedback process and permitting the therapist to use attributional strategies to mold the family member's attitude towards acceptance of the feedback. In addition, research has suggested that clients are more likely to accept and act upon intrinsic rather than extrinsic explanations of behavior (Valins & Nisbett, 1976). Unfortunately, indirect feedback is time consuming, intrusive, and difficult to administer in a skillful manner.

Our clinical rule of thumb is to rely primarily upon direct feedback during the early stages of communication training. When correcting subtle communication deficits in verbally sophisticated families during the middle and later stages of therapy, we are more likely to employ a Socratic approach to providing feedback. In extremely animated discussions of intensely conflictual issues, the therapist must exercise tight stimulus control over family members' verbalizations; at such times we always use direct feedback.

An excerpt from the evaluation phase of a discussion of cigarette smoking by the Snodgrass family illustrates the use of direct versus indirect feedback.

Example.
THERAPIST: Mr. Snodgrass, why don't you evaluate the next solution, that Sally be permitted to smoke as long as she earns the money to buy her own cigarettes.
MR. SNODGRASS: That is a bad idea because with her history of not doing homework, chores, or coming home on time, I don't see how Sally could ever hold down a decent job long enough to earn money . . .
SALLY: There you go again . . .

Direct Feedback.
THERAPIST: Mr. Snodgrass, the topic is smoking, and I hear you also discussing homework, chores, or curfew. I realize that these are important to you, and you will have a chance to discuss them during other sessions. But your changing the topic and talking about past problems sounds like you are putting Sally down and discounting her ability to improve her behavior. Sally's response indicated she obviously didn't like this. Let's stick to smoking and evaluate the solutions without put-downs.

Indirect Feedback.

THERAPIST: Sally, how did your dad's comment come across to you?

SALLY: It hurt. Like he doesn't trust me or think I can ever do anything right.

THERAPIST: Mr. Snodgrass, how do you react when Sally dredges up the past while you're trying to talk to her about the present?

MR. SNODGRASS: Well. I suppose I don't like it.

THERAPIST: Why? Some people feel that you can only judge a person's future actions by their past behavior. So it may be important to recite all of a person's past wrongs to motivate them to improve in the future.

MR. SNODGRASS: Yes, but it can be awfully distracting. I get so angry when Sally brings up the past that I can't stay rational about the present.

THERAPIST: Sally, how angry did you just get when your dad brought up homework, chores, and curfew while he was discussing smoking?

SALLY: Pretty annoyed. But more hurt.

MR. SNODGRASS: Sally, you know I meant to help you do better, not hurt you. I just want to do what's best.

SALLY: You could help me by sticking to one thing at a time—smoking.

MR. SNODGRASS: I didn't realize this was such a big thing for you. I guess I'll try.

Commentary. If the therapist wished to keep Sally and her father on task, direct feedback would have been clearly preferable. However, if the therapist wished Mr. Snodgrass to increase his appreciation of the effects of his behavior on his daughter and the complimentarity of their mutual tendency to digress from a topic with put-downs, the indirect feedback would have been preferable.

Latency is a second critical dimension in providing feedback concerning communication patterns. Feedback may follow the negative behavior immediately or may be delayed until the sequence of behaviors has been completed. The use of immediate feedback permits the therapist to interrupt and redirect a sequence of negative behaviors before it interferes seriously with the overall flow of the discussion. On the other hand, extensive use of immediate feedback can be frustrating for the parents and adolescent. The therapist is likely to use immediate feedback with high-frequency, intensely negative behaviors which, if unchecked, will sidetrack an entire discussion. Alternatively, delayed feedback gives the family an opportunity to catch and correct their own negative behaviors or at minimum to experience fully the effects of their negative behavior. Yet too much delayed feedback decreases the degree of therapist control in redirecting chains of negative behavior. Again, our clinical rule of thumb is to begin the correction of a particular negative communication skill with immediate, repeated feedback, and as the parents and adolescent learn to self-monitor and correct their negative behavior, to increase gradually the delay of feedback. Often a code word or phrase voiced as a question ("Evaluation?" "I-statement?") or a nonverbal gesture (raised eyebrows) can be used to signal the occurrence of a negative response.

To whom the feedback should be directed is a third critical dimension. Feedback may be given to a monad, a dyad, or a triad. Behavior therapists have typically been trained to think in monadic units, whereas family therapy requires analysis of dyadic and triadic units. Parents and teenagers have also been taught to think in monadic units; each blames the other for the problem. Rarely does a family conceptualize the problem in interactional terms. Consequently, when the therapist directs a remark to a particular family member, each will evaluate the remark as either favoring or not favoring his/her position. Family members can be viewed as keeping a metaphorical "bank account" in which they give the therapist "credits" or "debits" for aligning with or against them. The therapist's long-term goal is to maintain a "zero balance," although there may be short-term deviations in either direction.

Maintaining zero-balance feedback is a little bit like rowing a boat. There are two ways to row a boat forward. The first involves pulling both oars simultaneously. Alternatively, the rower can sequentially place the left and right oars in the water and pull. Similarly, balance in giving feedback on communication skills can be maintained in two ways: first, commenting on a dyadic or triadic interaction pattern; or second, by directing comments over a series of interactions to parents and then to adolescents. Consider the following intervention to correct a parental lecture and adolescent put-down.

Example.

THERAPIST: Fred, it's your turn to define the problem.

FRED: I get mad when you *(To Mom and Dad)* nag me 15 times a night about doing my homework.

MR. SMITH: We wouldn't have to nag you if you'd just get it done. *(Fred begins to fidget, stare at the floor, and act inattentive)* When I was your age my father would give me a good paddling if I didn't do my homework. You kids these days just don't understand the value of a good education.

FRED: *(Mimicking)* You kids don't appreciate anything. I've heard that one a million times!

THERAPIST: *(Interrupting Fred)* Fred, that was a good definition of the problem. Mr. Smith, I understand your anger because Fred can't just do the homework. It's natural to want to express that anger. But the way you expressed it was a lecture. Fred stopped paying attention halfway through it. And Fred, I know that you get turned off by your dad's lectures. But when you mimic him in a sarcastic tone of voice, and put him down as you just did, I would guess that simply confirms his opinion that you won't listen to him unless he nags you repeatedly. So you both lose. Lectures followed by put-downs are a pattern we need to work on.

Commentary. The therapist comments on both Mr. Smith's lecturing and Fred's sarcastic put-down, explaining how they were flip sides of the same coin. Alternatively, the therapist might have chosen to focus primarily on Mr. Smith's lecture, helping him to rehearse an alternative expression of his dissatisfaction. At a later time, Fred's sarcastic put-downs might have been corrected. The selection of a strategy for giving feedback will depend upon the therapist's momentary priorities during the session.

Instructions and Modeling

The second portion of the correction procedure for negative communication behavior consists of instructions and modeling. These two techniques are used to provide the parents and adolescents with positive responses to replace the negative behaviors. The behavior to be emitted is described and role-played by the therapist in a simulated interchange with the family. Because modeling permits the therapist to rapidly enact nuances of interpersonal communication that are hard to describe, it is a particularly efficient procedure for teaching communication skills.

Three important guidelines govern the use of instructions and models. First, the therapist should provide simple, clear-cut instructions and unambiguous models of the target behaviors. Second, the therapist should tailor the instructions and models to fit the educational level, verbal sophistication, and cultural background of the family; responses that are alien to the family's culture are unlikely to be employed outside of the treatment setting. It is particularly important not to use technical terminology or complex vocabulary that might not be understood by the adolescent. Third, the therapist should take steps to prevent the family members from simply imitating the model without actively integrating it into their repertoires. It is useful to ask family members to "say it in your own words." The following admittedly exaggerated excerpt from a naive therapist's first session with the Petusky family poignantly illustrates the importance of these three guidelines.

Example.

MRS. PETUSKY: I ain't goin' stand for no more bad behavior from ya! Billie, I want ya to sit straight, look me in the eye when I talk t'ya, and mind me when I tell ya to do stuff.

MR. PETUSKY: You said it, ma!

BILLIE: Bull!

THERAPIST: Mrs. Petusky, I empathize with your deep-seated frustration about Billie's noncompliant behavior. But the way you expressed it came across as a command. Commands elicit reciprocally negative responses from Billie.

MRS. PETUSKY: What?

THERAPIST: What I mean is I'd like you to express your opinions in a more adaptive manner. For example, you might want to say, "Billie, I'm upset with the high frequency of your inattentive behavior, by which I mean your slouching in the chair, your failure to maintain eye contact, et cetera. I'm also annoyed when you fail to comply with my explicit instructions to complete your chores." Now you put that in your own words, Mrs. Petusky.

(Silence)

BILLIE: What does that word "empathize" mean?

Commentary. Clearly, this therapist has displayed a severe communication deficit by failing to adapt his style to the family's educational and cultural level. The following response by the therapist might have been more appropriate.

THERAPIST: Mrs. Petusky, I understand how pissed you feel when Billie doesn't mind. But you ordered him to obey, and he got worse, not better. Maybe there is a better way to get him to do it.

MRS. PETUSKY: What?

THERAPIST: You might say, "Billie, I get really pissed off when you ignore my requests to do stuff and don't look at me while I talk to you. We are going to have to deal with this now." You say it to him in your own words like you mean it.

Behavior Rehearsal

The third portion of the correction procedure for negative communication behavior consists of behavior rehearsal. After providing feedback, instructions, and models, the therapist asks the family members to practice the positive communication skills. Behavior rehearsal is particularly important because it gives the therapist an opportunity to assess family members' acquisition of novel responses. Following an initial rehearsal, the therapist may choose to provide further feedback, instructions, and models, and require a second rehearsal. In this manner, behavior rehearsal sets the stage for shaping more complex communication skills.

In order to facilitate a realistic rehearsal of an alternative behavior, the family can be asked to "replay the scene"; for example, an adolescent may be asked to restate the remark that incited his father's accusatory onslaught, followed by the father's rehearsal of a less accusatory expression of his displeasure with his son's behavior. The following modified rerun of the earlier example of Mr. Smith's lecturing and Fred's sarcastic put-down illustrates the entire sequence of correction, instructions, modeling, and behavior rehearsal.

Example.

MR. SMITH: We wouldn't have to nag you if you'd just get it done. When I was your age, my father would give me a good paddling if I didn't do my homework. You kids these days just don't understand the value of a good education.

FRED: *(Mimics)* You kids don't appreciate anything. I've heard that one a million times!

THERAPIST: OK. Mr. Smith, I understand your anger at Fred for not just getting the homework done. But the way you expressed it was a lecture. Fred tuned you out halfway through. I imagine this increased your anger. And Fred, I know you dislike lectures, but when you mimic your dad and put him down, he is going to stay on your case. Mr. Smith, let's try a different way of making the same point. If I were you, I might say, "Fred, I become very angry when I repeatedly ask you to do your homework and you don't do it. I'm disappointed because I feel that I have worked hard to help you have a good education." Now, Mr. Smith, you put it in your own words to Fred.

MR. SMITH: Fred, I'm angry when the homework isn't done. I feel badly telling you over and over again to do it because I think I've done a lot to help you get a good education. I feel let down.

THERAPIST: Great job! Fred, now what would you like to say to your dad?

FRED: Ummm . . . Gee . . . I'm not sure.

THERAPIST: Go ahead. Tell him what you think of what he said. Before you had some strong feelings about it.

FRED: Well . . . Dad, it's true I don't like it when you tell me over and over to do my homework. But you're right. I don't like homework. I didn't know it hurt you, though, and that you wanted me to learn a lot in school. I just thought you wanted me to do my homework because your dad made you do it when you were a kid.

THERAPIST: Fred, it takes a big man to admit he was wrong. Now, I think the two of you are really on the right track. Let's list some solutions to this problem.

Commentary. After the therapist corrected Mr. Smith and modeled an appropriate expression of dissatisfaction, Mr. Smith was able to express his disappointment as well as his anger. Only then did Fred "hear" his father's expression of disappointment, which surprised and disarmed him. Instead of reciprocating one negative response with another, he acknowledged his father's disappointment and accepted responsibility for his own behavior. The therapist praised both of their efforts. It is often true that a pivotal correction of one family member's unfortunate remark disarms the others and breaks the reciprocal chain of negative communication, radically redirecting an entire interaction.

There is a word of caution, however: The compulsive practitioner can easily become bogged down by correcting too many negative behaviors too thoroughly during a problem-solving discussion. As a result, the family will not be able to solve the problem within the session. If the goal of the session is to resolve the disagreement, the therapist must correct communication patterns selectively and redirect the family when not-yet-targeted behaviors arise. However, some families do exhibit high rates of reciprocally negative interchanges, necessitating numerous corrections on a statement-by-statement basis. In such cases, several sessions can be scheduled exclusively for the intensive communication training. At the beginning of an intensive communication training session, the therapist should explain that the emphasis of the meeting will be on the way the family members talk to each other, and that the issue under discussion may not be completely resolved until a later session.

CONTENT OF COMMUNICATION TRAINING

Many of the communication targets in Table 8-1 are self-explanatory. In this section of the chapter we will comment in more detail on several of them. Readers interested in additional discussion of other communication targets should consult T. Gordon (1970), Jacobson and Margolin (1979), Piaget (1972), and Strayhorn (1977).

Talking through a Third Person

Talking through a third person is the most common communication pattern targeted for change, and in our experience the easiest to modify. "Talking through a third person" refers to a situation where a family member directs a comment, intended to be received by another family member, to the therapist. For example, when the therapist asks Mr. Jones to define the problem to his son, Mr. Jones may look at the therapist and say, "The problem is that Johnny doesn't do his chores." The task was to define the problem to Johnny with the therapist listening, not to define the problem to the therapist with Johnny listening. In many cases family members talk through a third person simply because they are unaccustomed to having a therapist ask them to interact directly during a treatment session. To correct this, the therapist may interrupt the family member and say, "But please tell Johnny the problem and I'll listen." During the initial problem-solving discussion, the therapist may have to make this statement repeatedly to prompt direct interactions between family members. Eventually, most parents and adolescents catch on.

If the family continues to resist instructions to talk directly to each other, then talking through a third person may represent more than a simple communication deficit. It may pervade family interactions at home, serving to detour conflict or reflecting a difficulty in family structure. In this case, the therapist should conduct a functional analysis by determining the frequency of the problem's occurrence at home and its antecedents and consequences. For instance, when an unassertive mother indirectly send messages to a "spoiled brat" son through the father, the parents may be afraid to confront their son directly. They are not working well as a team or are displaying a weak parental coalition. Their indirect communication may be a way of avoiding unpleasant conflict while discharging their responsibility to "discipline" their son. The therapist would then strengthen the parental coalition by teaching the parents to confront their son directly. Similarly, when an adolescent girl and her mother send indirect messages to the father by talking to each other, the indirect communication may serve several functions. In behavioral family therapy, the therapist should therefore assess factors related to the mother's failure to confront her husband concerning whatever is at issue. If the mother and father disagree about a variety of issues, for example, the mother may attempt to use her close relationship with her daughter to punish, to exercise control, or to avoid experiencing unpleasant interchanges with her husband. In this instance, the goal of the therapeutic strategy would be to push the mother and father to confront each other directly concerning their disagreements, without involving their daughter. In both of these examples, the therapist would repeatedly use the corrective strategy of insisting that the family members communicate directly with each other. At times, it may be necessary to ask the family member who is the "messenger" to either leave the room or move to a distant corner to facilitate direct communication between the other two. Strategies discussed in Chapter 10 may be needed to supplement communication training.

Accusing Defensive Statements

Accusing and defensive statements are another common communication pattern targeted for change in families. A parent will often make an accusatory, blaming remark, which sets the occasion for a defensive reply by a teenager. Or a teenager will attack a parent in an accusatory manner, followed by a counterattack from one or both parents. We treat accusations and defensive behavior as dyadic or triadic communication targets. Family members typically reciprocate accusations with either defensive behavior or additional accusations. The analysis of sequences of accusatory remarks and defensive rebuttals exemplifies the principle of contingent, moment-to-moment reciprocity in action. Sequences of counteraccusations and defensive rebuttals vary topographically, necessitating the development of keen observational skills for recognizing their occurrence. The most common form is a you-statement followed by a denial of responsibility.

Example 1.
MOTHER: Your room is a pigsty.
SON: I cleaned it up Sunday. It's my room so I can do what I like with it. Anyway, you and Dad never clean up your room.

Example 2.
DAUGHTER: You're always telling me, "You don't respect your parents." I can't stand that stupid talk.

FATHER: Young lady, you have no right to talk to us that way. I just can't understand why you always mouth off like that.

Example 3.

MOTHER: We've discussed your delinquent friends a hundred times. I've told you I don't want you hanging out with that crowd. They are a bad influence on you.

SON: I don't hang out with a bad crowd. You're always putting down my best friends.

FATHER: If they aren't a bad influence how come you always smoke pot with them.

SON: I never smoke pot.

MOTHER: Yes you do. . . .

Occasionally, accusations are "disguised" as seemingly innocent, quasi-positive remarks.

Example 4.

THERAPIST: Mr. Jones, please define the curfew problem.

MR. JONES: My problem is that Robert is an irresponsible teenager who comes home late when he has been told to get in by 11:00 p.m.

ROBERT: My problem is that my parents are living in the Stone Age.

Example 5.

THERAPIST: Let's list some solutions for the dating problem.

MOTHER: OK. One solution would be that Brenda stop acting like a 2-year-old and recognize that she could become pregnant if she isn't careful.

BRENDA: My solution is for my mother to start living in the 20th century.

When accusatory, defensive patterns are targeted for change, the therapist should interrupt the discussion with a correction as soon as an accusation is made. You-statements should be replaced with I-statements (T. Gordon, 1970). An I-statement begins with an "I" and tells the other person in what way his/her behavior is unacceptable to the speaker. The speaker may discuss facts, opinions, or feelings, but may not berate persons. Problem definition statements are a subset of the response class of I-statements. The following examples of I-statements are corrected versions of the accusations in the previous examples.

Example 1.

ACCUSATION: Your room is a pigsty.

I-STATEMENT: I'm very upset with the mess in your room.

Example 2.

ACCUSATION: You're always telling me, "You don't respect your parents." I can't stand that stupid talk.

I-STATEMENT: I become infuriated when I'm accused of not respecting you.

Example 3.

ACCUSATION: We've discussed your delinquent friends a hundred times. I've told you I don't want you hanging out with that crowd. They are a bad influence on you.

I-STATEMENT: I'm very upset by the friends you hang out with. I'm worried that they will influence you to get in trouble with the police, skip school, and smoke pot.

Example 4.

ACCUSATION: My problem is that Robert is an irresponsible teenager who comes home late when he has been told to get in by 11:00 p.m.

I-STATEMENT: My problem is that Robert comes home after 11:00 p.m. even though I thought we had agreed to an 11:00 p.m. curfew.

Example 5.

ACCUSATION: OK. One solution would be that Brenda stop acting like a 2-year-old and recognize that she could become pregnant if she isn't careful.

I-STATEMENT: Before I give a solution, I just want to tell you, Brenda, that I'm really scared that you might become pregnant, even though you don't mean to.

ACCUSATION: My solution is for my mother to start living in the 20th century.

I-STATEMENT: Mom, that makes me angry. I really don't want to get pregnant. I'm hurt that you don't have more faith in my judgment.

Occasionally, parents object to the use of I-statements because they doubt that they can genuinely convey the intensity of their affect in this format. In reality, there is no a priori limit to the intensity of affect that can be expressed through an I-statement. The trick is for parents to select a verb that accurately portrays their strong emotions. The affect that is expressed should match the affect that is felt. Of course, clinical experience suggests that parents may find that they experience less intensely negative affect when they cease blaming.

The recipient of an accusatory onslaught often feels like taking a defensive posture. However, if the attack can be construed as a natural result of an unfortunate deficiency in the attacker's skills rather than a personality defect in the recipient, it is feasible to respond assertively yet unoffensively. This cognitive set is particularly germane to adolescents who are commonly blamed for wrongdoing by their parents. We often make the analogy between an unskillful expression of dissatisfaction and missing a basket in basketball or some similar activity familiar to the adolescent. Three alternatives to defensive rebuttals are recommended: reflections, validations, and assertive I-statements.

Reflections are expressions of empathy and understanding. Empathy implies a direct apprehension of the speaker's words, especially the emotional component of the other's experience. While a paraphrase is a purely intellectual restatement of the meaning of a statement, a reflection is a restatement of the speaker's point with the addition of an inference about the speaker's underlying affectual state. Reflections can be double-edged swords. Since they are inferences about unobservable feeling states, they constitute attempts at mind reading, which may itself be a negative communication habit. However, when made in a skilled, caring manner, a reasonably accurate reflection can rapidly defuse the high level of emotional arousal inherent in a accusatory onslaught. Thus, reflections can help to bridge the generation gap.

We teach family members to make reflective statements by asking them first to paraphrase the content of each others' remarks. When they can paraphrase content accurately, we ask them to try to listen for the "feeling tone" in the speaker's remarks and add a "feeling" component to their paraphrases. It requires repeated, guided practice with modeling and feedback from the original speaker to learn to make reasonably accurate reflections. For family members with the prerequisite degree of verbal sophistication, the results are often worth the efforts.

Validation, a concept closely related to reflection, is discussed in detail in communication training manuals for couples (Gottman, Notarius, Gonso, & Markman, 1976; Jacobson & Margolin, 1979, pp. 204–206). A validating statement is one in which the speaker disagrees with another's accusing remark, yet explicitly affirms (1) the legitimacy of the opinion or feeling underlying the remark and (2) the intrinsic worth of the other person as a human being. The validating remark differentiates between the personality and the behavior of the individual; the person's opinions, feelings, or actions are deemed legitimate and understandable, even though the speaker clearly disagrees with them. To illustrate the notion of validation, consider the following response to one of the previously mentioned accusatory remarks.

Example.

ADOLESCENT: You're always telling me, "You don't respect your parents." I can't stand that stupid talk.

FATHER: I understand that you're upset when I suggest that you don't respect us. It's natural to feel that way. I feel put-down, though, when you express it by imitating me and calling my statement "stupid." This is the kind of thing I mean by "disrepect." It would be easier for us to deal with this issue if we both could find better ways of expressing our feelings.

Commentary. The father acknowledged the legitimacy of his daughter's frustration at being told that she is behaving in a disrespectful fashion, yet he disagreed with the way she expressed her frustration; in fact, he cited the expression of frustration as an example of the behavior that he labeled disrespectful. He concluded by accepting responsibility for his contribution to the shared negative interactional sequence and suggesting that they both need to work toward a change. The effect of the validating remark was to affirm his daughter's basic worth as a human being while assertively pinpointing the troublesome tone of her communication. Validation is an excellent response to a family member's hostile, accusatory remarks because it tends to interrupt cycles of reciprocal negative comments and defuse high levels of emotionality, permitting the other person to regain a rational composure without "losing face."

The last portion of the father's response to his daughter also illustrates the third tactic for responding to accusatory remarks in a nondefensive manner: an assertive I-statement. The father gave his daughter feedback about the aspects of her remark that bothered him, that is, the sarcasm and the use of the put-down, "stupid talk." The therapist can teach family members to pinpoint objectionable aspects of each other's communication. This tactic extends the general strategy of improving communication through the use of therapeutic correction by teaching the family to self-correct by giving each other feedback without the intervention of the therapist.

Validations combined with assertive I-statements are particuarly helpful strategies to teach adolescents to apply when their parents' accusations put them on the defensive. The adolescent, who is usually less verbally sophisticated and skilled than the parent and who invariably "loses" in a verbal "power play" of reciprocal accusatory comments, can now express his/her anger in a more adaptive manner. Adolescents find themselves left with residual unexpressed anger if asked to "swallow" a parental onslaught by responding with a straightforward reflection. In our experience, parents are more easily able to absorb an adolescent's accusatory comment, make a reflection, and not be left with undissipated anger.

Caution should be observed, however, when teaching family members reflection, validation, I-statements, and self-correcting feedback. Since most families have a long history of inappropriately giving each other feedback concerning communication, it is easy for them to distort the validation and assertive I-statement process into a continuation of their old, maladaptive patterns of communication. The following dialogue illustrates the potential for abuse of newly acquired communication skills.

Example.

DAUGHTER: My problem is that you bug me 15 times a day about doing my chores and homework, and I don't like to be called a lazy good-for-nothing.

MOTHER: So you're saying that you get upset when you don't complete chores or homework and feel like a lazy good-for-nothing.

DAUGHTER: No Mom, I'm saying I get upset when you call me a lazy good-for-nothing!

MOTHER: I can understand your anger. It's good to get it off your chest. But if you would only do your chores and homework, there would be no need to be angry in the first place. You have to learn to accept feedback better.

Commentary. The mother correctly decided to make a reflective statement. However, instead of reflecting her daughter's feelings, she rechanneled her own opinions and feelings into a quasi-reflective statement that was more critical than helpful. When the daughter attempted to correct her mother's "misunderstanding," the mother "validated" the daughter's expression of anger. Under the guise of giving feedback, she twisted her validation into another example of the nagging behavior to which her daughter had originally objected.

Seriously distressed families frequently distort positive communication skills into negative interactions. The therapist should anticipate the possibility of this type of distortion, model correct versus incorrect usage of reflection, validation, and I-statements, and monitor carefully their implementation. When a parent reports that an attempt to use a newly acquired communication skill at home backfired, the therapist should get a detailed account of the interactional sequence and check carefully for distortions.

Interrupting

A third, commonly corrected communication deficit is interrupting. Parents and adolescents often interrupt each other's conversation. Not only can interruptions break the speaker's train of thought, but they can also elicit angry counterattacks from the speaker. However, there is some evidence that interrupting isn't necessarily a negative behavior. Family interaction researchers have found that in several studies nondistressed families interrupted each other more than distressed families (Parsons & Alexander, 1973). The positive interruptions tended to be requests for clarification. In our own research validating the modified MICS, nondistressed mother–son dyads also emitted more interruptions (mean proportion = .08) than distressed dyads (mean proportions = .07), but this small difference was not significant. Working within a "matching-to-sample," functional family therapy philosophy, Alexander and Parsons (1973) reasoned that if nondistressed families interrupt more to request clarification than distressed families, then teaching appropriate interrupting skills should be one goal of an intervention program for distressed families. Although we do not teach our families to interrupt each other, we do believe, based on both the empirical research and our clinical experiences, that the therapist should conduct a functional analysis of the nature of the interruptions and the verbal style of the family before labeling interrupting as an a priori communication deficit in need of change.

Interrupting that functions to disrupt or sidetrack the conversation should be targeted for change, while interruptions that function to clarify or facilitate the conversation might be tolerated. If a daughter interrupts her mother to disagree or utter a put-down, then the interruption is a hindrance to effective communication. If she interrupts her mother to suggest a novel solution to the problem, then the interruption may be facilitative. How frequently family members interrupt each other may also determine the perceived valence of the interruptions. A father who repeatedly interrupts his sons with mind-reading comments is likely to elicit annoyance, while a father who occasionally interrupts his son to reflect his feelings is likely to elicit a sympathetic response. In highly verbal, intelligent families, members often interact at a frenetic pace characterized by multiple interruptions and a rapid flow of creative ideas. For such families interrupting is a well-established natural characteristic of their speech, not a communication deficit in need of remediation.

Occasionally, the therapist will encounter a family where members interrupt repeatedly to complete each other's thoughts. The mother may begin to express an opinion, but the adolescent will complete her sentence; the adolescent will begin to express his/her feelings, but the father will complete the expression. Members encourage, rather than object, to the pattern of "taking each others' voices," and the impression of an overwhelming degree of intimacy emerges. Consider the following example:

Example.
THERAPIST: Mr. Jones, please define the allowance problem.

MR. JONES: My problem with allowance . . .

MRS. JONES: Is that Mary wants more money than we think is proper.

MARY: I agree. My problem is that I need more money to buy . . .

MR. JONES: Clothes . . .

MRS. JONES: Records . . .

MARY: And books.

THERAPIST: You're a very close family. You talk for each other.

MR. JONES: We understand each other . . .

MARY: Very well.

If excessive, interrupting to "take each others' voices" may be diagnostic of more than a simple negative communication skill; it is often one manifestation of the functional interaction pattern that structural family therapists have dubbed "enmeshment" (Minuchin, 1974; see Chapter 2). With an enmeshed family, the therapist might target interrupting in order to disengage the family, permitting the adolescent to become more independent of the parents, not merely to correct a negative communication habit.

The therapist can teach a family several alternatives to interrupting. First, parents and adolescents can be instructed to look for natural pauses in the conversation as points of entry for the expression of opinions. Second, they can be instructed to raise their hands or otherwise gesture when they wish to enter the conversation. Third, they can be encouraged to keep their remarks succinct in order to prevent the need for interrupting; parents are particularly guilty of making long-winded remarks which their teenagers either interrupt or ignore.

Fourth, they can be instructed to interrupt with an "Excuse me, but there's something that I need to say right now" in "emergencies" where an immediate response to another's comment is called for.

Nonverbal Communication Deficits

Nonverbal communication has recently gained recognition as an important component of the overall communication process in families. In fact, some researchers have relied exclusively upon nonverbal behavior when attempting to encode affect as part of family interaction studies (Gottman, 1979). Parents and teenagers communicate nonverbally through their body posture, gestures, facial expressions, and gaze. Frequently, family members react strongly to each other's nonverbal messages, occasionally misinterpreting the meanings of particular gestures. The most common nonverbal communication targets during problem-solving communication training have been failure to maintain eye contact, excessive fidgeting, slouching posture, and incongruence between the verbal and nonverbal channels of communication.

Failing to maintain eye contact is primarily, although not exclusively, a communication deficit exhibited by adolescents. The darting sideways glance, the pattern of alternately staring at the ceiling or the floor, the stone-eyed glassy look, and the intense, inflexible stare at a trivial object in the far corner of the room are benchmarks of adolescent behavior familiar to many parents. Parents interpret lack of eye contact as a sign that the teenager is not listening, is bored, doesn't love the parent, or is hostile and defiant. Sometimes, the parents' negative interpretations are correct, particularly when an interaction is on a negative course. At other times, failure to maintain eye contact may be a behavioral representation of anxiety, shame, sadness, or embarrassment, or a nonverbal strategy used by the teenager to punish the parent. Occasionally, failure to maintain eye contact is a purely habitual response. Unfortunately, defensive and guilty parents who tend to overinterpret failure to maintain eye contact as a sign of defiance and disrespect react in an accusing manner, inevitably spurring continued lack of eye contact.

The therapist's goal is to encourage family members to establish and maintain eye contact comfortably during conversations, recognizing that at times factors interfering with eye contact may need to be explored before this goal can be attained. Several types of interventions have proven helpful. First, the therapist might give a verbal prompt such as "I would appreciate it very much if you would look at your parents while you talk with each other." Second, the therapist might give a humorous nonverbal prompt by moving into the contorted position on the floor necessary to establish eye contact with an adolescent who is staring at the ground. Third, the therapist may employ a reverse role-play by asking the parents to stop making eye contact with the adolescent in order to permit the adolescent to experience the consequences of this communication deficit.

Fourth, the therapist can functionally analyze the role of the lack of eye contact. One method for doing this involves making a reflective, empathetic remark to assess affective or cognitive variables underlying the adolescent's failure to maintain eye contact. For example, the therapist might say, "It sure can be embarrassing to talk about sex with our parents." Alternatively, the therapist can use a Gestalt enactment technique to assess the underlying variable. For example, the therapist might say, "Alesia, you know your eyes say it all. They are talking for you. Can you let your eyes talk? If your eyes had words, what would they say?"

In some cases, failure to maintain eye contact is a strategy for preventing tears from flowing (especially for males). Behaviorally oriented clinicians have typically not been trained to cope with crying during therapy sessions. Parents and teenagers will often wish to cry but may be inhibited because they feel that crying is an unacceptable behavior or a sign of weakness. The therapist must learn to be comfortable with family members' tears unless they are used manipulatively to distract from the issue under discussion. It is often helpful for the therapist to ask parents to give their son or daughter permission to cry during the therapy hour.

Excessive fidgeting or postural contortions are a second common nonverbal communication target. As with failure to maintain eye contact, fidgeting may be interpreted as a sign of inattention, restlessness, lack of concern, or defiance by family members. The therapist should intervene to determine the parents' perception of the adolescent's fidgeting. In some cases, restlessness may be a symptom of Attention Deficit Hyperactivity Disorder (Barkley, 1981) rather than a communication deficit, and parents can be guided to accept or circumvent it without drawing malicious conclusions. The parents should be prompted to verify the accuracy of their perceptions in a nonthreatening manner while the adolescent should be prompted to express any dissatisfaction with the parents' behavior verbally as well as nonverbally. Of course, it is crucial for the parents to be willing to accept verbal feedback from the adolescent before the teenager can be expected to translate nonverbal restlessness into verbal expressions of dissatisfaction. Prompts, role-plays, and Gestalt enactment interventions may be employed to clarify the function of unusual posturing. The following vignette incorporates these suggestions.

Example.
MR. HAGGERTY: Sam, I've told you a hundred times that I can't understand why you find it so difficult to complete your homework.
(Sam slouches in his chair, hands and legs outstretched and limp, slowly sliding towards the floor.)
MRS. HAGGERTY: Doctor, you can see for yourself what we mean when we say that Sam doesn't care about what we say. Look at the way he is slouching, as if he hasn't heard a word his father said. He never does that with his friends. Wouldn't you call that just plain rude?

THERAPIST: *(To parents)* I appreciate your annoyance with Sam's posture, but I wish to explore this further. Would you give him permission to say whatever is on his mind?

BOTH PARENTS: Why, of course. That's what this meeting is all about.

THERAPIST: *(To Sam)* Our bodies often speak for us. When I sit back like this *(Sits up rigidly with arms and legs crossed)*, I'm often feeling uptight. When I let it all hang out like this *(Slouches, like Sam)*, it could mean many things. If your body could talk, what would it be saying now?

SAM: *(Sits up more attentively)* That I can't stand being treated like a 2-year old and lectured about homework. . . .

MR. HAGGERTY: *(Interrupting)* But, we're . . .

THERAPIST: *(Interrupting)* You gave him permission to speak his mind. Please listen first and comment later. Go ahead, Sam.

SAM: My dad always lectures me about homework and this really bugs me.

THERAPIST: I appreciate your sharing this with us, Sam. I'd like you to try to tell him with your mouth, not only with your body. And Mr. Haggerty, I can promise the family more slouching if lecturing continues. But perhaps we can find another way of expressing opinions and feelings. Notice how Sam is sitting up nicely now. He has had a chance to speak his mind. And I want to thank you for hearing him out. All those negative feelings can weigh a person down to the point where they are ready to fall out of their chair, as Sam was. If you get them out, you can sit up straight again. Right, Sam?

SAM: Right.

Commentary. After validating the parents' annoyance with Sam's posture but circumventing the mother's attempt to win him over to her side, the therapist aligned himself with the adolescent and used a Gestalt enactment technique to encourage the adolescent to translate his nonverbal message into words. When the father interrupted, he was silenced. Each family member was praised for the positive aspect of his/her behavior. The family was left with the metaphor of slouching as a visual representation of being weighed down by unexpressed feelings.

The astute behavioral clinician might question the rationale for invoking a symbolic metaphor while correcting Sam's inappropriate posturing. The metaphor was not introduced because the therapist believed that Sam's slouching was truly a symbolic representation of "being weighed down by angry feelings" (although some therapists may adhere to such beliefs). Rather, the therapist wanted the family to attribute a positive function to the slouching in order to permit Sam to "save face" and gracefully stop slouching without the necessity for a confrontation over his parents' interpretation of the slouching as defiance and not caring. Metaphorical reframing statements can be powerful reattributional strategies during problem-solving communication training.

A third common nonverbal communication target relates to the incongruence between a person's words and nonverbal responses.

Example.   An attractive, 30-year-old divorced mother repeatedly smiled and laughed while telling the therapist how dissatisfied she was with her 13-year-old son's failure to complete his chores and follow her instructions. Meanwhile, her son gazed at her lovingly, returning her smiles and laughs. It became clear to the therapist from observing their mirror-image nonverbal interaction that this mother and son were extremely close to each other, yet the closeness made it difficult for the mother to express her disapproval of her son's behavior. Because of the incongruence between her glowing demeanor and critical statement, the mother was not making a convincing presentation of her dissatisfaction to her son. Later, she complained that "he doesn't take me seriously." The therapist pointed out the inconsistency in her behavior and asked her to rehearse a more serious presentation of her complaints.

When incongruencies between verbal and nonverbal behavior occur, it is appropriate to stop the discussion, assess the message that the speaker wishes to send, and teach the speaker a more consistent method of expressing the message. Sometimes this involves assisting the speaker in recognizing as well as expressing affective cues associated with the mixed message.

FINAL NOTE ON COMMUNICATION TRAINING

Throughout this section of the chapter, we have discussed in considerable detail common communication deficits and procedures for remediating these deficits. Behavioral clinicians working with families will occasionally encounter uncommon communication deficits idiosyncratic to a particular family. Feedback, instructions, modeling, and behavior rehearsal can easily be adopted for use with these idiosyncratic deficits. For instance, the way in which a father smiled was problematic for one sensitive 13-year-old girl. Her father was a jovial English teacher with an excellent sense of humor. Unfortunately, he spoke in a somewhat pedantic manner. His daughter objected to the excessive upward curvature of her father's lips when he smiled while talking with her; her father's "English teacher smile" meant that he was secretly making fun of her even though his comments appeared perfectly innocent. Her father was genuinely surprised to learn that his smile bothered his daughter, especially since he had a great deal of difficulty discriminating a "positive smile" from an "English teacher smile." The therapist asked the girl to interrupt the conversation whenever her father emitted an "English teacher smile." Then, her father was asked to clarify whatever he was saying to his daughter. It became apparent that she misinterpreted and responded to her father's nonverbal mannerisms when they were accompanied by sophisticated phraseology. As her father learned to temper his pedantic style, the daughter became more comfortable with his smile.

Whether the concern is an inappropriate tone of voice, an accusatory remark, or a poor problem definition, we emphasize a swift, directive intervention balancing structured behavioral training procedures with clinical flexibility. The supraordinate goal of problem-solving communication training interventions is to teach skills during therapy sessions that will restructure family verbal interaction. This chapter has presented a microscopic analysis of the skills to be taught and the methods for teaching them. However, in order to be a successful teacher, the therapist must encourage the family members to apply their new skills in the natural environment. They must also develop cognitive sets compatible with the acquisition and exercising of the skills. In the next chapter we will turn to the procedures that we have developed for fostering appropriate attitudes towards the skills.

CHAPTER NINE

Cognitive Restructuring

As outlined in Chapter 2, cognitive factors play an important role in parent–adolescent conflict. Family members' perceptions, expectations, beliefs, attributions, and information-processing styles mediate their affective and behavioral responses to each other and are closely tied to the observable reality of their interactions. When family members process information inaccurately, committing logical errors such as arbitrary inference or overgeneralization, they may become overly hostile and antagonistic toward each other, impeding positive communication and effective problem solving. Over time they may develop rigid, absolutistic beliefs that dominate their interactions and cause attempts at conflict resolution to grind to a halt. Rigid, negative belief systems, especially those centering around the themes of ruination, fairness, approval, perfectionism, obedience, self-blame, and malicious intent, contribute to the development and maintenance of circular, interlocking contingency arrangements whereby family members avoid or impede reality-based discussion of conflictual issues. Yet the developmental thrust of increased adolescent independence seeking confronts the family with a continuing need to resolve conflicts, producing bitter, negative interchanges. In some families who already have effective problem-solving communication skills in their repertoires, cognitive distortions are the primary factor promoting continued conflict.

This chapter is designed to outline how to use cognitive restructuring techniques to help parents and adolescents change problematic perceptions, beliefs, expectations, and attributions. Strategies for cognitive restructuring are derived from Ellis's rational–emotive approach (Dryden & Ellis, 1988; Ellis & Grieger, 1977; Goldfried & Goldfried, 1980) and Beck's collaborative empiricism (Beck et al., 1979; DeRubens & Beck, 1988). In Ellis's approach, the therapist challenges the validity of the beliefs and helps the client replace unreasonable beliefs with more suitable alternatives. The persuasive authority of the therapist is the basis for disconfirming absolutistic cognitions. In Beck's approach, the therapist collaborates with the family to design and execute "mini-experiments" that test and disconfirm the credibility of various beliefs. The data generated by the mini-experiments, rather than logical challenges provided by the therapist, serve to disconfirm beliefs. Although proponents of these two approaches differentiate carefully between them (e.g., Hollon & Beck, 1979, p. 192), we agree with those who found that they dovetail nicely (Meichenbaum, 1977). In our treatment, they are integrated.

Evidence attests to the effectiveness of cognitive restructuring for treating a variety of adult disorders (Dobson, 1988), including anxiety problems (Beck & Emery, 1985; Goldfried, 1979), assertion difficulties (Linehan, 1979), and depression (Beck *et al.*, 1979), and it has been suggested as a component of behavioral marital therapy (Doherty, 1981; Epstein, 1982; Jacobson & Margolin, 1979; Stuart, 1980). In addition, some forms of cognitive restructuring are similar to the family systems technique of reframing (Minuchin & Fishman, 1981), and we also draw from the family systems literature in cognitive restructuring.

In the pages that follow, we discuss two forms of cognitive restructuring. The first is used primarily to relabel negative attributions attached to the causes of other family members' behavior. The duration of this intervention varies, depending on the malleability of the attribution. The second, more complex form of cognitive restructuring is reserved for pervasive distortions that influence large classes of interactive behavior. Either, both, or neither of these approaches may be needed, depending upon the extent and type of problematic cognitions family members display.

DEALING WITH MISATTRIBUTIONS

Causes of behavior are important to people: as a species, we seek to understand the "whys" of our environment and the behavior of those around us. Family members frequently make inferences about why others in the family behave as they do. Unacceptable assumed causes may lead the attributing member to refuse to consider certain solutions. For example, some parents want teens to change their behavior, but only if their reasons for doing so are acceptable. Acceptable attributions vary, but might include "because she respects me," "because he loves me," or "because it's his/her responsibility." Any solution involving material rewards will likely be automatically discarded by a parent for whom these assumptions are activated, since the teen would be performing the desired behavior for the wrong reasons. Alternatively, misattributions may surface as mind-reading statements, impeding effective communication.

Several different strategies can be used to encourage family members to develop less restrictive attributions. When attributions are verbalized, they can be treated as communication targets, using methods outlined in Chapter 8. When the attributions are covert, the therapist can elicit them, then either reframe the attribution or ask the attributor to verify or correct the assumption.

Reframing Attributions

Reframing, or relabeling, is a strategy that involves providing the individual with an alternative benign or positive way of labeling a situation. It is most often used when a family member attributes a negative motive or malicious intent to another's behavior.

Example.

MRS. JOHNSON: I don't understand why John behaves the way he does. He is intentionally trying to hurt me. I can't believe I've raised such an insensitive kid.

THERAPIST: You know, from what I've seen of John, he doesn't seem like that kind of kid. I think he really wants to please, but doesn't know how to do it.

Commentary. The therapist relabels John's behavior as a skill deficit, shifting the mother's notion that he behaves negatively to torment her to a more adaptive hypothesis: that he wants her regard but lacks the skills to attain it.

Reframing is particularly useful for helping parents and teens understand the changes that accompany adolescence. Parent overprotectiveness can be reinterpreted as concern for the adolescent's well-being; negative adolescent behavior can be reframed as awkward attempts to complete a normal process of establishing independence. Angry adolescent outbursts interpreted as lack of respect can be relabeled as attempts to communicate. The therapist need not believe the essential truth of the new explanation. Rather, the key to successful reframing is to find an alternate explanation that neutralizes the problem attribution and is acceptable to the family member.

With certain forms of adolescent behavior disorders, judicious reframing assumes a special importance. The adolescent with Attention Deficit Hyperactivity Disorder (ADHD) (Barkley, 1981) is often absent-minded, disorganized, and impulsive. Such adolescents often forget to complete tasks which they have begun, ranging from simple tasks such as turning off lights to more complex tasks such as turning in homework assignments. The persistent, chronic forgetfulness grows out of their basic biological predispositions towards ADHD and is not simply a malicious act (although there are certainly environmental contingencies which influence forgetful behavior). It is helpful for the therapist to teach parents to reframe the ADHD adolescents' forgetful behavior as due in part to the teenager's basic biological predispositions, not simply environmental contingencies or malicious intent. Although the adolescents may be held accountable for their actions, the chronic repetitiveness of the ADHD individual's inattentive behavior infuriates even the most patient parent and spurs endless angry conflict unless parents develop realistic attributions.

Correcting Misattributions through Verification

Attributions can also be modified by eliciting the problem attribution, then asking the member to whom the intent is attributed to comment on its truth or falsity. Alternatively, the attributor can be asked to check it out directly. This, of course, only works when the second member is likely to correct the attribution and not endorse it.

Example.

MRS. JOHNSON: I don't understand why John behaves the way he does. He is intentionally trying to hurt me. I can't believe I've raised such an insensitive kid.

THERAPIST: It sounds like you think he's out to get you. John, is she right?

JOHN: No, of course not. It's just that she gets on my back so much, it makes me mad.

THERAPIST: So you get mad when she gets on your back, and you don't know how to get her to stop getting on you. So you do whatever you want, because you're mad.

Commentary. The therapist elicits that problem attribution, then asks the son to comment, trusting him to provide an alternate reason for his behavior. When he does, the therapist paraphrases and reframes the new attribution into an interactional formulation more likely to promote positive problem solving.

Additional reframing examples may be found in Chapter 4. Systems family therapy also relies heavily on reframing, and the interested reader might consult any of the numerous references from this literature cited throughout this text for further discussion and examples of these strategies.

DEALING WITH MAJOR COGNITIVE DISTORTIONS

The therapist begins the cognitive restructuring process by giving the family a rationale relating behavior, thoughts, and feelings. Common unreasonable beliefs are reviewed, and steps for cognitive restructuring are outlined. Then the family is told that whenever cognitive distortions arise during problem-solving discussions, the therapist will stop the discussion to help the family challenge and replace them with more realistic thought patterns. Homework is assigned to practice identifying and challenging absolutistic beliefs through didactic debate and experiential learning.

Six general steps are followed for correcting cognitive difficulties: (1) give a rationale relating thoughts, feelings, and behavior; (2) identify the inappropriate cognitions or cognitive process; (3) challenge them; (4) model a more appropriate alternative; (5) propose an experiment designed to test the validity of these beliefs or processes; and (6) help the family plan a strategy to complete the "experiment" and rehearse the alternative cognitions. The following outline describes for the family the last five steps of cognitive restructuring.

I. Identify the inappropriate belief.
   A. Define the problem: State what words and actions of the others are creating a problem for you.
   B. Define the cognition:
      1. Identify the unreasonable thought or inappropriate belief that may be operating in that situation.
      2. Use the table of unreasonable beliefs (see Table 9-1) to help identify your thoughts.
   C. State to the other person or write down the inappropriate belief.

II. Challenge the inappropriate belief.
   A. What is the worst thing that can happen?
   B. Does any situation in the past challenge your present belief?
   C. What is the logical basis for your belief?
   D. Are you exaggerating, overstating, or thinking in an all-or-none fashion about the situation?

III. Identify a more appropriate belief.
   A. What is the most realistic belief given the situation?
   B. What would most people think in this situation?
   C. What is a "middle-of-the-road" position on this issue?

IV. Design an experiment to test out the unreasonable versus reasonable beliefs.
   A. Conduct a survey of other parents or teenagers in similar situations.
   B. Try out a solution based upon the reasonable belief and see what happens.
   C. Collect information from books, movies, TV or other sources to confirm or disconfirm the beliefs.
   D. Consider how you felt about the same situation when you were a teenager (for parents only).

V. Plan a strategy to conduct the experiment and rehearse the appropriate belief.
   A. Decide who will do what, when, and where to conduct the experiment.
   B. Specify the situation in which your unreasonable belief occurs.
   C. Role-play the situation and challenge your belief out loud with the help of family members.
   D. Record situation, belief, challenge, and outcome on a standardized recording sheet.

Give a Rationale for Cognitive Restructuring

The therapist teaches clients the connection between thoughts, feelings, and behaviors, emphasizing how cognitions concerning relationship events may be as important in determining members' affective reactions to each other as the events themselves. The therapist also points out how absolutistic, negative cognitions can polarize parents' and teenagers' positions on specific issues, and how their resulting negative feelings then impede effective problem solving and increase the likelihood of accusatory–defensive communication. Themes such as ruination, obedience, perfectionism, and unfairness are introduced as examples of problematic cognitions. Interactive dialogue actively involving the family in imaginary exercises provides a salient rationale for cognitive restructuring.

Example of Rationale.

THERAPIST: We've talked about how your thoughts about each other sometimes get you angry or depressed. Then your feelings make it difficult to avoid big arguments and hassles. Let's talk some more about how the way we think influences the way we feel. If you have a lot of very negative thoughts about your relationship, you will feel angry or depressed, right? If you have a lot of very positive thoughts, you will feel warm and loving toward each other. I'd like you to try something now. Close your eyes and imagine that recent argument you had about Sally's riding in cars with older boys. Mr. and Mrs. Jones, focus your attention on how disobedient Sally was to violate your carefully presented rule. Sally, you think about how unfair it was for your parents to forbid you to ride in cars with older boys. OK, Mr. Jones, what are your thoughts now?

MR. JONES: Sally should have obeyed our rule. Her disobedience showed a basic lack of respect for authority.

THERAPIST: And how do you feel as you have this thought?

MR. JONES: Very angry. The more I think about it, the angrier I get!

THERAPIST: Exactly. It is the extremely negative thoughts that lead to the strong feelings. Sally, what were your thoughts?

SALLY: How could my parents be so unfair when all my friends get to go driving with whoever they like? My parents just don't want me to have any fun.

THERAPIST: How do you feel?

SALLY: Mad. Ready to let them have it.

THERAPIST: So your negative thoughts also make you feel angry, and when you get so angry, you are more likely to do things you get in trouble for. This points out the reason for us to focus on your extremely negative thoughts. Most of us get so upset by our extreme thoughts that we act irrationally, usually making things worse instead of better. I've noticed thoughts having to do with obedience and unfairness are common for your family, and we will talk about these in a few minutes. Now close your eyes again and think about a fun experience the family had together, perhaps going out to dinner or to an amusement park. Now, Mrs. Jones, what are you thinking?

MRS. JONES: About going to Cedar Point last week. We all had such fun, and Sally even thanked us for taking her.

THERAPIST: And how do you feel as you have these positive thoughts?

MRS. JONES: Happy. Pleased.

THERAPIST: Just as negative thoughts bring on bad feelings, positive thoughts can cause good feelings. We need to deal with the extremely negative thoughts so that you can feel better about your relationship. Then it will be easier to resolve your differences and grow as a family.

Commentary. The therapist presented a simplified overview of the cognitive–behavioral framework by involving the parents and teenagers in an "experiment" that illustrated the relationship among thoughts, feelings, and interactions. This rationale can be tailored to the particular distortions of each family. By enlisting parents and adolescent as participants in a cognitive–behavioral exercise, and by tying the rationale and exercise to the family's own patterns of thinking, feeling, and interacting, the therapist sets the stage for the process of collaborative empiricism, later used to challenge and modify unreasonable beliefs.

Note that at this point the therapist carefully frames thoughts as cognitive events and focuses on their role in family process, rather than examining their content. Family members who are wedded to the notion that they are "right" (i.e., their thoughts reflect truth) are often more willing to examine the validity and utility of their beliefs once they have seen how particular beliefs lead consistently to problem consequences.

Presenting family members with a list of common unreasonable beliefs and more realistic alternatives can enhance the cognitive restructuring rationale (see Table 9-1). The therapist can review the list, inquiring about recent situations where particular relationship events triggered particular thoughts, feelings, and resulting conflicts.

Identify the Inappropriate Cognition

The goal of this stage of cognitive restructuring is for the therapist to teach the family to identify and monitor problematic cognitive processes and unrealistic beliefs. A discrimination training format often is useful for accomplishing this goal. The therapist presents examples of interactions replete with verbalizations reflecting distorted thinking, and guides the family to discriminate appropriate from inappropriate cognitions. When a preassessment discussion of a specific dispute has been audiotaped, the therapist can play the tape and ask family members to reconstruct their thoughts and feelings. By referring to the list of problematic beliefs, the therapist can teach the parents and teenager to identify thoughts that reflect themes such as ruination, obedience, or unfairness. Alternatively, an audiotape of a simulated parent–adolescent discussion can be played, and the family can be asked to discriminate examples of reasonable versus unreasonable cognitions.

When the family is later engaging in problem solving, the therapist can occasionally stop the discussion and direct their attention to mediating cognitive

TABLE 9-1 Common Unreasonable Beliefs and Alternatives

Unreasonable Belief	Reasonable Alternative
Parents	

Ruination:
If my teenager is given freedom and/or rules are relaxed, catastrophic consequences will result, which will ruin the teenager's future.

Come on! Many teenagers are given additional freedom without any bad reactions. Am I truly being realistic?

Obedience:
My teenager should always do what I ask or demand, and it is catastrophic if s/he fails to obey me.

Did I always listen to my parents? Have I turned out terrible? What is the worst thing that can happen?

Perfectionism:
My teenager should always know the right thing to do and should always make the right decision.

Teenagers, like parents, make mistakes and have a right to learn from their mistakes. No one is perfect.

Self-blame:
It is my fault when my teenager acts bad or makes mistakes. If only I had raised the child differently, this would never have happened.

We can only guide our children. We cannot ultimately be responsible for all of their behavior. Many other people have also influenced my teen.

Malicious intent:
My teenager is misbehaving on purpose to annoy, hurt, and anger my spouse and me.

Teenagers don't generally plan their misbehavior in advance. What are some other explanations for why it appears as if my teen is trying to hurt me?

Adolescents	

Fairness:
It is terribly unfair for my parents to enforce rules.

Parents have a right to let me know how they feel. Who promised life will always be fair?

Ruination:
Parents' rules will ruin my life by stopping me from having a good time, having friends, or doing what other teenagers do.

When was the last time a parental rule interfered with my plans? Did everything fall apart? Did I lose all my friends? Come on! What is the worst thing that can really happen?

Autonomy:
I should be permitted total freedom to do whatever I want without any parental interference.

Does anyone really have such freedom? Don't I really want help sometimes? Parents have a right to guide me, just as I have a right to let them know how I feel. We need to respect each others' rights.

Approval:
It is terrible for me to do things that upset my parents.

I can't please everyone all the time. Sometimes I must say what I think, even if my parents don't agree.

processes. In some cases, family members will clearly express their beliefs, as when an authoritarian father boldly asserts that teenagers should always obey their parents, or the depressed mother of a pristine daughter tearfully reveals her anxieties that her daughter will behave promiscuously if she is permitted to stay out late. In other cases, in-session behavior will cue a therapist to hypothesize the possible interfering role of rigid cognitions, as when parents and teenagers staunchly resist negotiating compromise solutions or one family member displays inappropriately intense emotional reactions to a seemingly innocuous suggestion by another.

Clinically speaking, individuals who clearly articulate their unrealistic ideas frequently prove more resistant to change than those who are more reticent in revealing their beliefs. The former see nothing inappropriate about their rigid cognitions, but the latter guiltily hide thoughts of which they may be ashamed. To elicit statements reflecting problem cognitions, the therapist can engage the family members in a dialogue liberally sprinkled with humor, exaggeration, and/or Socratic questioning. Humor in particular helps to make the family aware of the unreasonableness of their thought processes in a disarming yet unoffensive manner. As the therapist elicits reports of distorted cognitions, s/he reflects back to the family a conceptualization of the belief. Two cases illustrate this procedure.

Example 1.   During a discussion of curfew, Mr. Levin insisted that his daughter, Kathy, should come home by 10:30 p.m. until she reached 16. His refusal to compromise bogged down the discussion. When questioned, he would not give additional reasons for his strong belief; he simply insisted that "she is too immature to stay out later." The therapist hypothesized that a cognitive distortion concerning ruination (e.g., the perceived catastrophic consequences of Kathy's staying out too late) underlay his resistant behavior. The following dialogue ensued:

THERAPIST: So, you said Kathy will be mature enough to stay out until midnight when she reaches her 16th birthday, right?

MR. LEVIN: Right.

THERAPIST: How long is it until your birthday, Kathy?

KATHY: Six months.

THERAPIST: Or about 180 days. Now, Mr. Levin, Kathy is 1 day older with each passing day.

MR. LEVIN: *(Puzzled)* Right.

THERAPIST: So she is 1 day more mature. Now, if she can stay out 90 minutes later when she is 180 days older and more mature, and if she does mature 1 day at a time, I think we should let her stay out ½ minute later per night. That would only be fair, since she is maturing every day, right? *(Kathy and Mrs. Levin begin to giggle.)*

MR. LEVIN: *(Turns red, averts his eyes, and stares at the floor)* Well, I guess so . . . Well, uh-ah, Doc, what's bothering me is . . . you know . . . the things these kids do out there at night, and my Kathy . . . you know . . . she is a follower.

KATHY: Dad!!!

THERAPIST: I know it's hard to talk about these things. If I were you, I might be afraid that if Kathy stays out later, she will get into trouble—maybe with sex, drugs, or booze. Is that it?

MR. LEVIN: *(Meekly)* Uh . . . yes, that's it. All three.

Commentary. Through relentless but humorous pursuit of Mr. Levin's logic, the therapist pointed out the flimsy foundation for his stated reason for resisting a compromise concerning curfew. Either he had to provide a better reason or look foolish in the eyes of his family; he chose the former option, and his underlying cognitive distortion became explicit. His was a case of an extreme belief in ruination, that is, permitting his daughter to stay out later would result in promiscuity, alcoholism, and drug abuse. In adhering to this belief, he was also committing logical errors of arbitrary inference, overgeneralization, and magnification.

Example 2: The Hortons (Part 1).   Mr. and Mrs. Horton brought Larry, their adopted 13-year-old ADHD son, for treatment. Ritalin was helping his attention problems at school, but at home he was exhibiting increasingly rebellious behavior. During the first three sessions, successful problem-solving discussions about spending his allowance, sibling fighting, and bedtime were conducted. During the fourth session, the family began a discussion of Larry's disrespectful behavior at home. When Larry stated that his mother asked him to do too many chores, Mrs. Horton exploded in a fit of rage culminating in tears.

MRS. HORTON: That ingrate! All I ever ask him to do is put his clothes away and not make too much noise. And he just keeps agitating me. I get so mad I could kill him. *(Crying)* Maybe I should never have been a parent, and God is punishing me for adopting kids.

MR. HORTON: Please, dear . . .

LARRY: Mom . . .

MRS. HORTON: Don't "please dear" or "mom" me. Any decent kid wouldn't be so disrespectful after all I've done.

THERAPIST: I can see how angry you get when Larry acts disrespectfully. It's as if your world is going to collapse. You're carrying a very heavy burden.

MRS. HORTON: *(Softly)* Damn right.

THERAPIST: When Larry talks back to you, what does this mean about you as a parent?

MRS. HORTON: I don't know. *(Tearful)* I just worry so much that I've messed him up and he won't amount to anything.

THERAPIST: When Larry talks back to you, you blame yourself for being a bad mother. Parents are to blame for their teenager's faults.

MRS. HORTON: I guess so. He seems like such a bad kid.

THERAPIST: And a boy who agitates his mother even a little has to grow up to be an antisocial, terrible adult. This spells ruination for him and you.

MRS. HORTON: That's it.

THERAPIST: It sounds like you believe kids like Larry should behave well out of gratitude for all of the sacrifices their parents have made.

MRS. HORTON: Well, don't you think so?

THERAPIST: Well, I can certainly understand why you are so angry, regardless of what I think. If I were thinking so extremely—that each act of disrespect means total failure and self-blame, I would also be upset each time Larry talked back or disobeyed a rule. You are a member of a special club—the 100% club. Things are either 100% right or 0%. Nothing in-between. Larry will either grow up perfect or a total disaster. Is the world really black or white, or aren't there really also many shades of gray?

Commentary. Mrs. Horton's emotional outburst was clearly an overreaction to her son's disrespectful behavior, which was well within the bounds of normality for a 13-year-old teenager with ADHD. Elements of overgeneralization, arbitrary inference, selective abstraction, and dichotomous all-or-none reasoning were evident in her comments. The therapist pinpointed her unrealistic assumptions about ruination and self-blame, linking them to her extreme affective reaction while simultaneously attempting to express empathy and defuse her emotionality. Because of her anger level, humor was inappropriate at this stage of cognitive restructuring. The metaphor of "the 100% club" has proven especially useful clinically to help family members understand the absolutistic nature of their thinking.

Challenge the Inappropriate Belief

The goal of this stage of cognitive restructuring is for the therapist to challenge the logical premises of the unreasonable beliefs. When challenging unreasonable cognitions, the therapist should proceed cautiously, making liberal use of humor, and checking to ensure that the family member retains enough objectivity to step back from and examine the belief. We often "blow up" the belief, exaggerating it to absurd proportions and examining its consequences. With families the caustic approach of early proponents of rational–emotive therapy often backfires because it is very difficult for one member to admit being illogical in front of the others, without humiliation. The others may rally to support the unreasonable position to protect the member from the therapist's attack, whether or not they agree with the belief in question.

One way to challenge the belief involves first stating it in an exaggerated form without specific reference to the family's circumstances; most families will readily agree that the exaggerated statement is absurd. Then the therapist can skillfully relate the absurd statement to the beliefs held by the family members. Since they have already agreed with the therapist about the absurdity of the general principle, they are more likely to perceive the unreasonableness of their own positions. To be successful, the therapist must have the agreement of the family members at each step of this attributional maneuvering. Alternatively, the therapist can ask family members to marshall evidence for and against the veracity of a particular belief, and let the members' inability to make a convincing case serve as the basis for the challenge. Other family members can be invited to help evaluate the evidence when the therapist is confident that they will support reasonable positions. We continue with the Hortons.

Example: The Hortons (Part 2).

THERAPIST: Let me get one thing straight. You said that if Larry talks back to you now, he will grow up to be an antisocial adult.

MRS. HORTON: Right. He may not respect authority as an adult. He could even break the law.

THERAPIST: Children who talk back to their parents grow up to be hardened criminals.

MRS. HORTON: Maybe not hardened . . .

THERAPIST: But that follows logically from your position. *(To Larry)* Do you know any children who never talked back to their parents?

LARRY: All my friends do it.

THERAPIST: *(To Mrs. Horton)* Do you think every single one of his friends will grow up to be criminals?

MRS. HORTON: I don't know. I suppose not, if you put it that way.

THERAPIST: Well, it sounds to me like your reasoning says that all children must grow up to be criminals if they act disrespectful to their parents. We would all be in jail!

MR. HORTON: I talked back to my father and I'm not a criminal.

MRS. HORTON: Maybe you're right, but it really hurts me when Larry acts this way.

THERAPIST: I understand, and I am not trying to minimize the hurt or make fun of you. But I am saying that maybe the pain would be less if you thought differently about the things he says. Being a member of the 100% club can have its disadvantages!

MRS. HORTON: I guess so.

Commentary. The therapist exaggerated Mrs. Horton's unreasonable beliefs to absurd proportions and gently pointed out internal inconsistencies in her reasoning, validating her feelings but preparing her to view the situation more realistically.

Identify a More Appropriate Belief

During this stage of cognitive restructuring, the therapist models alternative, more flexible beliefs and cognitions. Extremist phrases such as "should," "must," "have to," and "always" are transformed into more tentative phrases such as "it would be nice if," "I would like you to," "I would really be pleased if," and "as often as possible." Logical, evidence-based conclusions are emphasized instead of overgeneralized, arbitrary, absolutistic reasoning. The therapist can review examples of extreme versus nonextreme cognitions on the list of problematic thoughts, personalizing them to fit a particular family. Socratic discussion and brainstorming techniques can be used to generate a list of alternatives for rigid, absolutistic cognitions.

Example: The Hortons (Part 3).
THERAPIST: Now, I would like you to think of all the possible alternatives to your thought that "children who talk back to their parents grow up to be antisocial adults." Larry and your husband can help, but just as with problem solving, don't evaluate the ideas—just list them.

LARRY: All kids talk back to their parents; it's just normal.

THERAPIST: OK. Any other ideas?

MRS. HORTON: Well, maybe if Larry talks back to us, it means he is just going through a phase.

MR. HORTON: It could mean he is angry at us about something, without saying anything about the future.

MRS. HORTON: Maybe he thinks our rules are unfair?

THERAPIST: OK. Or it could just be impulsive behavior with no particular meaning.

LARRY: Mom talks back to Dad, too. I'm just doing what she does.

THERAPIST: That's another possibility. Now that you have some ideas, how are you doing to decide what to believe?

Commentary. By generating a variety of alternative beliefs, the therapist not only helps the family think more flexibly but also defuses the impact of the original, absolutistic cognitions. As with problem-solution listing, the therapist should use humor to lighten the mood during the brainstorming phase of cognitive restructuring. The interchange culminated with the therapist's prompt to move ahead to propose an experiment to test the validity of the beliefs.

Propose a Test of the Old and New Beliefs

With a clearly specified alternative to the unreasonable belief in hand, the therapist is ready to take the next step of cognitive restructuring—propose an "experiment" that pits the two beliefs against each other. The goal of this stage of cognitive restructuring is to arrange for the family members to convince themselves, based upon their personal experience rather than external persuasion, of the utility of adopting the more flexible cognitive set. The experiment typically takes the form of a task to be completed at home, with clearly specified outcomes that confirm or disconfirm the distorted cognitions for family members.

Several general types of experiments are possible.

1. For a trial period, implement a solution feared irrationally by a family member and determine whether the dire consequences predicted by illogical beliefs do in fact occur.
2. Survey other credible parents or adolescents to determine whether their experiences confirm or disconfirm the validity of the illogical belief.
3. Observe family members' behavior and collect evidence to confirm or disconfirm the unreasonable cognitions.
4. Read a book or collect other objective published data to assess the validity of the belief.

Of course, the proposed experiment and the confirming or disconfirming outcome must be credible to the entire family if the results are to prove convincing. The cognitive restructuring model (outlined above) incorporates these suggestions in terms understandable to families.

Example: The Hortons (Part 4).   The Horton family might consider one of the following experiments to disconfirm Mrs. Horton's unreasonable beliefs.

1. Mrs. Horton could survey 10 parents of recently grown adolescents and ask them whether their teenagers talked disrespectfully and whether they considered their children to have grown up to be antisocial adults.
2. Mrs. Horton could read a book on adolescent development to collect objective information on the relationship between adolescent disrespect and adult criminality, the normality of petty squabbling, and the adolescent's cognitive ability to take parental perspectives on issues.
3. Mrs. Horton could try to make a list of 25 logical reasons why teenagers should talk nicely to their parents to repay them for earlier parental sacrifices.

In some cases, simply discussing unreasonable beliefs leads family members to understand their illogic. When members wholeheartedly embrace a new belief after discussing it, an experiment may not be necessary. Instead, the therapist can proceed directly to the next step—helping the member to incorporate the new thought into daily activities.

Plan Rehearsal and Incorporation of Appropriate Cognitions

The goal of this last stage of cognitive restructuring is for the family members to plan a strategy to conduct the experiment and to strengthen their adherence to flexible, positive belief systems by practicing self-statements consistent with these beliefs. The therapist prompts the family members to specify who will do what and when, where, and how to conduct the experiment. Elements of the strategy may be rehearsed in the sessions to prepare the family. For example, if Mrs. Horton were going to survey 10 parents, the therapist might help her determine which parents, what questions to ask, when to conduct the survey, and so forth. Her husband might be assigned the task of reminding her to complete the survey.

To facilitate incorporation of new, possibly alien cognitions into daily thinking, the therapist helps family members develop rehearsal and cueing systems for thinking rationally in troublesome situations. Rehearsal of appropriate self-statements may be formal or informal. Formal rehearsal is facilitated by teaching the family members to self-monitor thought processes through the use of a homework chart (see Figure 9-1; Goldfried & Goldfried, 1980). The client records the date, situation in which the thought arose, the unreasonable thought, the rational reevaluation, the action that was taken, and the consequence of this action. The chart serves as a discriminative stimulus to challenge unreasonable thought processes and to replace them with more reasonable alternatives.

Portions of systematic rational restructuring may also be used to provide additional rehearsal of rational beliefs (Goldfried, Decenteceo, & Weinberg, 1974). With this approach, imagination is used as a means of controlling the training procedure. As with systematic desensitization, a hierarchy of situations is constructed to enable the client to proceed one step at a time. The hierarchy consists of the situations in which the family member thinks unreasonably, graded in terms of the intensity of the affect associated with the thought patterns. These situations may either reflect a single theme or multiple themes. During the session, the therapist describes a situation and the family member imagines himself/herself in that situation, noting how nervous (or sad or angry) s/he feels. Next, the family member stops and analyzes the irrational thought underlying the affect. Afterwards, s/he reevaluates the situation in more rational terms, noting the new anxiety (or depression or anger) level. The therapist describes each scene several times until the family member can readily reevaluate his/her unreasonable thoughts. Technical details concerning such procedures can be found elsewhere (Bedrosian, 1981; Goldfried & Davison, 1976; Goldfried & Goldfried, 1980).

Systematic rational restructuring has been incorporated into problem-solving communication training either by meeting with a family member individually or by asking one family member to help the therapist construct the hierarchy and present the scenes to another family member. Since arranging this sort of practice is a fairly intrusive procedure, systematic rational restructuring is

Date	Situation	Unreasonable thought	Rational reevaluation	Action	Consequence

FIGURE 9-1 Rational reevaluation homework chart.

reserved for situations where the family member needs intensive, guided practice challenging a salient cognitive distortion.

Example.   Thirteen-year-old Sonya and her mother, Mrs. Goldman argued about Sonya's clothing, hygiene, make-up, and other factors related to her appearance. Further analysis revealed that these arguments stemmed from the fact that Sonya was extremely self-conscious about being bowlegged. Sonya believed that because of this physical condition, she was unattractive and would be totally rejected by males. She filtered her social interactions with her peers through this cognitive distortion, repeatedly putting herself down. To compensate for her "ugliness," she tried to dress seductively and wear excessive amounts of make-up; her dress habits led to confrontations with her mother, who wanted her to dress more conservatively.

In reality, Sonya's bowleggedness was hardly perceptible when she walked. She had an active social life and was not teased or rejected because of her condition. In order to help Sonya challenge this cognitive distortion, the therapist used systematic rational restructuring. A hierarchy was constructed around the theme of Sonya's anxiety concerning rejection due to her bowleggedness. The items in the hierarchy were graded in terms of the increasing anxiety and the increasingly catastrophic self-statements that they elicited. Representative items were

1. You see a handsome guy walking down the hallway in school.
2. A guy you like sits down next to you in class.
3. You decide to go roller skating.
4. You see a guy you know at the skating rink.
5. You want to start up a conversation with a cute guy sitting at lunch.
6. You look at yourself in the mirror when you wake up.
7. You think that a guy you like noticed that you walk in a funny way.

Mrs. Goldman participated in the systematic rational restructuring session. At first, the therapist presented an item to Sonya. She was instructed to imagine her worst fears about the scene, challenge the validity of the self-statements mediating her fears, and rehearse alternative, more realistic self-statements. Later, Mrs. Goldman presented hierarchy items to her daughter.

Sonya was assigned the task of rationally reevaluating unreasonable beliefs in vivo. Each evening Mrs. Goldman prompted Sonya to relate the day's events and helped her daughter rationally reevaluate situations where her bowleggedness created anxiety.

In most instances elaborate procedures for the rehearsal of appropriate beliefs are unnecessary. The therapist can informally guide the client to rehearse replacing unreasonable with reasonable beliefs during the session. Plans for using cognitive restructuring in vivo can be discussed, and the client assigned a rehearsal task.

FINAL NOTE

The cognitive restructuring techniques outlined here are adopted from the cognitive behavior therapy of the 1970s and 1980s. As our understanding of cognitive processes and their relationship to affect evolves, we expect significant advances in technology for intervening with families. Recent developments in strategic family therapy also offer interesting new possibilities for integration with cognitive restructuring. Particularly promising trends include the reframing of negative cognitions as "protective mechanisms," which help families cope with stress, and the use of "pretend interactions" in sessions to permit nonthreatening experimentation with otherwise foreign attitudes and behaviors (Madanes, 1981).

CHAPTER TEN

Functional/Structural Interventions

Skills and cognitions are the atoms or molecules that join to produce functional/structural interaction patterns. A behavioral–family systems model conceptualizes functional/structural interactions in terms of repetitive sequences of behavior that break down into interlocking contingencies within the family. Earlier treatment chapters focused on the molecular level of intervention: how to teach problem-solving communication skills and how to modify cognitive processes. The present chapter focuses on the molar level of intervention: how to fuse the atoms and molecules to produce powerful but well-directed chemical reactions. The material contained in this chapter is particularly relevant to more severely distressed, rigid families. Many problems and solutions discussed here have traditionally fallen within the purview of family systems therapies, and we have integrated them into our behavioral–family systems conceptualization of parent–adolescent conflict.

Functional/structural problems are fundamentally problems of hierarchy, alignment, and sequence. Parent–adolescent arguments, rebellious adolescent behavior, family fights, and bursts of negative communication or inadequate problem solving are events that take place within the context of an ongoing sequence of interactions between family members. When faced with a family with problematic structural patterns, the therapist must analyze and intervene to change not only the discrete events presented by the family but also the structural arrangements those events combine to form. Here we discuss five of the common patterns that occur in treating parent–adolescent conflict: (1) weak parental coalitions, (2) cross-generational coalitions, (3) triangulation, (4) adolescent misbehavior preventing marital conflict, and (5) the overprotection–rebellion escalator. Analyses of these patterns demonstrate how, with more complex cases, functional and structural analyses promote comprehensive treatment planning.

WEAK PARENTAL COALITIONS

A weak parental coalition refers to the situation where a "spoiled," omnipotent adolescent manipulates two parents who cannot reach an agreement with each other about discipline, and achieves his/her way or escapes discipline with regularity. The following pattern typifies this: (1) the adolescent misbehaves or disobeys a rule, creating an aversive situation for the parents; (2) one parent attempts to impose discipline; (3) the second parent tries to discipline the adolescent differently; (4) the parents overtly or covertly disagree about whose disciplinary method is better; (5) the adolescent ignores both parents' interventions and continues to misbehave or rebel, creating a continued aversive situation for the parents.

The primary functions operating here are coercion (mutual negative reinforcement) and avoidance, compounded by parental skill deficits. The adolescent's misbehavior is an aversive stimulus. The parents' attempts to terminate this aversive situation through discipline lead to reciprocally negative exchanges where each parent denigrates the other because they cannot agree on a course of action. The adolescent encourages this, thus escaping or avoiding negative consequences, and continues to misbehave, coercing the parents to continue to attempt to intervene, which they can never do successfully. Eventually, the parents may give up in frustration, allowing the adolescent to do whatever s/he wishes, avoiding parental controls. By giving up, parents also avoid continued aversive interchanges with each other over discipline. Structurally speaking, the term "weak parental coalition" refers specifically to the inability of the parents to take effective, joint action against their out-of-control adolescent.

The therapist's goal is to strengthen the parental coalition by teaching the mother and father to reach and implement effective agreements on rules, regulations, and consequences, thereby short-circuiting the functions of coercive adolescent behavior. This involves departing from the usual democratic stance of problem solving by encouraging parents to use their authority while still listening to the adolescent. Parents can be required to solve disputes while the adolescent listens silently. Alternatively, the therapist can involve the adolescent but give the parents a "final say" over rules and consequences. The therapist must insist that solutions include clear rules and consequences for noncompliance.

The omnipotent adolescent frequently raises serious objections to the parents' attempts at united action, but the therapist must block these objections, reassuring the parents that they need to stand firm. The parents often find it difficult to reach agreements (often getting bogged down in philosophical differences), requiring the therapist to dissect parental disagreements and refocus their efforts onto areas of commonality. Through persuasion, directive prompting, and, occasionally, couple sessions focused on parent–parent communication and mutual support, agreements can be reached. Then the therapist must ask the parents to anticipate all of the ways in which their teenager may sabotage the agreement and try to manipulate them into arguing with each other, and prepare them to cope with resistant adolescent behavior. Afterwards, the family is sent home to implement the agreement, and at the next session the outcome is reviewed. If the solution proved successful, the therapist congratulates the parents for holding firm and helps them reach similar agreement on an additional issue. If the solution failed, the therapist assumes the parental coalition is still weak and redoubles his/her efforts to close whatever loopholes led to failure.

Example 1.   Mr. and Mrs. Rosenbaum were unable to control their 17-year-old son Mark. He skipped classes, stayed out all night, smoked marijuana, and came home drunk on weekends. He was the youngest of four children and had been spoiled for many years. When they attempted to discuss rule infractions with him, he cursed at them, threatened to hit them, and stormed out of the house, accusing his parents of "child abuse." Despite protracted discussions with each other, friends, and relatives, the Rosenbaums were unable to devise effective disciplinary strategies. Depressed and frustrated, they had given up hope of regaining any control. The following excerpt illustrates how the therapist might begin to help the couple regain reasonable control over their son's misbehavior.

THERAPIST: I'd like to deal with Mark's skipping school first. Your son is engaging in serious truancy. If he continues to skip school, he will be joining the ranks of the high school dropouts and end up an aimless, unemployed young adult. I'd like the two of you *(Directed to parents)* to talk to each other now about solutions and reach an agreement about how you are going to get Mark to attend school regularly. Mark, I'd like you to listen quietly to this discussion without participating.

MR. ROSENBAUM: Mark must start going to class or else . . .

MARK: I won't go if I don't want to . . .

THERAPIST: Please be quiet, Mark. This is your parents' discussion. It will be your turn later.

MRS. ROSENBAUM: My husband is too strict with the boy. If he would only spend more time with him, maybe Mark would respect him more and go to school.

THERAPIST: Mrs. Rosenbaum, the two of you must reach an agreement now about how to get Mark to go to class. That is the only task before us. What will you do tomorrow morning when Mark refuses to go to school?

MR. ROSENBAUM: I will drive him to school and drop him off.

MARK: The hell you will!

THERAPIST: Quiet, Mark!

MRS. ROSENBAUM: But, honey, you've always told me you can't be late for work.

MR. ROSENBAUM: Then you drop Mark off at school.

MRS. ROSENBAUM: I can't get him into the car. He runs away from me.

THERAPIST: So who will get Mark into the car and who will drive him to school? I'm still waiting for an agreement.

MR. ROSENBAUM: I'll just be late for work. I'll do it.

THERAPIST: Mrs. Rosenbaum, what will you do to help your husband?

MRS. ROSENBAUM: I guess I could call and make up a good excuse for his boss for why he will be late.

THERAPIST: But how do we know Mark won't avoid going to class after you drop him off at school?

MARK: Come on, I'm not a child.

MR. ROSENBAUM: If you want to be treated like an adult, act like one.

THERAPIST: Mr. Rosenbaum, please tell Mark to stay out of this discussion between you and your wife.

MR. ROSENBAUM: Mark, don't interrupt your mother and me.

THERAPIST: Now, how will the two of you make sure Mark attends classes once he is in school?

Commentary. The therapist purposely raised the parents' anxiety about the dire consequences of continued inaction to motivate them to get going. Then the therapist repeatedly pushed the parents to exercise authority in reaching a concrete course of action for a specific rebellious behavior. Mark's attempts to subvert the agreement were blocked, and when the parents' own disagreement surfaced, attention was refocused on reaching a joint course of action. Such "sledgehammer" interventions would need to be continued until the parents are successfully taking united action to decrease their son's negative behavior. Haley (1980) has many useful suggestions for therapists attempting to strengthen weak parental coalitions.

CROSS-GENERATIONAL COALITION

Although cross-generational coalition refers to any coalition that crosses generational boundaries, here we use the term to refer to a pattern where one parent consistently sides with the adolescent against the other parent. In single-parent families cross-generational coalitions sometimes develop across three generations, as when a grandparent consistently sides with an adolescent against a mother. To some degree, cross-generational coalitions are inevitable in family life. In all families a parent occasionally agrees with a child and is at odds with the spouse. All children occasionally manipulate one parent (or grandparent) against the other to get their own way, for example, by asking both parents independently for permission to do something and then following the more lenient response.

Cross-generational coalitions become problematic when they *persist rigidly* in the face of developmental changes that require flexibly restructuring relationship patterns to resolve conflicts and avoid psychological pain. The parents' effectiveness as disciplinary agents diminishes because they are divided, with the adolescent's influence thrown in one direction. The father who refuses to discipline his antisocial, acting-out son, claiming "boys will be boys" after listening to his son's explanations of problem incidents against his wife's protestations, is stuck in a cross-generational coalition that fuels the son's escalating antisocial behavior. The grandmother who repeatedly overrules her single daughter's firm discipline when her cute granddaughter complains that "Mommy is so mean to me" is contributing to a pattern where her granddaughter may behave inappropriately as an adolescent without the checks and balances of a strong adult authority figure. Of course, these coalitions serve important functions for the adults and adolescents who perpetuate them. In the first example, the father may be gaining his son's attention, avoiding negative responses from his son, or punishing his wife by encouraging his son to misbehave against her. In the second example, the grandmother may gain attention from the granddaughter or maintain control over her own daughter by sponsoring her granddaughter's misbehavior. Adolescents typically profit from these patterns by gaining extra privileges and avoiding negative consequences for misbehavior.

The therapist must break up the problematic cross-generational coalition while strengthening within-generational coalitions, particularly the mother–father coalition. A combination of in-session interventions and homework assignments, using problem solving, communication training, and cognitive restructuring techniques strategically, can assist in working towards this goal. Strategies used from strengthening weak coalitions can be useful, with modifications, to help parents cope with adolescent manipulations. When a mother and adolescent gang up on a father, for example, the therapist can stop the interaction, ask the mother to check with her husband before agreeing with her teenager, and require the parents to discuss the issue. When an adolescent attempts to enlist a father's support against a mother, the therapist can instruct the adolescent to sit quietly while his/her parents discuss the issue first. Rearranging the seating so that the parents sit together and the adolescent sits on a different side of the room or similar manipulations of the physical environment may prove helpful as discriminative stimuli for appropriate within-generational coalitions.

Homework assignments set the stage for appropriate changes in coalitional structure. For instance, if a father refused to discipline a son who was rebelling against the mother's rules, the therapist might encourage the father to support his wife, not his son, so that the parents can take immediate, effective action to resolve independence-related disputes with their son. The therapist might assign the mother to call the father at work when she is faced with specific "disobedient acts" of their son, and the father might be required to instruct his wife over the phone how to handle their son. This could be followed by a brief problem-solving discussion each evening in which the couple reviewed the outcome of any disciplinary actions suggested by dad to mom during the day and reached decisions about future rules and consequences. To make the task more acceptable to parents who endorse traditional ideas, the therapist might emphasize the father's role as the head of the family, the special nature of a father–son relationship, and the resulting special importance of the father's "advice" for his son. In this way, the father is urged to side with his wife and parental negotiation is encouraged, but the father is permitted to continue his "special" relationship with his son without needing to sabotage his wife's discipline.

TRIANGULATION

In this interactive pattern, two members of the family disagree over an issue or action, and each tries to enlist the support of a third member; the third member vacillates between supporting each of the others, not consistently taking one side (otherwise the pattern would be a coalition). There are three possible triangles: mother–father with adolescent in the middle, mother–adolescent with father in the middle, and father–adolescent with mother in the middle.

As with coalitions, triangulation occurs naturally in all families, but the rigid persistence of triangles promotes conflict and hampers family adjustment. In our clinical experience families prone to excessive triangulation tend to develop cycles of switching between each of the three triangles, with the transitions punctuated by family crises. Triangulation is especially likely to be a problem in blended families where the natural parent is caught between the stepparent/spouse and the adolescent.

Example.   Fourteen-year-old Glen came with his natural mother and stepfather for treatment of family conflict. Mrs. Columbus complained that she often felt caught between her son and her husband; Glen would refuse to follow her husband's rules, and both stepfather and son would appeal to the mother to resolve their disputes. Sometimes she supported her husband, recognizing the importance of a united parental front, but at other times she felt he was too harsh on Glen and overruled him, siding with Glen. Glen learned that he could occasionally get his way by forcing his mother to choose between his and his stepdad's position, and he used this tactic manipulatively. Likewise, when Mr. and Mrs. Columbus disagreed about whose fault something was, they would appeal to Glen to help them decide, triangulating him.

This long-standing triangulated interaction pattern had become a problem recently because, with Glen's increasing desire for freedom from parental restrictions, he began to disobey his stepfather's rules, turning then to his mother for help, thus avoiding the consequences of his disobedience. The angrier Mr. Columbus became with Glen, the more frightened his wife became that her husband would hurt the boy; when frightened, she was likely to support her son against her husband, thus decreasing her fear but creating marital tension.

The therapist's goal was to break the escalating chain of triangulated interactions so that the parents could reinforce each other's attempt to negotiate as a team with their son. This goal was accomplished in the sessions by targeting "triangular" interactions as a negative communication habit to be corrected. The detrimental effects of triangular interactions were explained to the family, and a problem-solving discussion of chores was begun. (In such cases any topic is suitable for discussion, since the interaction process, not the topic per se, is the focus of the therapist's attention.) Whenever triangulated interaction occurred, the therapist stopped the interchange, gave feedback, and required an alternative response. For example, consider the following interchange during the "evaluation" phase of problem solving:

MR. COLUMBUS: Glen, if you would only get the chores done without a big hassle, I wouldn't get on your case in the first place.

GLEN: Mom, Dad's not being fair. I do my part. He always asks me to take out the trash during my favorite TV show.

MRS. COLUMBUS: Well, I don't know . . .

THERAPIST: Excuse me, but Glen is putting you in the middle again, forcing you to take his side or your husband's. Don't get sucked in.

MRS. COLUMBUS: Glen, I understand how you feel, but I don't appreciate your placing me in the middle.

MR. COLUMBUS: My wife always takes Glen's side. She should stick by me!

GLEN: But, Dad, you're so unfair.

MRS. COLUMBUS: You, know, Glen is right . . .

THERAPIST: Mrs. Columbus, you are getting in the middle again.

MRS. COLUMBUS: *(To husband and son)* OK. Why don't the two of you work this out. Leave me out of it!

THERAPIST: Good. Mrs. Columbus, would you mind changing seats with Glen so that he and his dad could sit next to each other and discuss this?

Each time the mother became triangulated between her husband and son, the therapist intervened to change the interaction, forcing son and stepfather to confront each other directly. Homework assignments included daily stepfather–adolescent discussions of recent problems without the mother present, maternal monitoring of the frequency of triangulated interactions at home, and daily husband–wife reviews of discipline problems. Through repeated in-session correction of triangulated interactions and strategic homework assignments, the therapist eventually decreased triangulation significantly.

ADOLESCENT MISBEHAVIOR PREVENTING PARENTAL CONFLICT

In some families an adolescent's rebellious behavior functions by helping the parents (and the adolescent) avoid marital conflict, separation, or divorce. Marital conflict is aversive to all family members; behaviors that reduce these aversive stimuli are likely to be increased through negative reinforcement. By misbehaving, a child can refocus parents' attention onto the behavior and away from their marital disagreements. Elaborate interlocking contingency arrangements may arise as both the marital discord and adolescent misbehavior escalate. In less behavioral terms the child is being "sacrificed" to sustain the marriage.

Contingencies operative in enmeshed families train their members to make such sacrifices, and these families are likely candidates for the development of contingencies that operate to keep the family together and avoid overt hostility.

It is difficult to untangle interlocking contingency arrangements linking marital and adolescent conflicts. When the therapist successfully intervenes to reduce parent–adolescent conflict by teaching problem-solving communication skills, the mechanism by which the parents previously avoided marital conflicts is removed, the couple begins to experience aversive interactions, and resistance or sabotaged interventions quickly result. If the therapist attempts to focus directly on the marriage, the couple will probably deny their problems.

To circumvent resistance, the therapist may simultaneously address parent–adolescent and marital problems, usually in the guise of addressing parent–adolescent conflict. It is often useful to adopt the framework of functional family therapy (Alexander & Parsons, 1982; Barton & Alexander, 1981), which has been reviewed briefly in Chapter 6. The functional family therapist views all interlocking sequences of behavior as being maintained by the "functional payoffs" they produce for their participants; these payoffs are thought to be given and received in the currency of interpersonal contact, with denominations ranging from "intimacy" to "distance."

Functional family therapists do not attempt to change the functions served by interlocking sequences of behavior; instead, they try to teach families less aversive mechanisms for creating desired relationship outcomes of intimacy or distance; that is, they change the topography of behavior. For example, suppose a mother and daughter argue about the daughter's curfew violations, and the mother later gains closeness by discussing the problems with her husband. The therapist would not attempt to reverse the mother–daughter distancing or the husband–wife closeness. Instead, the daughter could be taught less aversive mechanisms for becoming independent from her mother while indirectly encouraging increased contact between her parents. Her parents would be taught mechanisms for increasing their level of contact following positive rather than negative mother–daughter interaction. The sequence of payoffs is maintained, but is now accomplished in a less aversive manner, and both parent–adolescent and marital goals are addressed simultaneously without the need to obtain an up-front commitment from the couple to work on marital problems.

When intervening within a functional family therapy framework to change interlocking parent–adolescent and marital contingencies, the therapist follows two general steps: (1) use of cognitive restructuring and reframing techniques to indicate explicitly how the presenting problem is really part of an interlocking sequence of behavior involving the entire family; and (2) use of problem-solving, communication, and contracting techniques to produce changes in the topography of the sequences of behavior while maintaining their functions.

Example.   Mr. and Mrs. Martin came for treatment with 14-year-old John because John was depressed, failing several subjects in school, behaving noncompliantly at home, fighting with his 12- and 9-year-old brothers, and arguing with his mother (but not his father). The IC, CBQ, Marital Satisfaction Inventory (Snyder, 1981), and several other questionnaires were administered, and the family was audiotaped discussing fighting with siblings and homework. All of their scores on the self-report measures were in the highly distressed range, with poorer communication in the mother–son than in the father–son dyads. Further evaluation revealed a long history of severe marital discord, including a near-divorce 5 years previously. John's home and school problems began around the time his parents almost divorced. Mr. Martin now worked 16 hours a day and had virtually no contact with his wife. Mrs. Martin was a housewife with few friends and a poor relationship with her alcoholic father and hostile mother. She stayed at home alone throughout the day, leading an isolated, depressing existence. She placed a strong emphasis on family unity, related to her children in a controlling, overprotective manner, and became extremely upset when they misbehaved (especially when they fought, since this shattered her image of family harmony).

The therapist determined that virtually the only communication between the spouses occurred when the children misbehaved and Mrs. Martin complained to her husband about their acting out. The therapist hypothesized that Mrs. Martin obtained most of her social reinforcement from her children, since her husband was unavailable and her social life was constricted. Although she verbalized a desire for more intimacy with her husband, he passively resisted her attempts to involve him in joint activities, sexual contacts, or conversations about topics of mutual interest. The therapist hypothesized that Mr. Martin preferred to distance himself from his wife, perhaps because of previously aversive intimate contacts. John displayed the normal teenage demands for independence and privacy, but when he tried to distance himself from his mother, his actions threatened her major source of social reinforcement. She responded in an authoritarian manner to stop his independence-seeking behavior, resulting in many arguments. These arguments indirectly increased contact between Mr. and Mrs. Martin, since she attempted to coerce her reluctant husband to help her with her son.

Although the interlocking contingencies connecting John's acting-out behavior and the marital discord were clear to the therapist, the family was not aware of them. To focus directly on the severe marital conflict would have resulted in strong resistance. Instead, the therapist intervened simultaneously on marital and parent–adolescent problems, using a functional family therapy approach. Part of the intervention focused on John's fighting with his brothers as an issue around which to change the topography of the central functional interaction patterns. Step one involved giving the family feedback concerning their problematic interlocking contingency pattern, reframing it in a more positive light. This was done by asking the parents to report all of the topics of their communication during the week before the session. They indicated that they had talked very little during the week and that most of the conversations concerned the children's misbehavior. The therapist pointed out how they seemed to interact more when John and his brothers fought. The audiotaped discussion of fighting with siblings was played for the couple, and specific interchanges where one spouse supported the other in dealing with this issue were pointed out as additional evidence of how the couple achieved "intimacy" when coping with their children's fighting. John was then asked to rate the quality of his parents' marriage, which he acknowledged was "crummy." It was a revelation to Mr. and Mrs. Martin that their son recognized the problems in the marriage. The therapist suggested that John and his brothers tried to "help" their parents in two ways: (1) fighting whenever their parents wished to spend time together, to keep them apart since they might argue if they were together; (2) providing them with opportunities to unite around a common cause, that is, disciplining the children. The family was skeptical but attentive during this reframing discussion. The therapist did not attempt to persuade them of the veracity of his interpretation but simply asserted that if the family wished to stop the sibling fighting, the parents would have to convince their children that they no longer needed "help and protection." The family was instructed to bring all of the children to the next session. At the next session, the functional hypothesis about the role of sibling fights was reiterated.

The therapist then proceeded to step two of the intervention—using skill training to teach the family a more adaptive topography for achieving desired functional payoffs. A brief problem-solving discussion was held, with the emphasis upon having the three boys generate and evaluate solutions that help their parents have more time together without having to worry that the boys would hurt each other in the parents' absence. John suggested a contractual agreement—if his parents went out together for several hours on the weekend, he and his brothers would refrain from fighting during their absence. His parents added that they would like him to take charge of his brothers during their absence. The family agreed to try this solution, and implementation details were negotiated. The solution worked moderately well and was the first of several similar solutions that were negotiated, also to change similar interlocking contingency patterns.

Commentary. With this solution, the boys were able to achieve distance from their parents because their mother could not monitor their interactions closely. In addition, by putting John in charge, Mr. and Mrs. Martin acknowledged his authority and independence as the eldest son. The boys' interaction continued to function as the discriminative stimulus for increased parental intimacy, but the topography of the stimulus event had changed from "fighting" to "not fighting." Mrs. Martin was able to have more contact with her husband, but the contact was limited to several hours per week, not violating Mr. Martin's preference for interpersonal distance from his wife. With the increased spouse contact, Mrs. Martin did not have to rely as heavily upon her children for social reinforcement, making it easier for her to refrain from nagging them about their private affairs.

The original sequence of functional payoffs was maintained, but the topography was altered in a more positive direction. Of course, this intervention would not by itself be expected to lead to a lasting improvement in the Martin marriage. However, with the issue of sibling fighting neutralized as a marital issue, the therapist could more directly approach the couple about other marital conflicts.

Many of the features of functional family therapy are compatible with our approach to parent–adolescent conflict. However, we also maintain that functions other than intimacy, regulation, and distance serve to perpetuate negative interaction sequences. While Alexander and Parsons (1982) eschew changing the actual function of interactions, we frequently attempt to do so if this change accords with what family members verbalize they want. This is most likely to occur when one or more family members (1) wish to stop avoiding certain situations such as marital conflict but are paralyzed by irrational thought processes and/or excessive anxiety, and/or (2) actively want more intimacy or distance, but lack requisite interpersonal skills for obtaining what they want. Nonetheless, the functional family therapy approach may prove particularly helpful when simultaneously addressing parent–child and marital issues.

In some cases the therapist may eventually be able to broach the topic of marital conflict directly without meeting resistance from the family. Clinical experience suggests that after progress in reducing parent–adolescent conflicts, the couple is often ready to acknowledge the need for marital sessions. They now trust the therapist, have seen some positive results of treatment, and no longer are experiencing intense conflict with their adolescent. In several cases the couples spontaneously mentioned to the therapist in about the third or fourth session that they no longer needed help with their teenager but really did wish to have help with their marriage. By teaching skills for effective resolution of parent–adolescent arguments and disagreements, the therapist may neutralize the avoidance function of rebellious adolescent behavior in the marital relationship, and some parents may react to the resulting "vacuum" by recognizing their need for marital therapy.

When a couple requests help with their marriage, the therapist can either conduct marital therapy concurrently with family therapy or gradually phase out family sessions in those cases where parent–adolescent conflict has been ameliorated. Interested readers might consult Jacobson and Margolin (1979) or Stuart (1980) for further information on behavioral marital therapy.

THE OVERPROTECTION–REBELLION ESCALATOR

The overprotection–rebellion escalator is an interlocking contingency pattern where two parents with a relatively stable, mutually supportive marriage panic at the first sign of young adolescent rebellion and tighten up the rules and regulations in an authoritarian manner; the adolescent in turn escalates the rebellious behavior, leading to further parental restrictions and further adolescent rebellion. As the teenager demands freedom from restrictions concerning specific issues, the parents balk, perhaps because of their fear of aversive consequences if they relax their rules. Angered at the parents' refusal to reduce restrictions, the adolescent reciprocates by intensifying demands, emitting aversive verbalizations, or ignoring the parental rules. The parents find themselves faced with a coercive situation. Reciprocity of aversive behavior escalates when the parents attempt to punish the teenager's coercive behavior and the punishment elicits higher intensity coercive behavior from the teenager. The cycle culminates in one of three outcomes:

- The reciprocity of aversive actions escalates until the teenager commits an antisocial act that leads to involvement of a social control agency such as the police, the school, or a mental health professional.
- The parents "give in" to the teenager's coercive behavior and relax their restrictions. The coercive behavior is positively reinforced, the parental "cave-in" is negatively reinforced, and the cycle restarts.
- The teenager "gives in" to the parents' demands. Independence-seeking behavior is punished, submissive behavior is reinforced, and the adolescent may lose access to important sources of peer reinforcement. The adolescent's loss of peer reinforcement may elicit depressive affect or further anger towards the parents. Afterwards, the cycle restarts.

This scenario we label "the overprotection–rebellion escalator." The specific issues vary from family to family but will often include curfew, going places with peers, selection of friends, sex, drinking beer, and taking drugs. As long as the mother and father agree with each other in their dealings with the adolescent, the therapist's major task is to use the problem-solving communication training approach to break the cycle of parental punishment for adolescent independence-seeking behavior followed by reciprocally punishing, escalating rebellious adolescent behavior. In order to break this cycle, the therapist will typically have to use cognitive restructuring to challenge the parents' distorted beliefs that if they grant their teenager additional freedom, catastrophic consequences will ensue. This type of distortion appears again and again with overprotective parents. Problem issues should be solved one at a time, with extensive correction of parental statements reflecting fears about unrealistic consequences. Either the parents or the adolescent will have to take the first "calculated risks." The parent will have to risk agreeing to less protective solutions to disagreements, on the condition that the adolescent will reciprocate by behaving responsibly. Alternatively, the adolescent will have to begin complying with parental requests, on the condition that the parents will reciprocate by granting additional freedom from restrictions. In our experience, it is easier to get most parents to take the initial risk, often in the form of a 1-week "experiment" to try a new way of solving the problem.

SUMMARY OF
FUNCTIONAL/STRUCTURAL INTERVENTIONS

While we cannot enumerate all of the functional patterns that the clinician will encounter, we can offer some general guidelines for developing functional/ structural interventions within the context of problem-solving communication training.

1. *Pinpoint the sequence of interaction that constitutes the problem* through informal observation, clinical interview, and many of the other techniques suggested throughout this volume. Pinpointing the sequence involves deciding upon the degree of molarity or molecularity that punctuates family interaction in a treatment-valid manner. An entire sequence has been pinpointed when the therapist can start with one member's actions and outline successive behaviors of the other members until the original response recurs at a later point in time. At what point in the sequence the therapist starts may not matter as long as s/he eventually returns to the same point, since interlocking contingency arrangements are circular. Diagrams of interlocking contingency patterns may prove useful in identifying sequences.

2. *Identify the functions.* Having chunked reality into repeating sequences of interaction, the therapist must next answer the question, "What does the family as a whole, and each member individually, get out of this sequence?" This is the question of functions—what combination of reinforcement, punishment, avoidance, and/or other functions maintain each member's behavior within the sequence. As discussed earlier, hypotheses about functions are generated throughout all phases of therapy. These hypotheses are ultimately tested when interventions are attempted and changes occur or do not occur in predicted directions.

3. *Decide upon a goal for change.* The therapist must decide whether to change the functions subsuming the conflictual interactions, or leave the functions intact but change the topography of the sequence of responses emitted in achieving these functions. We regard the former approach as "strategic–structural" and the latter approach as "functional family therapy." Under the strategic–structural approach, the therapist attempts to reorganize the structure of the family system and fundamentally alter contingencies of reinforcement, punishment, avoidance, coercion, and so forth, in interpersonal interactions between family members. For example, in a family where an adolescent boy engages in delinquent behavior in order to coerce his disengaged father to pay attention to his depressed mother, the goal of the strategic–structural approach would be an alteration of structure and function. The therapist might establish as a goal greater involvement of the father with his son and wife, decreasing paternal disengagement.

Under the functional family approach, as outlined earlier in this chapter, the therapist does not attempt to change structure or function. Instead, the therapist attempts to teach the family more adaptive mechanisms for fulfilling currently existing functions. The therapist would not attempt to engage the father in intense interactions with his wife and son; instead, he would attempt to help the father maintain reasonable interpersonal distance from his son while nonetheless providing the wife with some increased contact from other adults. Clinical experience suggests that the greater the family's resistance to change, the more likely the therapist will be successful with a functional family therapy approach compared to a strategic–structural approach. Changing the way we meet existing needs is easier than changing both the needs and the way we meet them.

4. *Plan and implement a strategy for change.* The skillful therapist will tailor the strategy for achieving functional/structural goals to the particular family. In this volume we have presented problem solving, communication training, and cognitive restructuring as the primary strategies for change. Often, the therapist will create strategic homework assignments based upon elements of these three interventions. To decrease triangulated interactions, for example, a husband and wife might be instructed to conduct a daily, brief discussion of any disciplinary problems that arose with their adolescent, before taking disciplinary action. They might be trained to use clear I-statements and reflective listening during these discussions. When a therapist wishes to increase contact between a disengaged father and his wife without the adolescent's having to misbehave, the wife might be instructed to leave a note for her husband daily summarizing her son's actions throughout that day; leaving a note prompts a husband–wife contact regardless of whether the adolescent misbehaved or followed rules, but permits the husband to maintain greater distance than if he was required to discuss his son's behavior with his wife daily.

At times the therapist may employ a variety of additional techniques to address functional/structural problems. These include behavioral contracting, enactment, restraining, paradoxical prescriptions, family sculpture, and/or other less direct approaches. It goes beyond the scope of this volume to discuss these techniques, but interested readers might consult Minuchin and Fishman (1981), Madanes (1981), Haley (1976), and Gurman and Kniskern (1981).

The extent to which the practitioner will need to target functional/structural patterns for change varies considerably from family to family. In clinical-research projects we have encountered primarily intact families whose skill deficits and unreasonable beliefs contribute to independence-related disputes. The primary functional/structural target has usually been the overprotection–rebellion escalator. In clinical practice we have encountered a variety of functional/structural problems. Severely distressed families often present with complicated, intertwined contingency arrangements requiring lengthy, indirect interventions to change. Hopefully, further research will begin to clarify which interventions are most effective for which patterns of interaction.

CHAPTER ELEVEN

Sequencing Intervention

To maximize therapeutic effectiveness, problem solving, communication training, cognitive restructuring, and functional/structural interventions must be integrated into a goal-oriented sequence that moves clearly towards mutually defined goals but retains sufficient flexibility to be responsive to idiosyncratic crises and needs of particular families. Chapters 7 through 10 provided a detailed cross-sectional look at the major components of our intervention for parent–adolescent conflict. This chapter examines longitudinally how to integrate these components into a comprehensive therapeutic package. This involves a more thorough examination of the four loosely grouped stages of intervention outlined in the beginning of Chapter 7: engagement, skill building, conflict resolution, and disengagement.

Part of building a comprehensive therapeutic package involves intervention components designed to maintain and extend changes initiated during sessions. The behavioral tradition emphasizes repeatedly that newly acquired skills and cognitions do not necessarily generalize to the natural environment without explicit programming (Stokes & Baer, 1977). Procedures that explicitly program generalization of skills, cognitions, and interactions across time and settings typically involve a combination of "homework assignments" (i.e., specific instructions to behave differently between sessions in the natural environment) and in-session discussion of generalization issues. Homework and in-session generalization tasks are sequenced with the other components of our intervention.

SEQUENCING OF TREATMENT

Although the exact composition of therapy differs for each family, the following outline shows the general sequence of treatment, broken down by phase and session, for a 10-session intervention with an average distressed mother–father–adolescent triad.

  I. Engagement (sessions 1 and 2)
      A. Assessment of presenting problems, interaction patterns, antecedents, consequences, and family history
          1. Interview
          2. Informal observation

     3. Structured interaction tasks
- B. Building rapport with family and gaining their commitment to participate in a therapeutic process
- C. Establishing rationales for treating the family, not individuals, and for approaching problems within a skill-training format
- D. Negotiating a therapuetic contract
- E. Homework following first and second sessions
     1. Self-report measures: CBQ, IC, PARQ
     2. Make a list of goals in a family discussion

II. Skill building (sessions 3–5)
- A. Session 3: introduction to problem solving
     1. Review homework—give feedback on scores on self-report measures
     2. Give rationale for problem solving
     3. Conduct problem-solving discussion, using moderately intense issue
     4. Give feedback on problem-solving discussion
     5. Assign homework
       a. Implement solution
       b. Complete written problem-solving exercise
- B. Sessions 4 and 5
     1. Review homework, praising compliance or dealing with noncompliance
       a. How did solutions work?
       b. How did home discussions go?
       c. What interfered with completion of assignment?
       d. How was past week in general?
     2. Give rationale for communication training (session 4) and select a negative communication habit to correct
     3. Give rationale for cognitive restructuring (session 5) and select an unreasonable belief to challenge
     4. Conduct a problem-solving discussion
       a. If earlier solution failed, renegotiate
       b. Otherwise, pick new topic
     5. Correct negative communication/unreasonable belief during discussion
     6. Give feedback on discussion
     7. Assign homework
       a. Implement all solutions
       b. Conduct a problem-solving discussion at home

III. Intense conflict resolution (sessions 6–9)
- A. Review homework, praising compliance or dealing with noncompliance

    B. Select a negative communication habit or unreasonable belief to correct

    C. Intervene to change functional/structural pattern

       1. Strategically select problem to solve

       2. Assign in-session task tailored to change interaction pattern

       3. Anticipate crisis situation at home

    D. Correct negative communication habits and/or unreasonable beliefs

    E. Assign homework (at least 2)

       1. Conduct problem-solving discussion

       2. Carry out interaction tasks using component problem-solving communication skills

       3. Implement all previously negotiated solutions

       4. Carry out interaction task related to in-session task for changing functional/structural patterns

IV. Disengagement (sessions 9 and 10)

    A. Increase interval between sessions

    B. Review homework

    C. Discuss strategies for self-correcting negative communication habits or unreasonable beliefs

    D. Conduct final problem-solving discussion

       1. Decrease therapist prompts and feedback

       2. Ask family to run discussion with therapist listening

    E. Establish internal attributional framework for changes that have occurred

    F. Assign homework: maintenance tasks

       1. Discuss maintenance issues

       2. Implement solutions

       3. Readminister questionnaire measures

    G. Last session only

       1. Review course of therapy

         a. Were initial goals accomplished?

         b. What problems remain?

       2. Plan for maintenance

         a. Anticipate crises and plan strategies

         b. Integrate skills in daily routines

       3. Leave family with view of therapy as coping strategy useful at various developmental points in family life cycle

ENGAGEMENT

The engagement phase has already been described in detail in Chapter 4. Here we simply add several comments about homework assignments to be given during this initial phase of treatment. Since homework is an intrinsic part of therapy, it is important to establish a pattern of regular assignments even at the first session. The early assignments are designed to facilitate assessment, reinforce the rationale for a family intervention, and prompt family members to operationalize their problems in terms of clearly specified goals for change. Following the first visit, we usually give the family selected self-report measures to complete at home. At minimum, these include the CBQ or PARQ (short form) and IC. Family members may also be asked to list their specific goals for change and/or to keep track of behaviors of the other family members that annoy them. Reviewing their assignments heads the agenda for the next session.

SKILL BUILDING

The skill-building stage of therapy typically begins during the third session. Skill building begins in a session with three goals: to introduce problem solving, to conduct one problem-solving discussion, and to send the family home with an assignment to implement a solution. The highest priority during this session is to complete an entire discussion of a single issue. The experience of successfully negotiating a solution to even a minor problem during the session may be the most powerful motivator a therapist can provide for a family to cooperate with the overall regimen. In order to complete a discussion, the therapist must ordinarily be quite directive and circumvent negative communication patterns via redirecting strategies, noting these patterns for intervention in later sessions.

Problem solving is introduced with a brief rationale clearly stated in simple language that the adolescent can comprehend. The rationale provides a context for the ensuing discussion, and typically emphasizes that (1) family members will be learning how to communicate more effectively by discussing one specific problem per session under the guidance of their therapist; (2) the discussion will be patterned after a five-step model of problem solving, which will be outlined shortly; (3) the therapist will interrupt to give feedback about the content of the discussion and the ways in which family members are talking to each other; and (4) the eventual goal is for the family to learn to use problem-solving communication skills on their own at home. The temptation to pontificate endlessly while giving the rationale should be avoided because the adolescent will be likely to tune out the therapist as "just another adult giving a lecture." Family members will learn what they need to know about each step of problem solving as they reach it; it is unnecessary and confusing to the family for the therapist to spell out the details of each stage of problem solving during the rationale.

A sample rationale follows:

We are going to begin to work on a new way for you to solve your problems today. We will pick a problem to discuss, and I will suggest five steps to follow to solve it. I'll be like a "stage director," describing each step and guiding you to follow it. I'll stop you to comment on how you are doing. At future meetings, we'll go through the five steps with other problems; eventually, you will solve the most important problems you have and also learn how to solve additional problems on your own. Any questions?

Following completion of the rationale, a topic is selected for the first discussion. Ideally, this topic should be a meaningful issue for both the parents and the adolescent, but not so intense that it will evoke strong negative emotional reactions which interfere with the acquisition of new interactional skills. It should also be specific and relatively uncomplicated, to maximize the chances of reaching a solution during the session. Whenever possible, the adolescent should want to see the topic discussed, in order to maximize his/her participation. Scanning the family members' ICs for topics with anger-intensity ratings of 2 or 3 provides a menu of possible topics. When a consensus cannot be reached on a topic to discuss, we ask the adolescent to suggest "something you want to see changed at home but not the biggest gripe you have with your parents." Topics such as chores, curfew, or bedtime are well-suited for initial problem-solving discussions because they are easily operationalized, lend themselves well to the generation of a variety of concrete solutions, and can often be resolved in a relatively short period of time. By contrast, topics such as marijuana smoking, sexual activity, homework, talking back, and lying are difficult to operational-ize, and are likely to provoke strong negative emotional and cognitive reactions, making them poorly suited for an initial problem-solving discussion.

While parents in particular may initially balk at setting aside their presenting problems, most families ultimately accept the treatment sequence after some discussion of its rationale. Practicing new skills with easier tasks makes intuitive sense to most people. In addition, problems that are long-standing can usually wait 2 or 3 weeks without ill consequences. However, the therapist should also be flexible enough to bend these guidelines if an acute, high-intensity crisis arises. Examples might include decisions about whether an adolescent remains in the parents' home or is placed in foster care, a pending court appearance, or a threat of suicide or violent behavior. In these cases, problem-solving training should be supplanted by one or two sessions of crisis intervention, and begun after the crisis has subsided.

The therapist uses modeling, instructions, behavior rehearsal, and feedback to guide the family through the initial discussion, adhering to the guidelines outlined in Chapter 7. After the problem-solving discussion has ended, the therapist should give the family feedback concerning their behavior during the session, elicit their reactions to the session, and assign homework. The thera-pist's feedback represents a summative impression of the outstanding strengths and weaknesses of the session, with suggestions for future improvement. This is an occasion to be liberal with praise, to reinforce effort even in the absence of solid achievement. The following types of statements might be appropriate.

Example 1 (Average Session with Successful Resolution of Problem).

You've really made a good start learning to problem solve. You've gone through the five steps and successfully reached an agreement on the curfew issue. I particularly liked the way you helped each other out when defining the problem. We will have to work hard to unlearn put-downs and accusations, but that will come later. I can see this family has a lot of love and really wants to straighten out some bad communication habits that have been learned over the years.

Example 2 (Difficult Session with Partial Resolution of Problem).

You've really tried to solve the curfew problem. I can appreciate that it isn't easy to change your habits of talking to each other. The first step is often the most difficult to take, but you've started, and that's great. Of course, we have a long way to go. We will have to pay particular attention to the seemingly small swipes you take at each other. Tonight these zaps threatened several times to sidetrack you into angry arguments, but you managed to avoid these several times. That's the beginning of real progress.

The therapist can also ask each participant to give feedback to the other family members on positive aspects of their discussion. This ends the session on a positive note, as well as encouraging positive communication among family members. The therapist should listen carefully for family members' reactions to the structured and democratically oriented approach that characterizes problem solving and communication training. Parents may be unaccustomed to receiving direct feedback and guidance concerning their behavior in the presence of their teenage children. It may also strike them as odd that an adult in a helper role treats seriously the "ridiculous" opinions expressed by their adolescent offspring. Adolescents may be unused to disagreeing in public with their parents. Parents and adolescents may react in a claustrophobic fashion to the high degree of structure during the discussion, yearning to ferret out the causes of their problems or discuss their feelings freely. (The former usually translates to "get the therapist to side with me in blaming the other member for causing the problem," while the latter usually means unbridled expression of put-downs, accusations, and criticisms.) The astute therapist will have anticipated and taken the steps to minimize these reactions but will also permit the family members to express concerns about the value of the therapeutic process. The therapist will then acknowledge these concerns, provide reassurance, and/or reiterate the rationale of the treatment approach. At the conclusion of the feedback discussion, the therapist can give the family copies of the following problem-solving outline to take home with them for future reference.

I. Define the problem
  A. You each tell the others what they are doing that is a problem and how it affects you.
  B. You each paraphrase the others' statements of the problem to check out your understanding of what they said.
II. Generate alternative solutions
  A. You take turns listing possible solutions.
  B. You follow three rules for listing solutions.

       1. List as many ideas as possible.
       2. Don't evaluate the ideas.
       3. Be creative and freewheeling; suggest crazy ideas.
    C. One person writes down the ideas on a worksheet.
III. Decide upon the best idea
    A. You take turns evaluating each idea.
       1. Say what you think would happen if the family followed the idea.
       2. Give the idea a "plus" or "minus" and write the rating next to the idea.
    B. You select the "best" idea.
       1. Look for ideas rated "plus" by all.
          a. Select one idea.
          b. Combine several ideas.
       2. If none are rated "plus" by all, look for ideas rated "plus" by one parent and a teenager. Then, negotiate a compromise.
IV. Plan to implement the selected solution
    A. You decide who will do what, when, where, and how.
    B. You write down the details on the bottom of the worksheet.

Assigning of homework is usually the last activity of the session. Following the first session, two tasks are commonly assigned: (1) implementation of the solution negotiated during the session; and (2) completion of a written problem-solving exercise. The problem-solving exercise (see Appendix C) has been designed to permit parents and adolescents to practice components of the first three steps of problem solving. Family members are asked to discriminate correct versus incorrect definitions of problems and to write out solutions and evaluations of solutions. The exercise is conceptualized as an approximation of the behavior of conducting a problem-solving discussion at home, which will be assigned following later treatment sessions.

If a family has not completed a discussion of a problem during the first session, the first part of the assignment is obviously inappropriate. Instead, the family might be asked to practice problem-definition statements for 10 minutes or to prepare a list of conflictual issues that arise during the week.

How the therapist introduces the homework assignments to the parents and adolescent will influence their willingness to cooperate and consider the assignments as an intrinsic part of the therapy. Haley (1976) provides numerous suggestions, germane to homework assignments throughout treatment, for giving directives to families. Haley points out that family members will be more likely to complete an assignment if convinced that the assignment will achieve the ends they want for themselves individually and in the family. Thus, as the session nears an end, the therapist should present the assignment as a natural extension of the business of the session, stressing the role of the assignment in maintaining and extending the goals for that session. It is important for the therapist to check briefly with all family members concerning their perceptions of the assignment and their potential participation in it. Since adolescents may associate homework with unpleasant, effortful school assignments, terms such as "homework" and explicit analogies between school and therapy assignments should be avoided.

"Practicing a new skill" is one way to orient the family towards the tasks to be completed between sessions.

Example.

THERAPIST: I'm really impressed by the way this family solved the room-cleaning problem today. We've laid the foundation for some important new learning about how you can solve all problems. It's really like learning anything new. Even like baseball or basketball. Bill, you told me that you play basketball, right?

BILL: Right.

THERAPIST: The first time you played, was it easy?

BILL: No.

THERAPIST: How did you learn to be a good player?

BILL: Well, I watched the other guys, and well, I guess I played a lot.

THERAPIST: Right. The other guys showed you the moves and then you practiced. Did it get easier after a lot of practice?

BILL: Yes.

THERAPIST: Same thing with family problem solving. It gets easier with more practice. We practiced here today, and I'm going to ask you to practice a bit more at home. Mrs. Jones, you want to have better communication with Bill, right?

MRS. JONES: I would like that very much.

THERAPIST: And Bill, you want your mother off your case?

BILL: Right!

THERAPIST: OK. This practice at home will help you accomplish these goals. I'd like you to set aside 20 minutes on one day this week to complete these written exercises. They will help you learn the steps of problem solving we did here today. I'd also like you to try out the solution you negotiated during our meeting today.

MRS. JONES: But what if we get into an argument when we try the solution?

THERAPIST: I don't expect perfection. Just as with basketball, you don't get every shot in. Especially at first. If you get in an argument or get stuck, it is not a catastrophe. It simply means we went astray at one of the stages of problem solving and need to renegotiate an alternative solution. Try not to panic but do notice where things broke down. We'll discuss it next week and work on fixing the solution.

Commentary. The therapist helps the family anticipate difficulties completing the assignment and prepares them for coping with these difficulties. In prescribing tasks to be completed at home, precision is paramount. Assignments should be given in clear, specific terms, rather than suggested generally. It is often helpful to write down the assignment for the family. The declarative "I want you to do . . ." is preferable to the interrogative "Would you be willing to do . . .?" Redundancy is preferable to misunderstanding. Finally, concluding the prescription of an assignment by asking the family members (particularly the adolescent) to repeat the assignment insures that they understand the task.

The remaining sessions during the skill-building phase of treatment divide roughly into three sections: (1) review of homework and troubleshooting; (2) problem-solving, communication, and/or cognitive restructuring discussion; and (3) feedback and assignment of homework. Specific guidelines will be given for each of these activities.

Review of Homework and Troubleshooting

Because of the importance of homework in fostering generalization, careful review of assignments is essential. At the end of this review, the therapist should be able to answer the following questions:

1. How much of the assignment was completed?
2. To what extent did each family member carry out his/her share of the assignment?
3. Did the assignment have the predicted impact on the family?
4. What difficulties arose?
5. If the family did not complete the assignment, why?
6. What could be done to increase completion of future assignments?

If the assignment was completed satisfactorily, the therapist should express pleasure at the outcome and give additional instructions for continuing relevant aspects of the assignment. Praising the family for completed assignments is important; it is very easy to take completed assignments for granted. Subsequent discussion of the homework should be framed to illustrate how the at-home tasks contribute toward the overall goals of therapy.

If the family has not completed the assignment, the therapist should assess the reasons why this failed to occur. With legitimate practical interferences, arrangements should be made for the task to be completed before the next treatment session. Interactional difficulties can also interfere with completing the assignments, indicating that the assignment may have required skills beyond the members' abilities or may have exacerbated the level of conflict to intolerable proportions. In such cases, smaller, more realistic tasks should be assigned until the family's newly acquired skills are robust enough to withstand the entire task.

Lack of cooperation, poor participation, or sabotage by one or more family members can also lead to incomplete assignments. The adolescent may refuse to participate in discussions at home. A family member who was dissatisfied with a solution negotiated during a treatment session may undermine its implementation. Siblings who are not participating regularly in therapy may interfere with solutions that are aversive to them. When lack of cooperation by the adolescent, the most common difficulty, is encountered, the therapist should assess whether (1) the adolescent objected to the assignment but failed to voice the objections earlier; (2) the adolescent felt that the parents were unfair and biased in their implementation of the solution; or (3) the lack of cooperation is a generalized manifestation of rebellious or independence-seeking behavior, directed this time towards both the parents and the therapist. In the first and second instances, the therapist can help the adolescent formulate complaints in precise, nonaccusatory language and then can prompt appropriate expression of these complaints when the problem is renegotiated.

The third instance requires more creative, individualized strategies. At times, the heavy-handed way in which the parents attempt to initiate completion of assignments sets the stage for noncompliance, and the therapist may ask the teenager to suggest preferred ways of initiating the assignment and then discuss these suggestions with the parents. Alternatively, the problem may need to be redefined. For example, the Jones family agreed to a solution to a cigarette-smoking problem that, in part, involved Tommy's looking for a part-time job to earn the money to purchase cigarettes. However, Tommy made no attempt to locate a job. During an individual session with Tommy, the therapist learned that Tommy believed his parents would force him to put most of the money he earned into a savings account, and that he did not consider the effort of working worth the meager return. The problem of who would control Tommy's money needed to be resolved before he could comply with the original solution to the cigarette-smoking problem.

Occasionally, families make no attempt to complete an assignment and do not present a reasonable excuse for their failure. How the therapist reacts to this situation is crucial. By excusing the family easily, the therapist diminishes the importance of his/her authority, decreases the likelihood that future assignments will be completed, and implicitly models for the family backing down in the face of a difficult challenge. By the same token, "lecturing" or "blaming" the family models an inappropriate response of an authority figure to noncompliant behavior.

We have found two strategies useful in these situations. The first strategy involves an open, direct discussion of the problem. The therapist can indicate that in his/her experience, when families do not complete assignments and have no reason for their noncompliance, they lack confidence in the therapist and the intervention. The family is then asked to express their concerns about therapy, and the therapist can attempt to address their concerns directly. It is important for the therapist not to get in the position of defending therapy against a long list of accusations and attacks. After a reasonable explanation of the rationale for the intervention approach, the therapist should simply ask the family to think about whether or not they wish to continue in treatment and call in several days with their answer. If the family indicates that they wish to continue, a new contract should be drawn up specifying the nature of future homework assignments and the contingencies for future noncompliance. These contingencies might include cancellation of a session, forfeiture of deposits, termination of therapy, or completion of the assignment during their session time, without the therapist present.

Second, the therapist might employ restraining, a mild paradoxical technique that involves telling the family to remain the same in order to spur them to change (Haley, 1976). The therapist restrains the family from completing the assignment by telling them that their failure to complete the task indicates that they are not ready for that type of change; that it is best that they not change since change could be a dangerous thing, and it was therefore a wise decision for them not to complete the assignment. They are told that the pace of therapy will have to be slowed down since they are not ready for certain assignments, the number of sessions and the cost required to overcome the presenting problems will need to be increased, and under no condition should they attempt to complete the assignment at this time. The assumption behind restraining is that by telling the family that they are not ready to complete the assignment, they will be challenged to complete it on their own the next week. Even if they do not complete the assignment the next week, restraining is helpful to the therapist in avoiding a power struggle with the family while maintaining control of the session when faced with a clear challenge to therapeutic authority. While we cannot point to any empirical evidence for the effectiveness of restraining, we have found it to be clinically effective.

Noncompliance with therapeutic directives that persists over several sessions will be discussed further in Chapter 12.

A review of homework blends easily into a more general review of parent–adolescent relations during the week. Family members frequently describe crises that occurred during the week when they are asked to report the outcome of their homework assignments. Parent–adolescent relations are so fluid that a major family fight over a single issue may set the stage for disruption of a wide variety of previously assigned therapeutic tasks. Such crises provide invaluable information concerning functional/structural interlocking contingency patterns and the degree of generalization of newly acquired skills. They also give the therapist an opportunity to troubleshoot currently problematic aspects of interaction at home.

In collecting this information, the therapist should seek to avoid common pitfalls. Eager to relate their latest tribulations, family members may attempt to seduce the therapist into lengthy discussion of these events. Certain families who thrive on theatrical antics will present new "crises" every week. Unless the therapist resists being drawn into prolonged advice-giving discussions, little skill training will be accomplished. It is important to listen briefly to the family's story, gathering assessment data relevant to treatment goals and making a judgment about the seriousness of the crisis. Often, the therapist can place crises in proper perspective through the opportune use of cognitive restructuring. Then, a smooth transition should be made to the planned agenda for the session by using the crisis to generate a particular problem to solve or a particular communication target to correct. Alternatively, the family's topic can be discussed after problem solving is concluded.

When the therapist judges the crisis to be of overriding significance, the planned agenda should be suspended while the therapist attempts to help the family cope with the immediate situation. Examples of two different types of crises follow:

Example 1. Mr. and Mrs. Smith had negotiated agreements with their son, Jimmy, concerning curfew, helping out around the house, and allowance. By the third skill-building session they were beginning to conduct successful home discussions. Then Jimmy brought home a report card with failing grades in English and math. A major argument erupted. The parents canceled the three previous agreements and grounded their son for 3 months. Later that evening Jimmy stole $50 from his father's wallet and stayed out all night with his girlfriend. Because of the family's previous steady progress, the therapist judged the crisis to be serious and dealt with it instead of beginning to solve another problem.

Example 2. At the beginning of the second, third, and fourth sessions, the Ludwicks reported the following crises: (1) Mrs. Ludwick had become very upset when she noticed a "hicky" on 15-year-old Sally's neck; (2) Mr. Ludwick had become very angry at Sally when she came home from a date 15 minutes past curfew; (3) Sally threatened to run away after her parents refused to let her go out with a new boy they had not met. On each occasion the family presented the crisis with flamboyant, hysterical fervor. The therapist judged the "crises" to be variations on the theme of parental overprotection of their pubescent teenage daughter. Instead of suspending planned problem-solving discussions to discuss each situation, the therapist empathized with their strong emotional reactions and then politely reframed them as a "loving family's need to protect their attractive daughter from the evils of a corrupt society." Necking, curfew, and dating were the problems solved in future sessions.

Skill-Training Portion of the Session

Following the review of homework and troubleshooting, the therapist conducts one or more of the following three activities: a problem-solving discussion; a communication training exercise; or a cognitive restructuring exercise. The decision as to which activities to emphasize depends both upon the initial assessment of the particular family and on the family's performance in the previous sessions. When problem-solving discussions are conducted, the content is generally drawn from: (1) topics from the IC; (2) unfinished topics from previous sessions; (3) topics that were unsuccessfully or incompletely resolved at home; and (4) renegotiations of solutions that were unsuccessfully implemented at home. These sessions decidedly emphasize skill acquisition. Although potentially successful solutions are desirable end-products of these sessions, it is more important at this stage of therapy to shape appropriate problem-solving communication behavior than to reach a solution to the topic during the session. Thus, the therapist should make as many corrections for deficient verbalizations as necessary, and not restrict correction to gross performance deficits. This should be balanced, however, with a concern not to overwhelm the family with too many targets for them to remember. More than two new communication behaviors per person per session will probably create confusion.

The therapist may decide to conduct special communication exercises for families with severe deficits in communication skills. For example, parents who lecture incessantly to a defensive, hostile teenager may be asked to engage in 10 minutes of reflective listening while their adolescent practices clear, nonaccusatory expressions of grievances. The therapist would monitor the interaction and interrupt the parents' natural tendency to inject their own ideas into their reflective comments. Egocentric adolescents who fail to understand their parents' point of view may be asked to engage in a reverse role-play; the parents can role-play an adolescent complaining incessantly and making coercive demands and the adolescent can role-play a parent attempting to deal with such a spoiled adolescent. Role-played exercises are extremely flexible and can be created to teach virtually any communication skill.

Cognitive restructuring might be introduced following the guidelines in Chapter 9, either in response to the expression of specific unreasonable beliefs in the session or as a general coping strategy. The therapist might pick one of the common distorted cognitions (e.g., ruination, obedience, unfairness, or malicious intent) and relate it to the ongoing interaction, beginning to teach family members to challenge their unreasonable thoughts. We find that for most families some combination of the three types of skill-training activities is beneficial.

Feedback and Assignment of Homework

During the last few minutes of the session, the therapist should give a summary of the earlier activities and assign homework. The summary should emphasize the family's strengths and weaknesses, leading naturally into the homework prescription. At this point in treatment, conducting problem-solving discussions at home is a frequent assignment, repeated often over the remaining sessions. Relatively mild topics, or portions of the problem-solving sequence (e.g., problem definition) are assigned first, with the selection based on the therapist's prediction of what the family can handle successfully at home. Later, more complex topics are assigned. A successful interaction can often be insured by asking a family to complete a discussion started during a session. It is also wise to designate a regular time for problem solving at home and one parent to initiate the discussion; otherwise, chaotic families are unlikely to complete the task. Asking the family to audiotape the discussion allows the therapist to assess the family's skill use directly, during or after the next session. Families with severe skill deficits should be instructed to curtail any discussions that deteriorate into bitter arguments, to avoid creating aversive homework experiences.

Home discussion assignments should also be adjusted to fit the lifestyle of the family. Families' daily routines vary widely in organization and formality. While some parents plan activities carefully and interact with their children in a routinized manner, others are extremely informal and spontaneous. With a highly organized, formal family, the therapist might designate one member to lead the discussion, ask the family to follow the written outline of problem solving closely, decide upon a time and place for the discussion, and assign a secretary to record solutions and evaluations. In the case of a spontaneous, informal family, the therapist might leave the time and place for the discussion unplanned and emphasize that a written outline is a general guideline rather than a "bible." If the therapist is aware of any cultural or ethnic factors that may impinge upon the assignment, these should also be taken into account. Although audiotaping home discussions is desirable, audiotaping should not be required if one or more persons object.

The therapist can also maximize generalization of communication training and cognitive restructuring through homework assignments. Families can be asked to practice reflective listening, clear I-statements, or challenging unreasonable beliefs at home. Parents can be asked to write down and challenge specific instances of absolutistic cognitions, as outlined in Chapter 9.

After several skill-building sessions, the therapist will usually be able to gauge the capabilities of the family members and map out many of the major functional/structural interaction patterns within the family system. Decisions can be made about the maximum level of skills likely to be attained by the family within the time-limited therapeutic contract, and the appropriate strategies to be employed as the therapist moves forward to the next stage of treatment resolution of intense disagreements. Highly sophisticated, verbally fluent parents and teenagers can be expected to master more subtle nuances of interpersonal communication than less sophisticated, verbally impoverished families. For the former, the therapist can plan to target subtle stylistic aspects of their communication for modification. For the latter, the therapist may have to accommodate the problem-solving communication model to their intellectual limitations. For example, some learning disabled teenagers may never really master the concept of a precise problem definition. Instead of spending 5 weeks teaching these adolescents how to operationalize their dissatisfactions precisely, the therapist should assess when the adolescent has attained maximum mastery of the skill and arrange compensatory contingencies to help the family resolve disagreements. For instance, parents might be taught to ask pinpointing questions to help the teenager translate vague statements such as "My problem is that I don't like curfew" into "My problem is that I feel embarrassed when I have to leave a party in the middle because I have to be home by midnight."

INTENSE-CONFLICT RESOLUTION

The shift from skill building to resolution of intense conflicts is gradual. The differences between these two phases have to do more with the therapist's cognitions about what is to be accomplished than with overt organization and activities within the sessions. During both phases, sessions consist of initial review and troubleshooting, problem-solving, communication, and cognitive restructuring discussions, and a summative review and prescription of homework. However, during the skill-building phase the therapist approaches choice points in the sessions with the cognitive set of "the teacher," while during the resolution-of-intense-conflicts phase the therapist's cognitive set changes to a "system restructuring engineer." In practice, the therapist may switch back and forth between these two modes of operating during sessions.

During the resolution-of-intense-problem phase, problem solving should center on severe, anger-producing issues that are exemplars of the central functional interaction patterns of the family. As the family discusses these issues, the therapist strategically guides them to change their basic patterns of interaction. Because the interaction patterns depicted in Chapter 10 (weak parental coalitions, cross-generational coalitions, triangulation, etc.) are most likely to surface now, these are a primary focus during this phase of treatment. Since the primary goal here is to deal with factors that impede the use of basic problem-solving skills, the therapist can depart from standard problem-solving communication correction procedures as necessary. In-session and home tasks can be constructed that address ongoing interaction patterns. Crisis situations can be anticipated, with an eye toward helping the family avoid their previously self-defeating behavior. Alternative strategies borrowed from other schools of therapy can be used as needed to modify the interlocking systemic arrangement that sustains high levels of conflict.

Example.   Mr. and Mrs. Bowman came for treatment because their 15-year-old son Rick had run away from home following a severe argument and physical fight between Rick and his father. Rick was also on probation for shoplifting, failing in school, and threatening his peers in school and the community. Assessment revealed that Rick and his father argued incessantly. Mr. Bowman was a critical, sarcastic man, expecting complete obedience and perfection from his son. He rarely praised Rick, afraid too much praise might spoil him. Mrs. Bowman felt that her husband was too strict with the boy and intervened whenever the father–son conflict became particularly heated. Usually, Rick would withdraw from the scene, leaving his parents to argue with each other about his conduct. Mr. Bowman also had a history of excessive alcohol intake. He worked 12 hours a day at a construction job, interacted very little with his family, and drank intermittently on weekends. His wife ran the household and raised Rick and his 19-year-old sister, who was not exhibiting any behavior problems.

The therapist began treatment with a focus on skill acquisition. Problems of chores, curfew, and homework were solved in sessions 2 through 4. Accusations, interruptions, and defensive remarks were the communication habits targeted for change during these sessions. The family reached solutions to the three specific issues with a great deal of redirection of negative communication by the therapist. In each case the family was able to implement the solution until a crisis arose; then the solution broke down completely. For instance, Rick stayed out 1 hour past the agreed-upon curfew and came home smelling of beer. His father, who was also drunk at the time, attacked Rick with an onslaught of sarcasm. When Rick called his dad a "drunken bum," his dad tried to strike Rick with a baseball bat. Mrs. Bowman stood between her husband and son, challenging her drunken husband to hit her instead of the boy. Mr. Bowman stormed out of the house and did not return for 2 days. Rick and his mother had a long talk about how Rick should realize that his father was under a lot of pressure at work and try to behave well to avoid upsetting his dad. The curfew solution ceased to work after this crisis, with Rick often staying out late.

By the end of the fourth session, the therapist hypothesized that the following functional/structural interaction patterns needed to be addressed during the resolution-of-intense-conflict phase of treatment:

1. Reciprocal punishing behavior existed between Rick and his father. Mr. Bowman was harsh and critical towards the boy, giving very little praise. Rick reciprocated by defying rules and misbehaving, thus obtaining attention and recognition from his father in the only way he could.

2. The parents' disagreements indicated a weak parental coalition: They were unable to take united action to consequate Rick's behavior.

3. When Rick and his father argued and fought, they triangulated Mrs. Bowman, who alternately supported her husband and son. The physically abusive behavior of Mr. Bowman, particularly when inebriated, forced Mrs. Bowman to step in and become involved.

4. Mr. Bowman adhered to rigid, absolutistic beliefs about obedience and perfection. Through his alcohol consumption and lack of contact with his family, he modeled behavior opposite to what he expected from other members of the family. His son imitated his actions, not his words.

5. The couple avoided marital intimacy by focusing on Rick's misbehavior.

6. Mr. Bowman's drinking helped him escape or avoid the problems in his family, and the negative interactions with Rick reduced the tensions associated with the family.

In the fifth session, the therapist brought up the failed curfew solution and decided to work first on the weak parental coalition. Noting that Mr. and Mrs. Bowman had different approaches to handling curfew noncompliance, the therapist asked the parents to solve the issue of how to deal with future noncompliance with the curfew solution, while Rick listened but did not participate. As his parents voiced their differences, Rick repeatedly attempted to interrupt them and the therapist repeatedly blocked his interruptions, urging the parents to reach an agreement. When Mr. and Mrs. Bowman agreed that Rick would be grounded for 2 days every time he violated his curfew, the therapist matter-of-factly noted that since family members consumed alcohol, could they reassure each other that they would stick to the agreement, even if under the influence of alcohol. Mrs. Bowman's attempts to raise her husband's drinking as the problem to be solved were blocked by the therapist, who noted they had sought treatment for conflict with Rick, not alcohol consumption. Seeing that the therapist did not simply blame all the family problems on his drinking, Mr. Bowman was relieved and agreed to stick to the grounding agreement under all circumstances.

The parental agreement strengthened the weak parental coalition and began to change conditions so that Mr. Bowman would not need to drink to avoid unpleasant interactions at home. Over the next week Rick violated his curfew one time and was grounded, to his great surprise. Mr. Bowman stuck to his agreement and in fact spontaneously decreased his drinking over the week.

At the next session the therapist decided to address the reciprocity of punishment in the father–son relationship and the lack of paternal reinforcement of prosocial adolescent behavior. Noting that the father–son relationship had vastly improved and that the dyad had had no serious arguments during the past week, the therapist asked Rick and his father to brainstorm a list of activities that they might enjoy doing together. During this discussion, they were asked to sit next to each other and Mrs. Bowman was asked to listen but not make suggestions. The list included items such as fishing, hunting, camping, working on the family car, and going bowling. Mrs. Bowman had a difficult time staying out of the conversation; however, the therapist carefully blocked her interruptions. In doing so, triangulated behavior was targeted, since she thrust herself into the middle between her husband and son even when they did not draw her in.

When the father–son dyad had a reasonable list, each was asked to tell the other which activities they thought the other did best. Critical comments were interrupted and redirected, and the father and son were able to be surprisingly positive. The dyad was asked to select one activity to do together during the next week and to plan the details of its implementation. They selected a fishing trip. Mrs. Bowman again interrupted, pointing out that Rick's father could easily become frustrated and hurt his son. The therapist asked Mr. Bowman to reassure his wife that he could handle himself. Rick expressed disbelief at his mother's worries. The session ended with the therapist asking the father–son dyad to go fishing together but predicting a less-than-smooth trip. The therapist expected the mother to try to sabotage the father–son interaction.

At the next session, the family reported that a crisis had arisen during the fishing trip. Mr. Bowman had drunk several beers while fishing and, while partially inebriated, had begun to criticize Rick's impatience with fishing. Rick then wandered off to another part of the lake, where he joined several other teenagers smoking marijuana. When he returned and his father realized that Rick was stoned, Mr. Bowman almost lost his temper and struck Rick. Rick reminded his father of what happened with the curfew crisis, and the dyad did not come to physical blows. However, they were still very angry at each other. Mrs. Bowman acted smug towards the therapist in the session. Upon further questioning, she revealed that she had placed the beer in the boat so that "my husband wouldn't get too thirsty." True to therapist predictions, she had sabotaged the increased positive interactions between husband and son. Interestingly, the curfew agreement continued to be followed.

What consequences might maintain her sabotage of increased positive interactions between her husband and son? The therapist hypothesized that increased father–son contact decreased both mother–son and mother–father contact, since her triangulated role in the father–son interactions kept her in contact with both her spouse and son. The therapist decided to develop a task that would maintain contact with her husband and son for Mrs. Bowman while simultaneously increasing positive father–son contact.

First, the parental coalition was strengthened by asking the spouses to agree with each other that each dyad within the family deserved to have special time together and that the entire family also deserved to have special time. The spouses were asked to list examples of appropriate activities for mother and son; father and son; mother and father; and mother, father, and son. The parents agreed with the therapist and listed several activities. Next, father and son were again asked to select a pleasant activity to do together. They selected bowling. The therapist noted that since Mrs. Bowman was also an expert bowler, perhaps she could sit down with Rick before he and his dad went bowling and give Rick some pointers. Also, the therapist indicated that she might reward her husband for being a good father by going out to dinner with him on the weekend. The family agreed to this series of activities.

Although Rick and his mother talked and Rick and his father bowled (without incident), the couple did not go out to dinner. They indicated that they stayed home because they wanted to make sure they were present to note Rick's compliance at curfew time. The therapist learned from this task that, while increasing mother–son contact was sufficient to prevent the mother from sabotaging father–son contact, the couple continued to use adolescent misbehavior as an excuse to avoid marital contact. The therapist had the family conduct a problem-solving discussion of how to monitor curfew compliance without the couple needing to stay home.

Commentary. In this example, problem solving is blended with selected functional and strategic family therapy approaches to plan a series of interventions and tasks over several sessions that address central functional/structural interaction patterns. This is the essence of the resolution-of-intense conflict phase of intervention.

During this phase of therapy homework assignments consist of problem-solving discussions, implementation of solutions, and tasks that utilize components of problem-solving communication training in daily interactions. The goals of assigning practice of component skills are both to accomplish strategic changes within the family system such as those outlined in the Bowman example and to prompt the use of the skills under naturally occurring environmental conditions. "Natural conditions" may also be simulated during the therapy session in preparation for the assignment. Thus, an interactional sequence designed to help a family avoid or cope with common crises can be developed and rehearsed in advance of the crisis, giving the family automatic responses to fall back on. An example of an interactional task follows.

Example.   Mr. Sharp lost his temper and interrogated his 15-year-old, unassertive son Timmy when he thought Timmy was lying about something. Timmy lacked the verbal skills to stand up to his father, denied the accusation, and then "played dumb." Timmy's response infuriated his father, who continued his verbal onslaught. The interchange culminated in Timmy's being punished, often for crimes that he had not committed. The therapist trained Mr. Sharp to state his displeasure with his son's behavior in a clear, nonaccusatory tone of voice. Timmy was trained to appraise his father's tone of voice and then respond with a validation and an assertive I-statement to give his father feedback. After simulated interchanges had been practiced during a treatment session, Mr. Sharp was instructed to make at least one critical remark a day to Timmy, attempting to speak in a nonaccusatory tone of voice. Timmy was instructed to validate the legitimacy of his father's anger while commenting assertively on the content and tone of his father's communication. Mrs. Sharp was asked to monitor the dyadic interaction between her husband and son.

Commentary.   In traditional clinical terminology, Timmy's initial response to his father's accusations would have been classified as "passive–aggressive." The assignment was designed to break the dyadic cycle of adolescent passive–aggressive and paternal aggressive responding, transforming it into a self-correcting, mutually assertive interaction pattern.

The resolution-of-intense-conflict stage of therapy continues until the family no longer reports serious disagreements in clinical practice, or for three to four sessions in research studies. Since all families have some conflict, the family should reach a point when they cope with conflicts on their own through the use of newly acquired skills and where functional/structural goals are accomplished without painful interchanges.

DISENGAGEMENT

As family members experience increasing success implementing solutions negotiated during treatment sessions, discussing problems on their own at home, and resolving the intense conflicts that brought them to therapy, the therapist begins to prepare for termination. Disengagement is a gradual fading-out process, involving gradually lengthening the interval between sessions. Increased responsibility is placed on the family for resolving disputes without the direct guidance of the therapist. Strategies whereby the family monitors and corrects communication problems themselves are planned, and the therapist reduces prompts during in-session discussions. Therapeutic gains are attributed to the family's coping skills rather than the therapist's interventions. More session time is devoted to monitoring of the family's efforts at home than to the resolution of new problems.

A useful "test" of readiness for termination is to ask the family to resolve a disagreement for 10 minutes either during a session or at home, while the therapist is absent. The discussion is audiotaped and reviewed later by the therapist. Reports of productive discussions at home are another indication that termination should be considered. When teenagers were involved in their parents' marital disputes, the ability of the parents to discuss marital issues directly without involving the adolescent is another sign of readiness for termination of regular family sessions (although marital therapy may still be indicated). Finally, individual and family goals set during the initial assessment can be reassessed, and preassessment measures readministered for corroboration of family members' self-reports.

The decision to move into the disengagement phase can sometimes be difficult. Some dependent families for whom therapy is a way of life may never want to terminate and, when the therapist begins to talk of possible termination, may suddenly encounter new problems and renewed crises, as if to avoid the loss of therapist attention. Other families may have only made partial progress towards initial goals, but the therapist reaches the conclusion that this family is unlikely to make much additional progress at the present time.

With therapy addicts, very gradually introducing the idea of termination may be helpful. The therapist can indicate all of the ways the family is exhibiting self-control and reframe termination as a thinning out rather than a cessation of therapy. It can be pointed out that since 90% of the changes occur between sessions anyway, therapy never really ends. Furthermore, access to the therapist never really ends (assuming the family and therapist remain geographically nearby), since the family can always increase the frequency of sessions in the future. Regular contact can be discontinued by framing the process as "long-term follow-up," with the therapist meeting with or telephoning the family every few months for a year. If the family has changed during treatment and is reticent to terminate primarily out of anxiety over possible relapses, gradual thinning of sessions generally works well. Such families frequently cancel 6-month or 1-year follow-ups, at which point the therapist can congratulate them on the maintenance of their behavior change and urge them to continue doing well on their own.

More difficult are those families whose progress is partial. Most therapists like to consider themselves successes and would be unlikely to suggest termination without complete accomplishment of initial goals. However, our clinical experience suggests that certain families are so entrenched in their interlocking contingency patterns, negative problem-solving communication habits, and cognitive distortions that only partial success is possible with our current technology. These families often give the therapist signs that termination should be considered. After a long plateau with little progress beyond earlier achievements, they begin to arrive late for sessions, come without certain members, skip sessions without calling, or fail to complete assignments. Normally, such behaviors would be considered resistance and handled in the manner discussed in Chapter 12. However, if these occur after a series of no-progress sessions, the therapist should consider as an alternative whether the family is likely to progress further or should be terminated. Examples of this type of situation include a multiple-problem family where the therapist has reduced parent–adolescent conflict but has not changed marital discord, or an enmeshed mother–adolescent single-parent family where the mother has learned to solve problems and be less overprotective but still intrudes too much at times. After deciding to move towards disengagement, the therapist should try to help the family solidify whatever gains they have made and clearly indicate to them the areas in which they need additional work in the future. Certain families need "breathing room" to assimilate change and after several months will contact the therapist to resume working on unfinished business. It is difficult to operationalize criteria for making this judgment; when in doubt, we recommend consulting with colleagues concerning the decision to terminate with a partially improved family.

Another real-world but sometimes difficult factor related to termination involves finances. In clinic and private practice settings, families who have third-party insurance reimbursement often have a limited amount of coverage. The therapist must take into account the number of sessions covered by insurance and the family's ability and willingness to pay for additional sessions. Often, in families with limited coverage and no ability to assume the financial obligation for therapy on their own, realistic, short-term goals are set and sessions are spread out over longer intervals earlier in treatment. The therapist must also exercise professional integrity about finances in deciding to terminate: termination means reduced revenue for the therapist, who could easily continue unnecessary sessions for some time. Obviously, ethical considerations require that the therapist not involve families longer than is beneficial for them.

A useful assignment for all families during the disengagement phase is to invite a sibling to attend a therapy session to discuss an issue involving the sibling (sibling fighting is a natural issue for this session). The adolescent client can be placed in charge of teaching a younger sibling the steps of problem solving. This task serves as a review of problem solving for the adolescent and as a source of recognition of the adolescent's new status as an "expert" on resolving disagreements. Siblings may also be invited to participate in problem-solving discussions conducted at home. Occasionally, several siblings have been invited to participate in problem-solving discussions at home or in the session. One of us

(A. R.) can recall a memorable session where a 13-year-old girl and her mother brought three sisters, aged 12, 10, and 8. A generally acceptable solution to the problem of chores was reached, which involved all of the girls. Any solution reached without the siblings present would otherwise have had to be renegotiated at home to take them into account. The sisters were also able to appreciate what their sister had been doing for 7 weeks and feel a part of the process.

Often, naturally occurring shifts in the seasonal schedules of the family and the therapist set the stage for phasing out treatment by stretching the interval between sessions, for example, summer vacations, therapist's out-of-town trips. Follow-up sessions include reviewing previously implemented solutions and tasks, helping the family solve any new crises, and providing positive reinforcement for continued maintenance of gains. We may also readminister questionnaires and behavior sample measures. During the final sessions we emphasize that coping with family problems is a life-long developmental process, and that as families develop over time they may get stuck in transitions. Therapy may be helpful in overcoming difficult transitions in family development at various times throughout the life cycle. At termination we leave the family with an open invitation to call in the future as needed.

CHAPTER TWELVE

Resistance

Resistance is a concept common to most schools of therapy. Individuals and families may fail to change established behaviors, despite consistent efforts by the therapist and the fact that they often voluntarily sought professional help to bring about such changes. Different therapeutic orientations have conceptualized resistance in very different ways. Within a psychoanalytic paradigm resistance is defined as conscious and unconscious emotions, attitudes, and behaviors that operate against the progress of therapy. Therapy emphasizes exploring resistance to produce insight and behavior change (Greenson, 1967). Within a family systems paradigm, resistance has been viewed as the family's attempt to maintain the homeostatic balance of functioning that has produced the presenting problems (Aponte & VanDeusen, 1981).

In a comprehensive guide for the practicing family therapist confronting resistance, Anderson and Stewart (1983) suggest a pragmatic definition, which offers a general framework.

Resistance can be defined as all those behaviors in the therapeutic system which interact to prevent the therapeutic system from achieving the family's goals for therapy. The therapeutic system includes family members, the therapist, and context in which the therapy takes place, that is, the agency or institution in which it occurs. (p. 24)

Thus, therapy may bog down due to therapist factors, family factors, external environmental factors, organismic factors within individual members of the therapeutic system, or any interaction of these. Behavior therapists specify what some of these factors may be, including our incomplete knowledge of the mechanisms controlling family interactions, the limited efficacy of current therapeutic practices, idiosyncratic influences of the therapist's style or the therapeutic relationship, the client's individual skills and style, and the client's interpersonal network (Lazarus & Fay, 1982). Meichenbaum and Gilmore (1982) ascribe resistance to clients' difficulties integrating "anomalous data" into their personal conceptualizations of themselves and their problems, while Jacobson and Margolin (1979) describe resistance as resulting from the high cost of change in terms of effort.

Five general types of implementation problems are commonly encountered with families: difficulties engaging family members in treatment, difficulties directing sessions and maintaining control, difficulties maintaining rapport with family members, noncompliance with therapeutic directives, and interference from other problems that interlock with and/or exacerbate parent–adolescent conflict. The following outline lists these difficulties in more detail.

I. Difficulties engaging family members in treatment
   A. Adolescent reluctant to participate
      1. Stigma of mental health services
      2. Perception of therapy as parental punishment
      3. Perception of therapist as aligned with parents
      4. Problem belongs to parents, not teenager
      5. Afraid of peer ridicule
      6. Afraid parents will punish teen at home for what is said in session
      7. Fear of revealing family secrets, discussing sensitive issues
      8. Need to "protect" family from disconcerting change
      9. Loss of time better spent in other activities
   B. Parent reluctant to participate
      1. Scheduling problems
      2. Perception of problem lying within teen or between spouse and teen
      3. Denial of any problem at all
      4. Anxiety about opening a "can of worms"
      5. Misconceptions or misinformation about the nature of treatment

II. Difficulties directing sessions and maintaining control
   A. Family members attempt to change topic
   B. Family members do not give each other sufficient opportunity to speak
   C. Family members refuse to answer questions
   D. One family member attempts to draw therapist into coalition with him/her
   E. Arguments erupt between family members
   F. Family members ignore corrections of deficient communication
   G. Family members ignore the therapist, attempting to control the session themselves

III. Difficulties maintaining rapport
   A. Family members challenge therapist's competence based upon
      1. Professional credentials
      2. Age
      3. Sex
      4. Experience
      5. Theoretical orientation
   B. Therapist dislikes one or more family members who
      1. Ignore corrections of communication deficits
      2. Exhibit excessive cognitive distortions
      3. Remind therapist of conflicts is his/her life

IV. Noncompliance with therapist directives
    A. Failure to complete homework
    B. Reticence to participate in behavior rehearsal
    C. Direct challenge to behavioral approach
    D. Missed appointments
V. Problems outside the parent–adolescent dyads
    A. Marital conflict
    B. Depression
    C. Anxiety
    D. Attention Deficit Hyperactivity Disorder
    E. Low self-esteem
    F. Psychosomatic ailments
    G. Drug or alcohol addiction

Throughout Chapters 4–11 we noted many specific examples of these difficulties and suggested strategies for coping with them as they arise. In this chapter we focus primarily on more pervasive sources of resistance that can repeatedly disrupt or terminate problem-solving communication training. Readers interested in further discussion of resistance and implementation problems in family therapy approached from a variety of theoretical persuasions might consult Anderson and Stewart (1983), Gurman (1981, 1982), or the research and clinical exchange section of the *American Journal of Family Therapy*.

ENGAGING FAMILIES IN TREATMENT

Mobilizing two parents and an adolescent to make a commitment to participate in 7 to 17 sessions of family-oriented treatment is no trivial task. Adolescents may be reticent to participate for a variety of reasons (see outline above). Parents may not appreciate the need to attend sessions, viewing either the adolescent to be in need of an individual "fix" or the other parent as the culprit responsible for the problem. Basic strategies for handling these difficulties were discussed in Chapter 4.

Reluctant Adolescents

When basic strategies fail to overcome the adolescent's reluctance to participate over several sessions, reexamination of the functions of the adolescent's reluctance may yield clues about the source of the problem. Resistive, withdrawn behavior may consistently produce parental attention, serving as a positive reinforcer. Alternatively, the adolescent may escape parental lectures, demands, and criticisms by withdrawing. Some adolescents' refusal to discuss issues results in family chaos (e.g., rules are nonexistent or go unenforced), leaving the adolescents to do as they please with no negative consequences.

These situations are particularly troublesome because the therapist can inadvertently recreate in the session the circumstances that elicit and maintain the teen's withdrawal. Behavior maintained by parental attention will also be richly reinforced by therapist attempts to urge the teen to speak. Escape and avoidance functions will be strengthened if the therapist allows the teen's silence to detour discussions or impede resolution of problems. It is therefore important for the therapist faced with the "silent treatment" to formulate and test hypotheses about the function of the teen's behavior. Meeting with the teenager individually to assess reluctant participation can sometimes assist in this assessment. In the absence of the parents, teens sometimes respond very differently to the therapist.

Withdrawal maintained by parental attention can often be changed by minimizing that type of attention in sessions and simultaneously increasing the reinforcers for alternative responses (i.e., participation). Sometimes sessions between the teen and therapist alone that focus on teaching the adolescent skills for direct self-expression serve as a useful link in this shaping process. The following example illustrates this strategy.

Example.   Mr. and Mrs. Johnson and their son Sam requested assistance for parent–adolescent difficulties. During the initial session, the parents recounted several situations in which Sam appeared to "feel bad" about something and moped around the house, picking on his brother. When asked by his parents (who were both highly verbal and articulate) what was the matter, Sam would repeatedly deny any negative feelings. Eventually, one of his parents would be able to "drag the problem out of him," and they would discuss it, improving the situation until the next time Sam encountered a personal problem. Sam was very quiet during the initial assessment sessions, answering questions in single words and phrases and protesting that he did not want to participate and that nothing was wrong with his relationship with his parents.

The therapist speculated that Sam's withdrawal and denial of problems, both in sessions and at home, was reinforced by parental attention. As preliminary steps toward dealing with this problem, the therapist arranged to meet individually with Sam and to strengthen an alternative to withdrawal: voicing his feelings and opinions directly, as they occurred. The therapist also helped Sam and his parents together negotiate a time-limited contract whereby Sam's attendance and participation in four family sessions earned him some new albums he had been wanting to buy. After two individual sessions, Sam and the therapist had established good rapport and Sam's ideas and answers to questions were more fully elaborated. The therapist then conducted family problem-solving sessions, working on "Sam's not talking when he feels bad" as one of the problems. Sam participated in discussions although he continued to be the quietest of the triad. Solutions were carried out at home, and Sam's withdrawal at home began to diminish in frequency. No contract was needed to elicit his participation in subsequent sessions.

A clue that silent behavior is maintained by escape from negative parental communication occurs when a teen refuses to talk whenever parents are present but speaks freely when alone with the therapist. In these cases, discussing the functions of the adolescent's behavior with the teen during individual sessions and making an agreement with the teenager to help the parents to be less negative if the teen will do his/her share by participating in sessions can sometimes produce more frequent verbalizations from the teen. Parental listening skills, put-downs, and lectures should be targeted for immediate communication training. During family problem-solving sessions, the therapist can coach, model, and support the teen's participation. Coupled with intervention when the parents respond negatively to the teen, this strategy can help the family overcome their ineffective patterns.

Teen resistance that functions to avoid parental discipline and thereby continue free access to potentially inaccessible outside sources of reinforcement (e.g., staying out late with friends) poses a more insidious, less easily handled problem. In these cases, the locus of the reinforcer is often at home or in the community rather than in the session. In some cases, encouraging the parents to negotiate stringent rules and telling the adolescent s/he must stay out of the discussion provokes the adolescent into speaking after 5 or 10 minutes. The adolescent can then be encouraged to suggest more lenient alternatives, and the parents can be urged to compromise, thus reinforcing an alternative to silence— offering alternatives—with the same reinforcer that maintains silent behavior (decreased strictness, more independence). This, in turn, allows the adolescent access to important reinforcers via less disruptive means.

Yet another insidious pattern surrounding adolescent resistive behavior occurs when that behavior serves a "protective function" for the teenager and the family (Madanes, 1981). As depicted in Chapter 10, parents may avoid negative marital interactions by devoting excessive attention to the discipline of a rebellious teenager. In behavioral terms, the teenager's argumentative, defiant behavior may be negatively reinforced by the reduction of parental fighting and the removal of a threat of parental separation or divorce; the parents may be coerced to attend to the teenager's defiant behavior to reduce the aversive situations created by the teenager. Concentrating on the adolescent's problematic behavior also helps the parents avoid discussion of their own marital conflicts. If this circular pattern of interactions is interrupted by a therapist, the adolescent resists participation, to "protect" the parents against cessation of their avoidance behaviors. Such "protective resistance" is also common when the teenager is afraid of revealing a family secret such as incest, child abuse, or spouse abuse.

To overcome protective resistance, the therapist must make it explicit to the teenager that the parents' marital conflicts or the family secrets will be handled competently and that the family will not be permitted to fall apart. In an individual session with the adolescent, the therapist can frankly discuss the teenager's anxieties about separation and divorce, providing direct reassurance that marital problems will be addressed. Alternatively, during a family interview, the therapist can reframe the adolescent's rebellious behavior as "helpful," noting the "great sacrifice" made by the teenager to "help" the family. The high costs of this help can be highlighted, and reassurance can be provided that the therapist will use his/her expertise to help the family find more adaptive mechanisms of "protection" that exact a less costly personal sacrifice by the adolescent. In cases of severe marital conflict with potent avoidance contingencies involving adolescent misbehavior, we have found it is best to indicate that therapy will focus on parent–adolescent, not marital problems, unless the family specifically requests a shift in emphasis. Later, the therapist may be able to use functional family therapy tactics to address simultaneously the two domains.

If, after all attempts, the adolescent is still unwilling to participate, we choose one of two options. The first is to see the parents alone, which we do only under circumstances in which the parents wish to continue and it appears that skill training or some other form of behavioral intervention could benefit them even in the adolescent's absence. The second option is to terminate and refer the parents for a therapeutic approach that does not involve the adolescent.

A final comment on reluctant adolescents: Some therapists find it more difficult than others to work with adolescents and have consistent problems engaging adolescents in treatment. In cases where the therapist has nearly uniform difficulties relating to teenage clients, examining one's own therapeutic style may prove more fruitful than focusing solely on the adolescent's behavior. Therapists who come across as authoritarian or judgmental, who try too hard to be "with it," and who inadvertently discount the teen's opinions may have difficulty establishing rapport with teenagers. In these cases, honest examination of one's therapy patterns (e.g., by self-monitoring or listening to audiotapes of previous sessions) and feedback, discussions, and role-played practice with colleagues and supervisors can help locate and correct the source of the problem. We will talk more about dealing with negative therapist attitudes towards families later in the chapter.

Reluctant Parents

Another common difficulty engaging families in treatment arises when one parent and an adolescent attend sessions but indicate that the other parent is unable, unwilling, or not needed to participate. Practical difficulties such as scheduling and extensive job-related travel may be cited, or the cooperative parent may report that there is an agreement within the family that the conflict is primarily between him/her and the adolescent. In our experience fathers are more likely than mothers to be the absent parent. The therapist must decide whether to treat only the dyad, refuse to treat the dyad, or attempt to involve the absent parent.

Family systems therapists often assume that the child's behavior problem is an expression of generalized conflict in the family involving the marital dyad (Minuchin, 1974). From this perspective the absent parent is inevitably part of the problem, and therapy cannot proceed without his/her attendance. But since social-learning theorists do not assume an inevitable relationship between child behavior problems and marital conflict (see Chapters 2 and 3), therapy may proceed under certain circumstances without the participation of both parents.

One investigation has examined the impact of the absent parent on the outcome of an intervention similar to problem-solving communication training. Martin (1977) recruited families experiencing mild to moderately severe parent–child problems with first- to fifth-grade children and assigned them to a father-included treatment condition, a father-not-included treatment condition, or a wait-list condition. The two treated groups received a brief intervention consisting of training in conflict resolution, communication, and contingency management skills, drawn from Parent Effectiveness Training and behavioral theory. Both treated groups showed greater reductions in rates of problem behavior at postassessment than did the wait-list controls, and these changes were maintained at 6-month follow-up. However, improvement in mother–child problems was the same whether or not fathers were included. The results suggested that at least with mild to moderately distressed parent–child relationships, it may not be necessary to include fathers in a treatment program designed to improve mother–child interactions.

Martin carefully pointed out, however, that in particular cases (those characterized by extreme marital conflict over child rearing), the absence of the father impeded progress. In drawing inferences from Martin's study, several additional cautions should be observed: (1) since all of the fathers in the study were willing to participate in therapy, although some were assigned to the father-absent condition, the results may not be generalizable to families where fathers are unwilling to participate; (2) improvement in the mother–son dyad, and neither the father–son nor marital dyads, was assessed; and (3) preadolescents were treated, and parent–adolescent conflicts may differ qualitatively and quantitatively from conflicts between parents and preadolescents. Further, the finding in our research (see Chapter 3) that parents with parent–adolescent difficulties have higher scores on the Conflict over Child Rearing Scale of the Marital Satisfaction Inventory than parents without parent–adolescent conflict (Rayha, 1982) also implies that in at least some circumstances both parents' participation may be necessary.

The decision to treat or not to treat a dyad must rest with the therapist, not the family. A careful assessment of the circumstances surrounding the absence of the spouse should be conducted during the initial interview. If the spouse is opposed to therapy or unwilling to participate, our clinical experience suggests that s/he is usually a part of the problem. If the spouse is favorably predisposed towards therapy but unable to participate because of genuine practical difficulties such as scheduling, the therapist may agree to treat the family with intermittent participation by the spouse. (See Chapter 13 for a successful case example of this.) Assignments such as completing self-report questionnaires, listening to and writing comments on audiotapes of therapy sessions, and coming in for a single assessment session at a convenient time are good tasks for assessing the genuineness of the absent spouses's commitment to helping improve family relations. If the therapist elects to treat a dyad but predicts that the outcome may be limited since both parents are not participating regularly, this should be stated explicitly when formulating family goals.

In one evaluation of problem-solving communication training (Robin, 1981), five triads, three mother–adolescent dyads, and two father–adolescent dyads participated. In the therapists' opinions, the absence of the second parent hampered the course of treatment in three of the five dyads. In each of these cases the nonparticipating parent either sabotaged the solutions to problems that were reached during training sessions or created additional problems at home. In the three dyads where treatment was successful, the overall level of family conflict was mild to moderate and the presenting problems were primarily negative adolescent reactions to overprotective behavior by the participating parent. In addition, there was minimal evidence of marital conflict.

When the therapist judges that the participation of an unwilling spouse is essential for progress, s/he should make active attempts to involve that individual. Either the mother can use her power to get the father to attend or the therapist can make a direct contact with the father. In our experience, the most effective approach is the latter. The therapist can telephone the father and invite him to attend the next session without making any commitment to attend regularly. The request should be phrased in terms of the therapist's need to understand everyone's perspective on the problem in order to be helpful. A direct request for participation from the therapist is preferable to an indirect request transmitted through other family members because the family members may have a vested interest in discouraging the spouse from attending the session. It also helps for the therapist to be flexible with respect to scheduling a session with the reluctant parent, even if this is a slight inconvenience to the therapist.

Most fathers respond positively to a direct invitation from the therapist. When they do attend a session, it is important for the therapist to avoid accusatory comments directed towards the father, to indicate clearly the rationale for attendance by all family members, and to treat the father's views respectfully. Strategies suggested in Chapter 4 for reframing issues to highlight the contribution of all family members can also be used to help the father appreciate the importance of his role in family change.

Occasionally a parent will continue to resist attending sessions, despite a nonthreatening overture from the therapist. In such cases Doherty (1981) outlines several useful suggestions. If the presenting problems are chronic and the family is stablized, therapy can be terminated until both parents agree to attend. If the family is in an immediate crisis, work with the mother–adolescent dyad should continue. However, the issue of whether the mother wishes to remain married to a man who refuses to help his family in times of crisis can also be raised.

On rare occasions, the therapist may decide that it is better to work with a parent–adolescent dyad or even an individual adolescent, despite the opinion that presenting problems involve both parents and the teenager. One such dramatic case is described below.

Example. Mr. Mallman was an authoritarian father and husband who insisted that his ways be followed in trivial as well as significant matters. Mrs. Mallman was, in her own words, a "recently liberated woman" who was now rebelling against her husband's tyrannical methods, more like a teenager than an adult. Many of their arguments revolved around 14-year-old Jim, who had recently been apprehended by the police for shoplifting. Jim had grown up in an atmosphere of severe family strife and, in the therapist's judgment, was acting out in order to unite his parents on his behalf, helping to reduce their own marital fights.

The family had been seen for five sessions of family therapy by another therapist prior to the referral to one of us (A. R.). During these sessions, the parents came to physical blows and traded vicious accusations. Following the third session, Jim took an overdose of sleeping pills as a suicide gesture, which temporarily reduced his parents' fighting. Their fights resumed when Jim returned home from a short stay in a psychiatric hospital. Family therapy was terminated at the request of the family following the attempted suicide episode. Shortly thereafter, the shoplifting incident transpired, and at the family lawyer's suggestion, Jim was referred for individual therapy.

Given the long history of parental violence and physical abuse, triadic family sessions threatened physical danger and almost certain ineffectiveness. Yet the therapist felt that Jim was basically a nice teenager who was the victim of unfortunate family circumstances. Therefore, it was decided to see him individually and in dyadic sessions with one parent at a time. The goals of therapy included strengthening Jim's autonomy from his parents, helping him remain aloof from their marital struggles, and using problem-solving communication training to decrease Mr. Mallman's authoritarian overcontrol of Jim's decision making. It was made explicit that resolving marital conflict was not a goal of therapy. While these goals were admittedly limited, it was not judged feasible to conduct sessions with both parents present.

Therapy produced modest gains over a 1-year period. Jim's self-esteem was bolstered through individual sessions. No further delinquent behavior in the community occurred, and Jim began to learn how to get his needs for freedom met without becoming embroiled in his parents' endless marital conflicts. Attempts to teach the father to change his style of communicating with his son failed. His beliefs were too rigid to change. Marital conflict continued unabated until Mr. Mallman's sudden death from a heart attack. Jim was the first to find his father dead in the shower, a very traumatic experience. The therapist was able to help Jim mourn his father's unexpected death. Interestingly, Mrs. Mallman changed her attitude following her husband's death: finally freed from his "tyranny," she became extremely depressed and guilty about her failure to resolve marital conflicts before he died. Her depression quickly turned to anger when she discovered that 2 days before his death he had changed his will, left her nothing, and left everything to his sons and brother. She challenged the will in court in a long, drawn-out lawsuit. Even after death, marital conflict continued.

Commentary. If the therapist had refused to treat the case because the family could not be seen together, Jim might well have gone on to develop more serious problems. In addition, the therapist would not have been able to help Jim following his father's unpredictable death. This case emphasizes the importance of remaining flexible in choosing alternatives to family intervention, even if these alternatives appear to imply acceptance of less-than-ideal goals for change. Indeed, Szapocznik, Kurtines, Foote, Perez-Vidal, & Hervis (1983) found that strategic family-focused treatment involving only one family member can be as effective as similar treatment with larger family units.

This discussion has emphasized the problems of absent parents in intact marital units. Problem-solving communication training does not require a two-parent family to be effective, however. The treatment approach is equally applicable to single- and two-parent families, as long as presenting problems revolve around parent–adolescent conflict.

DIRECTING SESSIONS AND MAINTAINING CONTROL

Because problem-solving communication training is a highly structured, goal-oriented intervention, the therapist must maintain relatively tight stimulus control over family members' verbal behavior during treatment sessions. "Relatively tight stimulus control" means that (1) the discussion focuses on tasks deemed appropriate by the therapist; (2) if the discussion is not task-oriented (i.e., light, recreational conversation), then the therapist has allocated time for such activity; (3) the therapist can stop or start the discussion at all times, and loud, hostile arguments do not persist unless the therapist wishes to assess briefly the nature of such interchanges; and (4) the therapist is able to intervene and provide emotional protection for family members who may be scapegoated, attacked, or put down excessively by others.

In earlier chapters, we reviewed various difficulties directing family interviews and suggested appropriate strategies for therapists to extricate themselves from runaway interviews. When arguments persist despite the therapist's preventive actions (see Chapter 4), the therapist should forcefully intervene to insure that ground rules for decent interpersonal conduct prevail. Then the therapist should formulate hypotheses about why these patterns continue.

As with other forms of persistent resistance, the functional analysis provides a vehicle for formulating these hypotheses. Thus, the therapist begins with the assumption that arguments are functional; that is, they serve some important purpose for the individual(s) in the family. Understanding and overcoming the behavior entails clearly specifying the nature of the resistant response, its current and historical antecedents, and its consequences, both within and outside the session. These hypotheses can then be tested through direct questioning or small AB experiments, introducing changes in session procedures and noting their effects.

In our experience one factor that sometimes maintains persistent arguments over several sessions is the therapist's failure to enforce the ground rules consistently. Beginning family therapists in particular often are reluctant to be directive with families whose interactions move quickly, fearing to be thought "impolite." It is important to realize, however, that without structure, sessions are unlikely to accomplish much.

In other cases, families seem to be participating willingly in treatment but explode with anger at the slightest provocation. These families will readily admit when they are calm that they have difficulties with their "short fuses." These cases probably should not be thought of as resistant, because they are generally compliant with directives and participate actively in therapy. Instead, it may be useful to conceptualize their arguments as elicited by the experience of intense anger, in turn elicited by something in the interaction process. Thus, emotion-laden interchanges can be treated as communication problems. Anger-control interventions such as those developed by Novaco (1975) may also be useful. In one family, for example, two sessions were devoted to solving the problem "what to do when we get really angry with each other and aren't calm enough to discuss anything." After working out strategies to avoid destructive explosions, the therapist can catch early cues preceding explosions and use these to coach family members in how to implement the strategies they have committed them-selves to using.

When neither of the above seems to apply, the therapist should carefully look for what the family accomplishes or avoids by disrupting sessions. Once having formulated a hypothesis, the therapist may be able to devise a series of strategic maneuvers to allow family members to accomplish the same end without arguing so viciously. In some cases, a paradoxical intervention can be useful, at least temporarily: The therapist tells the family (using a sincere tone of voice) that obviously they prefer to pay their therapy fees to argue, and since that is their preference, s/he will gladly sit back and relax (or leave the room) while they argue, requesting to be informed when they have finished. Alternatively, the therapist may regain control by reframing arguing as the family's style of communicating how much they care about each other and playfully helping the family plan and execute an argument in a step-by-step fashion. By guiding the family in conducting the "argument," the therapist can indirectly prevent them from avoiding the issue under consideration, while also maintaining session control. Finally, as with the Mallman case described earlier, the therapist can elect to see family members individually or in smaller units. From a behavioral perspective, though, those individuals whose arguments function to avoid some aspect of therapy would be expected to produce different avoidance strategies when seen individually. Regardless of the strategy employed to reduce persistent arguing, hypotheses about the function of such arguments should be consistently considered.

After an argument laden with heavy negative emotions has subsided, the therapist may decide to review what has happened, adjourn the session, or meet with family members individually. Immediately after an out-of-control argument is usually not the best time to resume calm, rational problem solving, either inside or outside of sessions.

We have discussed only a few of the ways in which family members can sidetrack sessions. The sensitive therapist should constantly be on the lookout for creative diversionary tactics and be prepared to cope with them. Feeling lost or wondering how the original topic resolved into the current discussion is a good clue that a diversion was successful and should be identified and corrected to prevent similar problems in the future.

DIFFICULTIES MAINTAINING RAPPORT

Chapter 4 offered suggestions for facilitating the establishment of strong rapport between therapists and families. These included liberal use of reflective, empathetic comments, appropriate maintenance of eye contact and other nonverbal gestures, avoidance of one-sided statements, and so forth. Despite the best efforts of sensitive clinicians, situations occasionally arise where problem-solving communication training bogs down because of poor rapport between family members and the therapist. Family members may challenge the therapist's competence based upon professional credentials, age, sex, experience, or theoretical orientation, or may simply express personal dislike of the therapist. Therapists may begin to feel animosity or dislike towards one or more family members. From a behavioral perspective it is paramount to pinpoint the elements of the therapeutic interaction that interfere with maintenance of rapport.

Direct challenges to the therapist's competence usually take the form of one or more of the following themes (Anderson & Stewart, 1983):

1. "You are not a psychiatrist; how can you really understand us?"
2. "You only have a master's degree; we need a more experienced person."
3. "You look too young [too old] to understand."
4. "You're too male [female]."
5. "You don't have teenage children."
6. "Are you successfully married?"
7. "You don't understand our religion."

8. "You haven't had a child with this problem and can't understand."
9. "You're too behavioral."
10. "You talk to us in strange language."

Anderson and Stewart have written extensively about how to cope with such challenges, and many of their suggestions form the bases of the recommendations that follow.

Such challenges may reflect misconceptions about therapy, lack of information, defensiveness on the part of the family, lack of faith in therapy or the therapist, attempts to triangulate the therapist, or resistance to difficult material being dealt with in therapy. It is crucial for the therapist to try to assess further the reasons for the family's concerns rather than reacting defensively, even though the reasons may seem obvious. Giving the family permission to raise objections to therapy or the therapist and probing for further information is often a helpful first step. The therapist might say, "Many families have questions about whether therapy can really help them. That's OK; let's discuss your questions." The therapist would follow up with a series of more specific questions designed to pinpoint the source of the family's concerns.

Often challenges are based upon misconceptions. Family members may unrealistically believe that in order to be effective a therapist must be a perfect human being who has overcome all of life's obstacles, is successfully married, has raised several brilliant, well-adjusted children, and has no personal vulnerabilities. Alternatively, they may believe that only a therapist who has undergone the same life experiences as they have can really appreciate their situation and help them. If the therapist is not similar to the family member in age, sex, marital status, religion, race, and so forth, how could s/he possibly appreciate their situation or even begin to help them change it?

Providing information in a nondefensive, straightforward manner often goes a long way towards correcting misconceptions. The therapist can explain that therapists, like clients, are fallible human beings with strengths and weaknesses, but that they have had extensive special training in helping families and in not permitting their personal fallibilities to interfere with their professional work. The family can be asked whether they know any physicians or lawyers who are less-than-perfect human beings. Usually, they will respond affirmatively, permitting the therapist to point out that a surgeon who yells at his teenage children too much may still be highly competent in the operating room.

Misconceptions related to age, sex, experience, or parenting status can be handled in a similar manner. When older parents challenge the young, inexperienced therapist's ability to understand their position on the grounds that the therapist has not raised teenage children, the therapist can describe his/her training. The dangers of too much personal experience with a phenomenon might also be noted: Therapists who have had a great deal of conflict with their own teenagers may not be as objective as those who have not raised children. Finally, the physician analogy might again be invoked: A physician does not have to experience a disease to treat it effectively.

An alternative approach involves acknowledging that the difference between the therapist and the family member might become a legitimate problem and enlisting the family member as an ally who is asked to help bridge the gap by giving the therapist feedback if that member thinks an important issue is being misunderstood: "No, I've never been a single, Hispanic mother raising three teenage boys in the inner city. If you think I am not understanding you because of this, please let me know so we can discuss it and you can teach me to understand better. Good communication is, after all, the goal of our work together."

When challenges represent indirect attempts to sabotage the direction of therapy or avoid difficult material, additional steps need to be taken. The therapist should try to answer the question, Why now? What has transpired recently in therapy that the family is finding difficult to deal with? Is the family being asked to emit behaviors that are not in their repertoires? Does adherence to a cognitive distortion underlie the challenge? Has the therapist touched upon a central functional/structural pattern that the family is trying to disguise or avoid? Reviewing earlier assessment information, questionnaires, and tapes of the session in which the challenge occurs may help to pinpoint the answers to these questions. Since the therapist becomes a part of the system by engaging the family in treatment (Haley, 1976), the family can be expected to generalize the way they interact with each other to their interactions with the therapist. Parents who avoid marital conflict by becoming embroiled in endless arguments with their adolescents over independence-related issues may be expected to attempt to avoid the therapist's attempts to discuss marital conflict by picking an argument related to the therapist's personal characteristics. Couples who triangulate their children may be expected to triangulate the therapist. Family members who are unable to communicate negative affect without accusations in the home are likely to communicate with accusations to the therapist.

When the therapist identifies why the family is indirectly challenging him/her at the present time, there are several strategies that may be taken. If a communication deficit or cognitive distortion underlies the challenge, identifying the deficit and providing immediate remediation through modeling and behavior rehearsal is likely to prove effective. For example, an authoritarian, accusing father may put down a therapist's suggestion because the therapist appears inexperienced or young. The therapist may treat the father's put-down as an example of the same type of negative communication that elicits defensive reactions from the adolescent; s/he might point out the negative response and how it made him/her feel, acknowledge the father's disagreement with his/her suggestion, and model a more constructive way for the father to express dis-agreement with the therapist.

If a central functional/structural interaction pattern underlies the challenge to the therapist, planning a sequence of strategic moves to address the pattern is preferable.

Example. Dr. Meyers was a neurosurgeon attending therapy together with his wife and 16-year-old, out-of-control daughter. During the engagement phase of treatment, he began to challenge whether a nonphysician therapist could really help his family. The therapist gave a standard informational response, but the challenges persisted. Therapy was being conducted in front of a one-way mirror and several colleagues were watching (the family had agreed to this procedure). The colleagues telephoned in a request for the therapist to step out of the room for a momentary consultation. When the therapist went behind the mirror, his colleagues pointed out that Dr. Meyer's challenge to the therapist's credentials had been made at the moments when the therapist was beginning to assess marital relations, raising the possibility that the husband was trying to avoid a discussion of his marriage. The colleagues, who included two psychologists and a pediatric resident, also suggested that the therapist tell Dr. Meyers that "the group behind the mirror recognizes that it takes special expertise to understand difficult areas of family life, and that the group, particularly its physician member, agree with the stance taken by the therapist and encourage the family to do the best they can talking about difficult areas; after all, the therapist cannot treat a 'disease' without a correct 'diagnosis,' and a full 'history' is necessary to make a correct diagnosis." When the therapist gave this message to Dr. Meyers, he ceased challenging the therapist's credentials and permitted limited discussion of marital relations.

Commentary. Essentially, the technique of appealing to a higher, credible authority figure, discussed in Chapter 7, was used to help bolster the therapist's position. The use of colleagues behind a one-way mirror as a "Greek chorus" that calls in suggestions and comments, helping the therapist orchestrate strategic maneuvers, is sometimes useful with resistant families (Papp, 1980).

In responding to challenges to competence, therapists must not only examine the client's behavior but also look inward to determine the extent to which their own behavior may be actively eliciting challenges. Therapists can easily review whether their feedback to the family has been unbalanced, possibly causing one member to conclude angrily that the therapist has aligned with another member. If so, the imbalance can be corrected. Alternatively, therapists can assess how their interpersonal style may be contributing to the negative interaction with the family member. Goldstein and Myers (1986, pp. 54–60) has summarized a variety of therapist behaviors that may elicit negative affectual reactions from clients: unusual exclamations of surprise, moralistic judgments, criticisms, false promises, threats, burdening the client with your own problems, displays of impatience, arguing, ridiculing, blaming, rejecting, displays of intolerance, dogmatic utterances, premature deep interpretations, and unnecessary reassurances. In addition, stylistic factors such as voice tone, speed of talking, accent, and so forth, may be problematic. In fact, any of the negative communication habits that we target in families should be examined as contributors to negative interactions between therapists and families.

Posture, physical distance from the client, and eye contact also contribute to rapport. Research has suggested that sitting close to the client, leaning forward, maintaining frequent eye contact, and facing the client directly may enhance rapport (Goldstein *et al.*, 1986). In our experience, however, some families prefer more interpersonal and physical distance from the therapist than others. The effects of brief physical contact also vary from person to person. Since violations of the families' tacit preferences for interpersonal and physical boundaries may interfere with the maintenance of good rapport, proxemic factors warrant careful assessment. A pat on the shoulder may be a helpful relationship enhancer for parents or adolescents, but the therapist should evaluate the interpersonal style of the family carefully before touching them. However, even interpersonally distant parents may respond to physical contact within their boundaries of acceptability. One of us (A. R.) can recall several rigid, authoritarian fathers who shook the therapist's hand at the end of each session for 15–20 weeks.

The therapist's own strong, negative affectual responses to family members can also interfere with the maintenance of rapport. Feelings of defensiveness, anger, or anxiety during treatment sessions traditionally have been considered "countertransference" issues, to be worked through in the therapist's own therapy. In contrast, a social-learning model postulates that the same principles that characterize family relations also operate between family members and therapists, who have "joined" the system in their roles as change agents. Just as therapists observe family interactions to pinpoint troublesome patterns, they should self-monitor interactions with the family and pinpoint the discriminative stimuli for their personal reactions. Reviewing audio- or videotapes of sessions with colleagues is a useful way to enhance such self-monitoring.

In our experience, therapists react negatively to family members when (1) the family member repeatedly tries to manipulate the therapist's response to a situation to achieve a personal goal; (2) the family member is unresponsive to numerous corrections of deficient communication skills; or (3) the family member's interpersonal style is reminiscent of the behavior of a significant individual in the therapist's family of origin or an individual with whom the therapist has unresolved conflicts. The first situation is essentially a control problem, and all of our earlier suggestions for coping with runaway sessions apply here. In the second case, the therapist must reexamine whether the skills currently being taught exceed the capability of the family or whether a cognitive distortion is mediating the unresponsive behavior. A new sequence of skill training or greater emphasis on cognitive restructuring may be needed.

The third case involves inappropriate generalization from personal to professional interactions. Everyone has areas of personal vulnerability based upon past experiences, particularly in their families of origin. When clients respond to a therapist like the therapist's parents, siblings, or significant others used to, the therapist may unwittingly react inappropriately or ineffectively due to stimulus generalization. For example, an inexperienced young therapist who is still struggling to resolve autonomy issues with his/her own parents may overreact with defensiveness and anger if attacked by an older, authoritarian father. Through self-examination and consultation with colleagues and supervisors, the therapist can learn to recognize personal responses to family interactions, to monitor when they are interfering with therapeutic effectiveness, and to develop self-instructional, attributional strategies for coping with them. Thus, the young therapist just described might learn to recognize that an ambivalent relationship with his/her own father might mediate defensive, angry responses to this client. Having recognized this interactional pattern, self-statements like "I know I am overreacting here because this father is just like my Dad; I have to calm down and think about how I should respond to this" may decrease his/her anger toward the client. When irreconcilable differences between the therapist and family persist, a switch of therapists may be desirable.

NONCOMPLIANCE WITH THERAPIST'S DIRECTIVES

Noncompliance with a therapist's directives is a multifaceted construct that subsumes a variety of client behaviors, including (1) failure to complete homework assignments; (2) lack of cooperative behavior during behavior rehearsal and problem-solving discussions; (3) direct challenges to rationales or procedures introduced by the therapist; (4) missed or late appointments; and (5) rigid adherence to distorted belief systems incompatible with therapeutic change. Earlier chapters discussed examples of noncompliant behavior, providing suggestions for coping with them.

With persistent noncompliance, as with other forms of ongoing resistance, the behaviorally oriented therapist should search for the functional role noncompliance serves for the individual(s) in the family. In our experience the following classes of variables frequently contribute to the maintenance of resistant behavior (Weiss, 1981).

1. *Dislike of behavioral approaches.* One or more family members may enter treatment with a preconceived negative cognitive set towards behaviorism. Although problem-solving communication training is not presented to a family as an explicitly behavioral approach, members may nonetheless object to its structure or social-learning philosophy. Usually, provision of explanatory information, couched in terms that the family can understand, is sufficient to overcome these objections. For example, a family may object to the assignment of homework because they do not believe they should have to work to produce change between sessions but rather that the therapist should magically facilitate change. The therapist can review the metaphor of learning a new skill, noting the contribution of practice to skill acquisition as a means of justifying the value of homework.

2. *Cognitive distortions.* As elaborated in Chapter 9, distorted belief systems and faulty attributions may mediate resistant behavior. Family members may fear that compliance with the therapist's directives would lead to catastrophic consequences. Some parents believe they never should compromise with their adolescents because compromise is a sign of parental weakness; if the parents

"give in," the teenagers will escalate their demands to unreasonable levels and eventually grow up to be spoiled, irresponsible adults. Some teenagers believe that their parents cannot possibly understand the complexities of growing up in today's society, and it is therefore fruitless to discuss important issues with their parents. Given such rigid cognitive sets, these family members may not comply with a therapist's assignment to conduct problem-solving discussions at home or may even balk at problem solving during treatment sessions. Guidelines given in Chapter 9 to change such inappropriate attitudinal responses can assist in altering the resistant behavior that results from counterproductive beliefs.

3. *Systemic factors.* Family members may resist therapeutic directives because of interference with self-maintaining, interlocking interactions within the family system. These forms of resistance reflect the "politics" of the relationship and can be understood only by assessing the function of problematic behavior in maintaining patterns of reciprocity and coercion within the parent–child and marital dyads. A functional analysis of interlocking sequences of behavior, outlined in Chapter 6, is a prerequisite for planning a strategy to change the sequences constituting the "resistance." Strategies may include direct behavioral techniques or indirect, paradoxical suggestions (Haley, 1976). Many of the suggestions for interventions outlined in Chapter 10 are applicable here.

Our attempts to overcome resistant behavior do not always prove successful. To analyze the function of the resistant behavior by specifying its antecedents and consequences is the most effective strategy we know. Understanding function, however, does not guarantee the success of strategic interventions designed to alter interactions. In a minority of severely distressed families, therapy has been terminated by either the therapist or the family when it was clear that the interlocking pattern of behavior promoting resistance to therapeutic change was beyond our abilities to change. We do not yet have empirical guidelines as to which cases are unlikely to be successfully treated by our methods, so at present we recommend trying a full range of strategies to overcome resistance before deciding to terminate.

PROBLEMS OUTSIDE THE PARENT–ADOLESCENT RELATIONSHIP

While the presenting problem with many families is ostensibly parent–adolescent conflict, a thorough behavioral analysis may reveal the presence of associated marital conflict and/or personal problems of individual family members. These associated difficulties may in some cases be major contributing variables accounting for parent–teen disagreements. If marital conflict, depression, substance abuse, or other forms of individual psychopathology are significant problems, the therapist must assess to what extent the marital or individual problems and parent–adolescent conflict are intertwined (as in triangulation). As noted earlier, behavioral marital therapy or individual treatment may be undertaken concurrently with or prior to problem-solving communication training.

Two other types of individual problems sometimes interfere with commitment to and participation in problem-solving communication training: anxiety and the Attention Deficit Hyperactivity Disorder. Anxiety is viewed as a multifaceted construct including cognitive, motoric, and physiological components. Chronic anxiety can be expected to influence interactions within the family at home and in treatment sessions. To assess the possible influence of these difficulties on family interventions, the therapist should determine whether anxious behavior is an antecedent or consequence of the parent–child conflict. If it appears to be a consequence, family-oriented interventions that teach conflict-resolution skills would be expected to alleviate the anxiety indirectly. If, on the other hand, the anxiety is an antecedent of poor coping with normal striving for independence and is a significant clinical problem apart from parent–teen conflict, family-oriented intervention would probably be insufficient unless the anxious member also received individual behavior therapy, cognitive therapy, or medication.

Transient performance anxiety can also create difficulties during problem-solving discussions. When an adolescent balks at participating in behavior rehearsal of communication skills, anxiety may be the mediating variable (Witkin, 1981). The therapist can help alleviate the anxiety by providing reassurance, asking the remaining members to give the adolescent permission to behave however s/he wishes, regardless of how "foolish" it appears, conducting a brief relaxation induction, or "doubling" for the adolescent, that is, modeling his/her role in the discussion. Usually, individual behavior therapy for performance anxiety is unnecessary.

Attention deficit hyperactivity disorders are among the most common behavior disorders of childhood and adolescence. The Attention Deficit Hyperactivity Disorder (ADHD) consists of a pervasive, cross-situational deficit in attentional processes, self-control, and concentration; a high level of distractibility, often accompanied by excesses of impulsive behavior; restlessness; overactivity; conduct problems; and learning problems (Barkley, 1981; Ross & Ross, 1982). Follow-up studies of ADHD children have demonstrated that during the teenage years overt overactivity decreases, but inattention and impulsivity persist (Weiss & Hechtman, 1986). Thus, the normal teenage rebelliousness and independence seeking are likely to be more intense with the ADHD teenager. Depending upon earlier family and school responses to the ADHD child, antisocial, aggressive behavior may be a difficulty during adolescence. Our recent research comparing ADHD teens and their parents to nonclinic families suggests that these families have major deficits in problem-solving communication skills, rigid beliefs characterized by malicious parental attributions, and disengagement (Robin, Kraus, Koepke, & Robin, 1987).

Two interventions are commonly used to treat children with ADHD: stimulant medication and behavioral intervention. While stimulant medication helps

75% of ADHD children to increase short-term self-control, attention, and learning, the long-term impact is less clear (Barkley, 1981). Behavioral interventions in the classroom, community, and at home have been effective in reducing disruptive behaviors and increasing completion of academic work; most of these interventions, designed for children under the age of 12, involve contingency management.

We routinely treat with problem-solving communication training a number of ADHD teenagers in conflict with their parents. The training is usually part of a more comprehensive intervention for the families. The outcomes have been positive, but the therapist must adjust the intervention to meet the special needs of this population. First, the therapist must establish reasonable goals for change, based upon an understanding of ADHD and adolescent development. Problem-solving communication training will neither "cure" ADHD nor provide a primary vehicle to control the central deficits in attentional processes; medication is often necessary for control of inattention. However, this training can help to increase ADHD teens' self-control and organization while simultaneously providing their families with a vehicle to resolve conflict. Cognitive restructuring can be helpful for guiding parents to develop reasonable expectations for an ADHD teenager (see example in Chapter 9). Finally, therapists need to keep in mind that when severe acting-out conduct disturbances characterize the ADHD teen's relations with his/her parents, the therapists may need to emphasize parental control through building a strong parental coalition (see Chapter 10) before moving to a democratic problem-solving process.

Second, the therapist and family must decide whether to place the adolescent on stimulant medication in conjunction with problem-solving communication training. In our clinical experience adolescents whose poor attention, inadequate organization, and excessive impulsivity interfere significantly with school learning benefit greatly from stimulant medication. If school achievement is not currently an area of difficulty, we would recommend stimulant medication primarily for control of social behavior in severe cases of ADHD characterized by delinquency, antisocial–aggressive behavior, and extreme impulsivity. In fact, clinical experience suggests that problem-solving communication training or any related intervention may fail unless the therapist moves quickly after the initial session to establish an appropriate medication regimen coupled with clear parental control strategies. Out of six cases of such severe ADHD–conduct disordered teens treated by one of us (A. R.) over the past 3 years, only three were successful. In these three cases medication was started immediately by a responsive pediatrician trained to deal with such teenagers, and parental controls were clearly established early in treatment. In the three unsuccessful cases, either an appropriate medication regimen was not established quickly or the parents were unable to respond to the therapist's demands to exercise strong, authoritarian controls. Readers interested in further discussion of stimulant medication with ADHD adolescents should consult Brown, Borden, and Clingerman (1985), Safer and Krager (1985), and Varley (1985).

Third, the therapist must keep problem solving concrete and take liberal opportunities to insure that the adolescent has attended to and understood what is being said in sessions. Assignments should be written down, and the formal, organizational framework of problem-solving communication training should be emphasized.

If these guidelines are followed, the therapist will find that problem-solving communication training can be helpful as part of the treatment of the ADHD adolescent. Research is sorely needed to validate our suggestions, and Barkley (1987) has recently begun a controlled outcome study comparing problem-solving communication training to parent training and nonspecific family therapy with ADHD teens.

In addition to marital conflict, depression, anxiety, and ADHD, family-oriented practitioners will encounter other personal problems of family members that impact upon parent–teen relations but require special, added components of an intervention. Examples include unassertiveness, low self-esteem, alcoholism, drug abuse, and anorexia. The astute clinician will conduct a thorough behavioral assessment to determine the functional relationship of these problems to parent–adolescent conflict. Then a truly comprehensive treatment program can be designed for each family.

FINAL WORD ON RESISTANCE

Despite the previous discussion, major resistances do not always arise during the implementation of problem-solving communication training. However, neither is this intervention a panacea for all difficulties between parents and adolescents. A more realistic appraisal suggests that our intervention is one type of skill-acquisition program for teaching families to resolve conflicts revolving around the developmental stage of family life where young adolescents begin to seek increased autonomy from their parents. In clinical practice it is often blended into a multidimensional therapy program tailored to the needs of each family. The practitioner is likely to encounter several but not all of the sources of resistance discussed in this chapter in the average clinical case. Through the judicious use of our suggestions and good clinical common sense, most of these problems can be prevented, anticipated, or overcome.

As we have noted, there is a great need for empirical investigations of resistance. A recent study by Chamberlain *et al.* (1984) illustrates an approach to operationalizing and assessing resistance in behavioral family therapy. These investigators developed a molecular observation system to measure client resistance in behavioral family therapy. Each parent response to therapist verbalizations was coded as being resistant or cooperative. Clear-cut definitions were written in a coding manual for resistant behavior, including interruptions, negative attitudes, challenges to therapist competence, changes of agenda, and not tracking. Trained observers reliably coded videotapes of therapy sessions for

27 families in the early, middle, and late stages of parent training for child management problems.

Results indicated that families displayed higher levels of resistance in the middle than the early or late phase of treatment, families who dropped out of treatment displayed more resistant behavior than families completing treatment, and agency-referred families were more resistant than self-referred families. Finally, low resistance was correlated with positive treatment outcome. Of course, the relationship of resistant verbal behavior in sessions to general resistant behavior (missed appointments, failure to complete assignments, etc.) remains to be established. Nonetheless, Chamberlain *et al.* have taken an important step in advancing the empirical analysis of resistance by developing and beginning to validate a molecular coding system for resistant behavior. This study raises the exciting possibility that sequences of therapist and client verbalizations constituting resistance and strategies to cope with it will soon be able to be examined behaviorally.

We hope that we have demystified the concept of resistance, in keeping with recent advances in behavioral conceptualizations (Lazarus & Fay, 1983) and family approaches (Anderson & Stewart, 1983). We would like to leave the reader with the impression that resistance, like any other construct, can be operationalized and targeted for change through empirically based, clearly specified procedures.

CHAPTER THIRTEEN

Case Studies

Throughout this volume we have presented examples of parts of treatment with numerous families. In this chapter we describe two case studies illustrating the course of problem-solving communication training from start to finish. The first case, the Holly family, included a moderately distressed father–adolescent dyad who participated in one of our clinical outcome studies (Robin, 1981). This case illustrates relatively straightforward parent–adolescent conflict difficulties and was successfully treated using primarily the skill-training components of the intervention. The second family case, the Millensons, involved a severely distressed mother–father–adolescent triad treated in private practice. This case illustrates the complexity of difficulties faced by severely troubled families. The Millensons' treatment was only marginally successful, and the multifaceted nature of their problems required various intervention strategies in addition to problem-solving communication training.

CASE ONE: THE HOLLYS[1]

Mr. Holly, a 41-year-old English teacher, and his 13-year-old daughter Sandi responded to an advertisement offering free communication training in return for participation in a clinical research project. They sought treatment because of (1) disagreements concerning issues such as dating, chores, television, and school-work; (2) Sandi's recently increasing defensiveness in response to many attempts at communication by her father; and (3) the father's apprehension about his inability to talk with his daughter without antagonizing her.

During the initial interview, Mr. Holly displayed a sophisticated, overly intellectual interaction style punctuated with a dry sense of humor that occasionally turned to sarcasm. He displayed genuine warmth towards his daughter but was unaware that his pedantic "English-teacher style" of communicating elicited negative reactions from her. Tolerant of the whims of a growing adolescent, he was generally flexible concerning decision making, but was convinced that in certain areas he knew what was best for Sandi.

Sandi's style made her appear both defensive and hypersensitive, lacking in self-confidence and easily upset by criticism. She had no history of delinquent, antisocial behavior, but she was receiving barely passing grades in school despite above-average intellectual ability. She felt she had a much closer, mutually understanding relationship with her mother than with her father. She described her mother as a person who related with tact and empathy and her father as a person who "tells it straight," often with biting humor. Wishing to please adults yet unsure of herself, she failed to let her dad know when his actions or words upset her. Instead, she brooded angrily until she exploded at him during a minor disagreement, taking him by surprise. She also noticed and interpreted minute details of her father's verbal and nonverbal responses.

Our decision to treat a father–daughter dyad in the absence of the mother illustrates a major divergence between the social-learning and more traditional approaches to family therapy. Many family therapists would regard this decision as inappropriate, since they would assume that the adolescent's problem behaviors are symptoms of general family distress and/or marital discord. Father–daughter conflict might be considered to reflect latent mother–daughter or mother–father problems. Treating one dyad within the system would be expected to result in incomplete change because improvement in the treated dyad would be predicted to upset the overall homeostatic balance, leading to resistance and/or sabotage by members who did not participate in treatment.

By contrast, the social-learning approach makes no assumptions regarding the relationship between conflict in one dyad and broader family relations. As outlined in Chapter 2, it is possible that difficulties between two members of the family interlock tightly with other members' behavior, but we believe this connection is not inevitable and needs to be established through a functional analysis of the family's presenting problems. Such a functional analysis is conducted during the assessment phase of treatment as discussed in Chapter 6. Clearly, if there is a functional link between father–daughter, mother–daughter, and mother–father conflict, the entire family needs to be treated. However, if no such link is established during the assessment phase, treatment might proceed with a subgroup of the family. If ongoing assessment indicates the presence of such a link during therapy, the entire family can be brought into therapy sessions as needed. For example, if Sandi's negative behavior towards Mr. Holly was related in part to her mother's negative reactions to her spouse, we would consider mother–daughter coalitional behavior a central difficulty. In that case, the father–daughter dyad should not be treated without the mother. No such links were found during the assessment phase, and since the mother traveled frequently on business, we agreed to treat the father–daughter dyad with minimal formal involvement by the mother. We did, however, arrange for Mr. Holly to review the sessions with his wife on a regular basis, and we included Mrs. Holly in a later session.

Assessment revealed excessive negative communication in the father–daughter relationship, an expressed desire by both father and daughter to work on their interactions, and an overall moderate degree of conflict. The daughter, being hypersensitive as many young teenagers are, was unable to deal with her dad's somewhat biting style, while the father felt helpless to adjust his style to his daughter's developmental changes. The central problem was conceptualized as a developmental crisis in the father–daughter relationship in the presence of relatively positive spouse and mother–daughter interactions, and thus treating the dyad seemed appropriate for both practical and conceptual reasons. Furthermore, although dyadic treatment is more likely to involve mothers and adolescents, the issues addressed in this case are very similar to those involved in typical mother–daughter crises. This fact, together with the detailed quantitative data available for the Hollys, made the case particularly suitable for presentation.

In accord with the research design of the study, Mr. Holly and Sandi attended a screening and preassessment session, seven treatment sessions, and a postassessment and feedback session. Eight weeks after the postassessment, they returned follow-up questionnaires by mail.

Preassessment Measures

The Hollys completed the IC, the CBQ, and two audiotaped discussions coded with the PAICS during the screening and preassessment meeting. At preassessment Sandi reported higher anger-intensity scores (3.0) and fewer issues discussed on the IC (7) than did her father (1.9, 16). On the CBQ both the father and daughter appraised their communication moderately negatively (19 and 18, respectively). Analysis of the PAICS data revealed higher proportions of positive than negative behavior for both Sandi and her father. Interruptions characterized both Sandi's and her father's negative behavior. Mr. Holly made frequent positive facilitative remarks, and Sandi's positive communication consisted mainly of assent–agreements. These data were consistent with the therapist's impression that the family was moderately distressed.

Session One: Engagement

The therapist began the first treatment session by asking the dyad to specify their goals for therapeutic change. Sandi indicated that she would like to improve communication with her dad, while Mr. Holly wished to learn to talk to his daughter without making her feel uncomfortable. He believed she harbored unexpressed, negative feelings towards him which caused her to "blow up" at slight provocations. Even during this exchange of goals, Sandi pointed out how her father's smiles annoyed her because she felt he was laughing at her. He considered his smiling innocent.

The dyad accepted the rationale for problem solving without resistance. The therapist guided the dyad into a discussion of chores. Sandi defined the problem as "when I'm busy doing other things, Dad over and over again asks me to take out the trash and do chores; this bothers me." Her father defined the problem as "you say you will complete some chores and then don't; that's a source of great irritation to me." The therapist elicited these definitions with little prompting and few corrections of more negative statements of the problems. However, Sandi overreacted to her father's definition, interpreting it as a put-down and then clamming up. After extensive therapist modeling, Sandi finally was willing to paraphrase her father's definition of the problem.

They then generated seven solutions:

1. Dad waits until Sandi is free to request she do a chore.
2. Sandi records jobs to be done on tape as a reminder and plays the tape after coming home from school.
3. Sandi does her chores before her homework.
4. Sandi places a sign on the basket of dirty clothing reading "Wash these clothes."
5. Sandi tapes Dad's mouth shut.
6. Dad pays Sandi $100 for each chore completed after the first request.
7. Sandi and Dad negotiate a contract for chores.

Session time ran out after solution listing. The dyad was assigned two tasks for homework: (1) to complete the problem-solving exercise sheet (see Appendix C) and (2) to list additional solutions for chores and evaluate the solutions but not to select a solution to implement until the next session. Because of the dyad's verbal sophistication, the therapist was comfortable assigning this abbreviated home discussion, a step usually reserved for later sessions.

Sessions Two through Four: Skill Acquisition

Sandi and her father completed both assignments. The therapist began the second meeting by reviewing the problem-solving exercise (identifying several problem definition statements as satisfactory or unsatisfactory, then correcting any unsatisfactory statements in writing). Mr. Holly correctly completed the homework, while Sandi incorrectly judged blaming, accusatory statements to be satisfactory. The therapist reviewed the criteria for problem definitions with Sandi, presented her with additional examples to discriminate, and gave tactful feedback that did not make her react defensively. The therapist used Sandi's reaction to point out to the dyad how well she was able to handle appropriate negative feedback.

At this point, the therapist introduced the rationale for communication training and targeted two negative communication habits: Mr. Holly's smirking laugh and Sandi's interruptions to make mind-reading statements about her father. These turned out to be the two most recurrent communication problems for this dyad. Sandi was prompted to give her dad feedback concerning any laughs she judged critical. She rehearsed ways to do this, and Mr. Holly attempted to modify his laughter in accord with her feedback. Mr. Holly in turn gave his daughter feedback when he noticed her interrupting and mind reading.

Communication training became somewhat convoluted as the dyad gave each other frequent in-session feedback on more and more detailed, minute aspects of their behavior. The therapist praised their efforts but redirected them to avoid getting bogged down.

Afterwards, the list of solutions and evaluations for the chores problem was reviewed. Sandi and Mr. Holly negotiated an agreement whereby Sandi would earn the privilege of going roller skating in 1 week if she (1) emptied the kitchen garbage daily and other trash containers Tuesdays and Thursdays; (2) helped her brother wash the dishes on weekends; (3) did her own laundry; and (4) got a positive report from school (her father had arranged for weekly written reports. As became apparent later, the school issue should have been handled separately, but at the time the therapist went along with their agreement).

Based on the high level of participation and verbal sophistication of both participants, the therapist hypothesized that the Hollys were capable of conducting at-home problem-solving tasks. Accordingly, homework consisted of implementing the solution to the chore problem, conducting an audiotaped problem-solving discussion of the use of the television, and giving each other feedback on laughs, smirks, and mind reading.

Session three continued to emphasize skill training. The dyad again completed their homework. Mr. Holly had noticed a definite improvement in Sandi's completion of chores and her school report, but a leg injury had prevented her from going skating. Since Sandi expected her leg to heal so that she could go skating the next week, the dyad planned to continue to implement this solution.

A review of the audiotaped home discussion of television use revealed that the father had dominated the talk, with Sandi too readily assenting to everything he proposed, recalling her high rate of agree–assent responses on the preassessment audiotaped discussion. During the home discussion she had agreed that if she completed all of her homework for 1 week, she could watch shows he deemed appropriate on the weekend. The therapist pointed out how Mr. Holly dominated the home discussion even though both had participated in discussions during treatment sessions. Sandi indicated that she was afraid to displease her dad by challenging him at home. Her father encouraged her to speak up if she disagreed and indicated he felt her lack of assertiveness was a general problem. Nonetheless, Sandi indicated that she was not yet comfortable contradicting his ideas and offering her own.

Later in the session the dyad began to solve the problem of Sandi's cleaning up her room. Although Mr. Holly defined the problem clearly, Sandi again got stuck stating her ideas. Modeling, behavior rehearsal, and gentle persuasion were used to prompt her finally to say, "He bugs me about cleaning up my room, and I'm satisfied with the room the way it is now." Time ran out partway through solution listing. The therapist asked the dyad to complete the discussion at home and also to talk about a concern Mr. Holly had voiced earlier in the session, Sandi's unwillingness to ask questions of her teachers. As in the second session, mind reading and paternal smiling were the communication skills targeted for change.

The dyad arrived for the fourth session with an audiotape of their homework discussions. They reported continued implementation of the chores agreement, but Sandi's weekly school report was unsatisfactory, again delaying the roller skating. Although they had not talked about room cleaning, they had talked about a variety of other issues, including Sandi's lack of assertiveness in school.

The second tape revealed a dramatic improvement in communication skills. Instead of dictating his ideas, Mr. Holly had used problem definition statements and had asked Sandi to use her paraphrasing skills to help her understand his viewpoint. The following excerpt illustrates this process:

MR. HOLLY: One of the things we talked about was the thing about you reacting to me or other adults as if you couldn't say what you really wanted to me or them just because they are adults. Do you know what I mean?

SANDI: No. You mean I wouldn't talk to you the same way I would talk to Sally or someone?

MR. HOLLY: No. Of course, you would talk differently, but, for instance, something might be wrong or you need something, and you would be afraid to ask. Like at school, if there's something you need cleared up with the teacher, you just let it go rather than talk to the teacher about it. But in my case, you know this thing we've talked about, where you assume I think or feel a certain way?

SANDI: Uhum.

MR. HOLLY: That's part of it. You won't say something to me or clarify something. You think I automatically think one thing even if I say something different because you don't hear me . . .

SANDI: *(Interrupting)* Yeah, I do.

MR. HOLLY: Because you think I'm thinking something when . . .

SANDI: *(Interrupting)* Something else?

MR. HOLLY: Yeah. That's something I'd like to resolve. It's a problem for me because it causes you to misunderstand me and others. Can you say what I think the problem is?

SANDI: Something like I'm afraid to ask you or any adult or my teacher anything because you think I would misunderstand?

MR. HOLLY: Let me say it again. The problem for me is that when you think I or other adults feel a certain way about something, you won't ask us about it because you assume you know how we feel. That leads to misunderstandings. Can you say that back?

SANDI: You're saying that I assume what you or other people are feeling and never really clarify it. Because of this, I misunderstand you or them.

MR. HOLLY: Right.

Later in this tape, Sandi gave her father feedback concerning a smirk that she interpreted negatively. He clarified his intent, and she perceived his mannerisms more benignly. The therapist was pleased to see the dyad self-correct a communication problem and the father make genuine efforts to reach out to his daughter.

The remainder of the fourth session was devoted to completing the discussion of the room-cleaning issue. An agreement was quickly reached: (1) Sandi would reorganize her room with her dad's help in a major spring cleaning; (2) afterwards, she would conduct smaller, weekly cleanups. Unfortunately, the discussion bogged down during planning of the implementation details since father and daughter had to reconcile their different interpretations of "clean." Mr. Holly was long-winded and picky about details, eliciting a defensive, restless response from his daughter. After therapist feedback about his lecturing style, the details were ironed out, and the dyad was assigned the task of implementing the solution.

Sessions Five and Six: Resolution of Intense Problems

Prior to the fifth session, treatment had proceeded in an ideal fashion. Skills were taught and acquired, homework was completed, and no major crises occurred between sessions. During the fifth session, a seemingly innocent remark by Mr. Holly unleashed a torrent of tears, sadness, and self-derogation from Sandi. The therapist was thus able to confront directly a central concern for the dyad—Sandi's absolutistic negative cognitions concerning disapproval and criticism, which mediated a variety of avoidance behaviors at home and at school, such as failing to complete homework and chores, denying responsibility for her mistakes, and shying away from assertive questions.

Searching for a topic to discuss, Mr. Holly suggested Sandi's interactions with boys. Asked whether she was willing to discuss this topic, she responded, "I don't care," a typical teenage response. Mr. Holly interjected that he thought his daughter's "I don't care" really meant "I care a lot but am afraid my dad and the therapist will be angry if I say I don't want to talk about boys." He inquired about the accuracy of his hypothesis. She responded that "I don't care means you adults are crushing in on me to make me do things your way."

A sudden change came over her face; there was a moment of silence, then she burst into tears. When she regained her composure, she revealed that she had a flashback to the beginning of fourth grade. The family had recently moved, and she was attending a new school for the first time. As the teacher introduced her to the class, they all began laughing because her last name (which has been disguised here) was homonymous with a word having common negative connotations. This experience had set the stage for protracted ridicule and teasing at school, shattering Sandi's already fragile self-concept. Peer taunting had continued to be a major problem for her since that episode. The proposed topic for discussion—boys—touched off this memory because boys teased her more than girls, and she believed that she had to be accepted by males before females would befriend her. She felt "crushed" by peers as well as adults.

Over the next 30 minutes Sandi remained tearful as she continued to reveal her sensitivity to ridicule. The therapist and her father aligned to provide reassurance and support while preventing Sandi from avoiding this painful but important topic. It became clear that Sandi adhered to the irrational belief that she must please all adults and peers. When anyone disapproved of her actions, she took it as evidence of her basic worthlessness. She related how she had told her father lies many times to avoid his disapproval, and how she reacted either aggressively to peer provocations or not at all. Behaviors that at first appeared rebellious now were understood as mechanisms to avoid anticipated disapproval. Interrupting to mind read adults, for example, was one strategy for softening the impact of disapproval by anticipating it.

After reframing Sandi's hypersensitivity as a positive characteristic that might help her to have a special understanding of others, the therapist gently shifted the discussion in a solution-oriented direction, that is, generating alternative behaviors she might emit when peers gave her dirty looks, bumped into her on purpose, or teased her verbally. Proposed solutions included (1) ignoring them, (2) fighting them, (3) coming back with assertive remarks, or (4) asking them to stop teasing her. The dyad evaluated the third solution as most likely to succeed, and as homework they were assigned the task of preparing Sandi to respond assertively when teased.

The theme of peer interactions also dominated the sixth session. Sandi was now able to talk openly and without tears about this problem. The experience of the fifth session, where she discovered adults would listen seriously to her concerns, appeared to desensitize her to the topic.

During the previous week the dyad had reviewed a variety of strategies for responding to teasing. Sandi related a series of recent teasing incidents. In one case a boy started calling her names and making obscene gestures at her; she ignored him, and her peers supported her and judged him inappropriate. Mr. Holly wondered whether he was really trying to express heterosexual interest in Sandi. Her female friends confirmed this hypothesis, permitting Sandi to view the situation realistically. The therapist used these incidents to challenge the belief that peer provocations confirmed Sandi's basic worthlessness. They then generated a list of common taunts and rehearsed possible verbal retorts; for example, if a girl were to say, "You're so short I can hardly see you," Sandi might reply, "At least my height is greater than your IQ." Sandi and her father reverse role-played peer provocations and assertive verbal responses to help prepare her for coping with them. Mr. Holly pointed out that Sandi's visibly hurtful reactions to teasing probably cued others that she was easily victimized, encouraging them to continue teasing her. Taking this new perspective on the problem, she began to realize why she encountered more teasing than did her friends.

The dyad also reported that all previously negotiated solutions were being implemented successfully and that a fruitful problem-solving discussion of the use of the telephone had been conducted at home during the previous week. The dyad had agreed that (1) Sandi could make 50 minutes of phone calls per day; (2) the maximum time per phone call was 30 minutes; and (3) Sandi would keep a written record of her calls.

As homework, the therapist asked the Hollys to discuss Sandi's relationship with boys and to implement the additional solutions to the peer ridicule problem. The family was also invited to bring a third member to the seventh session; they chose to bring Sandi's mother and requested the opportunity to talk about schoolwork.

Seventh Session: Disengagement

The mother–father–daughter triad attended the seventh session. Although the therapist was apprehensive about how easily the mother would be integrated into an ongoing therapeutic process, his fears were groundless. Mrs. Holly appeared to be a flexible, ebullient person, able to enter strong alliances with her husband in matters of control and discipline without jeopardizing her ability to align with Sandi to provide empathy and support. She had familiarized herself with the problem-solving outline prior to the session and had kept in close touch with the events of the previous sessions. The seventh session proceeded smoothly, almost as if Mrs. Holly had participated in all of the previous sessions.

A review of previously implemented solutions revealed that Mr. Holly and Sandi were generally satisfied with their outcomes. When asked about the use of the telephone, they responded that although Sandi forgot to keep a written list of her calls, her father had noticed a decrease in the overall amount of time she spent on the telephone.

Sandi showed considerable progress in the area of peer ridicule. She presented a list of reasonable proposed retorts to particular taunts, and indicated that she now attributed teasing to external factors (deficiencies in the attacker or environmental circumstances) rather than internal factors (her own inadequacy). Ignoring or assertively responding were her two most common weapons for fighting ridicule, exemplified in one case, when she was talking to a boy and a "big-mouthed" girl strutted over and asked the boy why he would want to be friendly with a "creep" like Sandi. The boy laughed, but Sandi ignored this provocation. Later, she asked the boy why he laughed and was pleased to learn he laughed at the girl's stupid question, not at Sandi, and had thought Sandi's response was mature. The therapist and Sandi's parents praised her confident reactions to situations that would have devastated her previously.

Following the review of homework, the family conducted an abbreviated discussion of playing the stereo too loudly. The therapist asked the family to run their own discussion. The discussion proceeded smoothly, with minimal interference from negative communication habits. The Hollys reached an informal agreement that Sandi and her father would be more tolerant of the other's taste in music. The discussion indicated that at least with manageable topics, the dyad had mastered basic problem-solving skills.

The final portion of the seventh session was devoted to a discussion of schoolwork. It quickly became apparent that this was a difficult issue when Sandi balked at discussing it. With hesitation, she indicated that she wished to complete her homework without interference from her parents and resented their intrusions into her academic affairs. In particular, she disliked her weekly school–home progress reports and her parents' requests to check her homework.

Mr. Holly acknowledged that ideally Sandi should complete homework without parental interference, but that her borderline grades and lack of candor about assignments suggested she was currently unable to work independently. He wished to monitor her progress closely until he was confident that she was prepared to succeed academically on her own. Just as Sandi had been unassertive with peers out of fear of disapproval, he hypothesized that she had been unassertive with teachers when she failed to understand material because she was afraid to appear stupid. Concurring with her husband, Mrs. Holly added that it was difficult to understand how Sandi had failed physical education, because of the reputation of this course as an "easy A." She speculated that Sandi lacked confidence in her athletic abilities and gave up without trying. She worried that the same pattern occurred in academic subjects.

Sandi protested that her parents were ganging up on her. Although defensive, she continued to talk with her parents and tried to produce evidence of recent improvement on tests. Her manner of responding to parental criticism revealed increased self-confidence. Unfortunately, time ran out before the discussion could be concluded. The therapist suggested working out a gradual process whereby increases in academic progress were accompanied by decreases in parental monitoring and to continue the discussion at home. In retrospect, schoolwork should have been addressed earlier in treatment, especially since the constraints of the research design prevented an additional session or two to finish resolving this issue.

Postassessment and Follow-Up

The dyad completed the postassessment measures during the next week and mailed back the follow-up measures 8 weeks later. On the IC the anger-intensity score decreased from preassessment to postassessment for father (1.9 to 1.2) and daughter (3.0 to 1.7). The quantity-of-issues score decreased slightly for the father but increased nearly 50% for the daughter. These changes indicated that, while the amount of conflict over specific issues had decreased, the amount of discussion reported between father and daughter appeared to have increased, at least in the daughter's eyes. On the CBQ, the dyad's appraisals of each other's behavior and their relationship improved substantially from pre- to postassessment (Mr. Holly, 6 to 3; Sandi, 11 to 5). These data suggested that relations at home had changed in a positive direction following treatment.

Examination of the PAICS data reveal that verbal productivity increased 38% and 75% for Mr. Holly and Sandi, respectively, from pre- to postassessment. Taken together with the daughter's self-reported increase in the quantity on issues on the IC, the verbal productivity data suggested that the dyad had attained their initial goal of increased communication. The frequency of positive behaviors increased, with the greatest gains on facilitation and humor. Although frequencies of negative behaviors also increased, the changes were primarily in interruptions. While this behavior is not necessarily a negative behavior in highly verbal families, it would be important to further analyze this pattern to ensure that Sandi's interruptions did not involve mind reading, a major problem for her initially.

Follow-up data revealed additional gains on the CBQ, with some backsliding on the IC; nonetheless, follow-up scores on the IC remained below preassessment levels. Inspection of individual items on the follow-up ICs revealed that several of the issues discussed during treatment (telephone calls and use of the television) remained mild sources of disagreement, while others (low school grades and cleaning up the room) were no longer problems. In general, the follow-up data suggested therapeutic gains were maintained over the 8-week interval.

Sandi and Mr. Holly were also asked to list anything learned during treatment that they had continued to use since termination and to rate family relations during the follow-up interval. Mr. Holly indicated that he continued to use feedback, problem definition statements, requests for reflections, and negotiation of solutions. He believed that family relations had remained stable since termination. Sandi indicated that family relations had improved since termination, but did not list any techniques that she continued to use. There were no further contacts with the family after follow-up.

Conclusion

This case nicely illustrates the interplay between the various components of intervention and, equally important, between the therapist's structuring and relationship skills. The therapist relied extensively upon problem solving to help the dyad resolve specific disputes. Not only did the dyad successfully implement specific negotiated solutions, but they also integrated the problem-solving approach into interactions at home. Formal homework assignments appeared to enhance this integration process. Communication training was interwoven throughout treatment as needed to correct misunderstandings and problematic interaction patterns. Despite the highly structured format of treatment and the constraints of the clinical research project, the therapist maintained sufficient flexibility to respond to crises—particularly the peer ridicule problem. When this problem arose, cognitive restructuring was introduced and two and one-half sessions were devoted to it, continuing to address the problem until gains were made.

Most of the specific disputes and communication deficits represented variations on a single theme—the daughter's reticence to express herself to others because of unreasonable fears of disapproval. In the early sessions, a skill-training approach was taken to this thematic problem. Later, a more cognitively oriented approach was emphasized. By termination, the daughter had begun to change both her attitudes and her behavior. The objective data corroborated the clinical impression of a successful treatment outcome.

The therapist was able to work successfully with this family in relatively few sessions for a number of reasons. First, the overall level of conflict was moderate. Second, the father was a reasonable, caring person who was not too threatened by his daughter's antics and was able to distance himself from situations and view them as problems in daily living, not catastrophic situations. Third, no marital conflict interfered with treatment. Fourth, the dyad complied with directives and completed homework assignments. Fifth, the therapist and dyad had good rapport, and most of the sessions were conducted in a light-hearted, humorous manner. Finally, there was a basic match between the "cerebral" style of the family and the "cerebral" nature of the therapist's cognitive–behavioral approach. In short, therapy was fun for everyone.

With respect to our behavioral–family systems model of parent–adolescent conflict (see Chapter 2), this case emphasized most strongly skill training and cognitive restructuring. Developmental changes set the stage for Mr. Holly and his daughter to have increased conflict around specific disputes and negative communication. The father's tendency to be verbose and critical, coupled with his daughter's dire need for approval and hypersensitivity to criticism, promoted conflict. He pursued her lapses in following rules, and she became increasingly defensive; reciprocal sequences of negative interaction escalated.

However, the family did not display significant structural problems, and functional/structural interventions were not emphasized during treatment. The parents worked as a team and there was little triangulation. Father–daughter conflicts did not disrupt the marriage but were handled within the father–daughter dyad, with the mother taking a supportive but nonintrusive stance. The case illustrates well how the clinician tailors intervention to the family, emphasizing only those treatment components that are relevant.

CASE TWO: THE MILLENSONS

The Millensons came to the clinic for treatment because of difficulties with their 15-year-old son Bill. Bill had recently been apprehended by the police on charges of stealing an automobile from a shopping center, going on a joyride, and accidently hitting a 10-year-old riding a bicycle. Bill fled the scene of the accident, and the 10-year-old was hospitalized with a concussion and a broken leg. Bill was released to his parents under house arrest until the case came to juvenile court. He had a recent history of school truancy, deteriorating grades, and disciplinary conflicts with his parents and teachers. He was also on probation for two instances of shoplifting at a shopping center near his home. Bill was the eldest of two adopted children and had a 10-year-old sister, Susan.

Case Description and First Session

It was apparent during the first session that the Millenson family was severely distressed and had multiple parent–adolescent, individual, and marital conflicts. Bill and his mother reported arguing incessantly about curfew, chores, home-work, school attendance, grades, and various other independence-related issues. Arguments erupted during most descriptions of their disagreements. Mrs. Mil-lenson, the primary disciplinarian, established rules for her son, which he openly defied. Afterwards, she yelled and lectured him. To reciprocate, Bill talked back, cursed, and rebelled even more against his mother's rules. Mother and son displayed clear excesses in negative communication and deficits in positive problem solving.

The mother voiced strong beliefs that Bill was totally irresponsible and likely to ruin his future. Bill believed his mother was terribly unfair, arbitrary, and out to persecute him. Their rigid adherence to these absolutistic cognitions of ruination, obedience, and unfairness aggravated conflicts already punctuated by skill deficits.

While Bill and his mother were enmeshed in an antagonistic relationship characterized by frequent negative exchanges and absolutistic thinking, Mr. Millenson maintained a distant, disengaged stance within the family. A success-ful programmer in a computing firm who often worked late and on weekends, he did not typically become involved in the day-to-day rearing of his children unless coerced by his wife. Relatively passive by nature and ineffectual as a dis-ciplinarian, Mr. Millenson was more lenient towards Bill than his wife was and did not support her efforts to cope with Bill's rebellious behavior. He spoke frequently in an intellectual, logical fashion and tended to ignore his own and others' feelings, while his wife frequently talked about her feelings and re-sponded impulsively and emotionally to a variety of issues. He avoided conflict at all costs, while she wished to bring disagreements out into the open and discuss them in depth.

A family history revealed that Mr. and Mrs. Millenson had disagreed over how to react to Bill's misbehavior for many years, with disagreement worsening at the onset of adolescence. Bill's early medical and developmental histories were normal. However, during preschool and grade school years, he behaved in a coercive, aggressive manner at home and was difficult to control. His mother had disciplined him sternly while his father had counseled reason and calm. Bill exploited their differences to get his way. At age 6 he was told he was adopted and began to display anger toward his mother. As time went on he began to talk about how he could not trust adults because his natural parents had given him away. During the first session he cited being adopted as the worst thing that had ever happened to him in his life.

The adoption theme played a prominent role in the present mother–son conflict. Bill believed strongly that neither his natural or adopted mother really wanted him, and that rules were imposed on him to drive him out of the home. He also talked about his adoption in ways that led him to obtain sympathy from others and to anger his mother. Occasionally, during the heat of an argument, Mrs. Millenson would make comments such as "maybe you should live somewhere else," confirming Bill's beliefs about his adoption.

The parent–teen conflict became heated once Bill reached junior high school. Mrs. Millenson had always objected to her husband's long hours, maintaining that Bill "needed a father." Mr. Millenson claimed he loved his job and that he could not cut his hours and maintain his position. As Bill approached adolescence, Mrs. Millenson became increasingly afraid that her son would be corrupted by delinquent, drug-taking peers. As Bill's increasing rebellious behavior had seemed to confirm her worst anxieties, she had become increasingly depressed and isolated, with few close friends to confide in and an unsympathetic husband who was rarely home. Her anger at her husband for what she saw as creating the problems with Bill set the stage for significant marital distress. Naturally, Mr. Millenson, a conflict avoider, withdrew further rather than confronting his wife's dissatisfaction. Her absolutistic, distorted perceptions of the threats posed by suburb-raised teenagers set the stage for her to impose strict regulations on her son in order to "protect" him from ruination. Bill recalled, for example, having a later curfew and more freedom to associate with peers at age 11 in his earlier neighborhood than at age 15 in his current environment. Bill interpreted the restrictions as rejections stemming from his adoption rather than maternal protective sanctions, adding yet another cognitive distortion to the family's array of difficulties.

Following the family session, Bill was interviewed individually. He came across as an angry, defensive youth with a poor self-image and a low tolerance for frustration. He indicated that when he wanted something, he acted to obtain it in the quickest, most direct manner, without considering the consequences. The automobile theft was a perfect example: He saw a car he wanted and took advantage of the situation without thinking about the repercussions. He was, however, reticent to talk about this incident, as well as his limited relationships with his peers. His impulsive behavior was evident in other areas of his life, such as the shoplifting, stealing money from his sister, evading rules, cutting classes, and lying to delay punishment. When asked about his inappropriate actions, he either denied them, explained that they were attempts to punish adults for unfair restrictions or putting him up for adoption, or acknowledged them with a great deal of self-denigration.

Together, this information revealed a clear-cut, circular pattern of interlock-

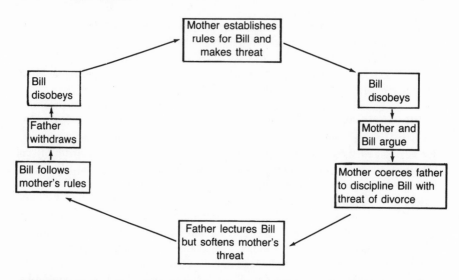

FIGURE 13-1 Sequence of interlocking contingency-related events for the Millenson family.

ing contingencies depicting serious functional/structural problems (see Figure 13-1). Bill's rebellion against his mother appeared to function to avoid limitations on his freedom while also indirectly resulting in positive reinforcement in the form of brief attention from his father, following severe disobedience against his mother. Mrs. Millenson's coercion of her husband to discipline was negatively reinforced by temporary reduction in conflict with Bill and positively reinforced by brief contact with her husband. Mr. Millenson avoided separation and divorce by eventually helping his wife with his son and avoided guilt by entering the family as a peacemaker. His intervention was also negatively reinforced by temporary suspension of mother–son conflict.

Overlying these functional interaction patterns were troublesome structural configurations. Bill and his father consistently formed a cross-generational coalition against his mother, with the father having the ability to increase or decrease his son's rebellion against his wife. Mrs. Millenson was overinvolved with her son, increasing his natural developmental tendency to rebel against her to achieve age-appropriate autonomy. The spouses had a disengaged, distant relationship characterized by clear marital disagreement about how to manage Bill, showing little indication that they had ever been able to work together as a team in this area.

Standardized Self-Report Measures

The family completed the CBQ, the IC, and Marital Satisfaction Inventory at home between the first and second treatment sessions. The triad's scores on the CBQ and IC were clearly consistent with extreme distress. On the CBQ both parents reported very poor dyadic communication with Bill (mother, 17; father, 13) and appraised Bill's communication behavior very negatively (mother, 36; father, 30). Bill reported slightly better communication and less conflict with his father (18) than with his mother (21). The IC data showed a similar pattern. The Millensons' scores were above normative means for distressed triads.

On the Marital Satisfaction Inventory, the parents' t scores of 64 to 71 on global distress, affective communication, problem-solving communication, and time together reflected excessive marital conflict common in couples seeking marital therapy (Snyder, 1981). The t scores of 69 and 78 on Conflict over Child Rearing reflected serious spouse disagreements over how to discipline Bill, while the discrepancy between Mrs. Millenson's high score and Mr. Millenson's low score on Dissatisfaction with Children reflected the difference in their perceptions of the severity of Bill's problematic behavior. Relatively little marital conflict was evident in specific areas of finances, sex, and families of origin. The low score on the Conventionalization scale suggested that the assessment was unlikely to have been biased by a social desirability response set.

In general, the self-report measures corroborated the therapist's impressions that (1) the overall level of parent–teen distress was severe; (2) mother–son relations were much more conflictual than father–son relationships; (3) the spouses were dissatisfied with their relationship, which was characterized by poor communication and inadequate problem solving; and (4) the spouses disagreed seriously over child-rearing issues and discipline.

Treatment Plan

The therapist recognized that the family's multiple parent–teen, marital, and personal problems predicted new crises erupting regularly. In addition, Bill's legal status was subject to change when his court hearing took place. The family's lawyer had advised them that if Bill went to therapy, attended school regularly, increased his grades, met his responsibilities at home, and did not get into further trouble in the community, the court might take a more lenient stance towards him.

Multifaceted interventions were obviously needed, but the upcoming court hearing and its uncertain outcome meant that long-term family treatment might not be possible. Therefore, the therapist decided to assign highest priority to reducing current conflicts between Bill and his parents concerning rules, based on the hypothesis that this might result in improvements in Bill's behavior at home and at school. Individual problems would be addressed (at least initially) within the context of family therapy. The therapist and the Millensons contracted for 10 sessions of family therapy, with the therapist spending an additional 30 minutes per week with Bill individually. The therapist hoped to use problem-solving communication training to change current conflict-resolution patterns and daily communication between family members. Cognitive–behavioral techniques might also be useful in helping Bill modify impulsive behaviors.

Sessions Two and Three: Skill Acquisition

Because the hostile interactions between Bill and his mother during the first family session had required frequent therapist interruptions to stop arguments, the therapist departed from standard procedures and trained the triad in basic communication skills before introducing problem solving. During the second session, the therapist used issues that arose over the course of the previous week as material for practicing clear, nonaccusatory expressions of affect, opinions, and verifications of meaning. The therapist modeled I-statements, then prompted the triad to rehearse similar statements and to paraphrase the speaker's content, checking for accuracy of understanding.

Put-downs and sarcasm continually crept into family members' attempts to state nonaccusatory opinions. Numerous corrections of inappropriate accusations and subtle sarcasm were necessary to teach positive behavior. Family members tried to "trap" each other, scoring put-downs, as in the following exchange:

BILL: I don't like it, Dad, when Mom is so strict.

THERAPIST: Mr. Millenson, please paraphrase Bill's statement.

MR. MILLENSON: You say Mom is strict, but what about the time she let you stay till midnight, and you came home high at 1 a.m.?

BILL: No, I didn't . . .

THERAPIST: Stop the action.

Bill attempted to state his opinion without an accusation, but his father's paraphrase culminated in a blaming question challenging the son's perceptions and dredging up the past. Bill also had great difficulty paraphrasing his parents' remarks accurately. Mr. Millenson repeated several times, "I insist he listen to me and consider what I say, but not blindly obey me." Bill understood his dad to require blind obedience, despite clarifications.

By the end of the session, the triad was beginning to make nonaccusatory statements of opinions and accurate paraphrases. Homework consisted of an assignment to practice such statements informally in daily interactions.

The week between the second and third sessions was uneventful: Bill tried to please his parents by following their rules and refraining from talking back to them. Although he felt his parents didn't appreciate his efforts, no major crises erupted. Family members reported predominantly neutral or positive interchanges with each other and had completed their homework. The rationale for learning a problem-solving strategy was given at the beginning of the third session, and the family chose to discuss Bill's cigarette smoking. On the IC, smoking had received higher anger-intensity ratings in the mother–adolescent (both mother and Bill scored their discussions as 5) than father–adolescent (father, 3; Bill, 1) dyads, as was typical for the Millensons.

The problem-solving discussion proceeded relatively smoothly for a first attempt with a severely distressed family. Bill defined the problem as "my

parents bug me about smoking and I want to smoke." Mrs. Millenson emphasized three aspects of the problem in her definition: (1) the high cost of
cigarettes, leading Bill to steal money; (2) the interference of smoking with
schoolwork, since he skipped classes to smoke; and (3) the "bad crowd" of peers
with whom Bill associated while smoking. Mr. Millenson objected to smoking
because of the health risks and Bill's hostile attitude when anyone attempted to
change his opinion about smoking.

They generated nine solutions:

1. Bill and his parents compromise on smoking.
2. Bill quits smoking.
3. Bill thinks about whether to smoke or not.
4. Bill smokes only outside the house.
5. Bill gets a job to pay for his cigarettes.
6. Bill stops cutting class or getting to class late in order to smoke.
7. Bill smokes only on weekends.
8. Parents ignore Bill's smoking.
9. Bill changes his attitude when parents talk to him about smoking.

Solutions one, five, and six were evaluated positively by everyone. An agreement was reached for (1) Mr. Millenson to accept Bill's smoking without
crusading to convince him to stop; (2) Bill to look for a part-time job to pay for
his cigarettes; (3) Bill to get to classes on time; and (4) Mrs. Millenson to
overlook smoking on the school grounds if Bill wasn't late for or missing classes.
As in session two, the therapist intervened repeatedly to correct accusatory
comments and prompt clear problem definition statements. Towards the end of
the meeting, Mr. Millenson expressed general pessimism about the possible
effectiveness of treatment, despite the successfully executed problem-solving
discussion. He indicated that Bill might promise to follow through with a
solution but would probably fail to live up to his promise. The family was
assigned the task of implementing the solution at home.

Sessions Four and Five: Resistance and Crisis

The Millensons appeared for the fourth session glum and angry. Mr. Millenson's
prediction of failure at solution implementation had come true, in part due to
parental sabotage fueled by the long-standing history of mutual mistrust. Bill had
read the help-wanted advertisements but had not applied for any jobs. His parents
decided that since he had not kept his agreement to look seriously for a job, they
would confiscate all his cigarettes. They searched his room and clothing in his
absence, infuriating Bill. Mrs. Millenson stated that Bill lacked the self-
confidence to seek a job and hadn't applied because he was afraid of being
rejected. Bill vehemently denied this and pointed out how his mother was again
persecuting him because she really hated him. Frequent and strong therapist

interruptions were necessary to short-circuit the mother–son accusatory–defensive interchanges.

Through judicious use of reflective listening, the therapist elicited Bill's fear that if he did find a job, his parents wouldn't permit him to spend his earnings as he wished. He therefore felt it was pointless for him to look seriously for work. Unfortunately, his parents confirmed his fear, indicating that they thought Bill could never be trusted to spend money wisely. In taking this position, they failed to understand how they were sabotaging the previous week's agreement, yet they then interpreted Bill's failure to look seriously for a job as further evidence of his basic untrustworthiness, placing their son in a classic double bind.

This crisis exemplifies the type of resistance encountered in behavioral family therapy. A seemingly positive change that would have given the adolescent increased autonomy and the parents evidence of increased teenage responsibility was resisted by everyone. The therapist examined carefully the "politics" of the family, illustrated in Figure 13-1, in search of a possible explanation for this resistant behavior.

If Bill had made a genuine effort at finding a job and his parents had supported the effort, the entire interlocking contingency pattern of the family would have been interrupted. Bill might have become more independent of his mother, decreasing mother–son conflict and leaving a vacuum in her life. Mr. Millenson would no longer have had an excuse to maintain a distant relationship with his wife and would not have been needed to enter the family as a peacemaker. The parents might have had to face their marital problems directly without adolescent misbehavior to distract them. While no one openly admitted to or discussed these interaction patterns, they served as hypotheses to guide the therapist.

Clearly, the therapist had not addressed this central functional/structural pattern effectively. The therapist decided to back off and treat the failure of the solution as an implementation problem, defuse extremist attitudes through cognitive restructuring, and negotiate in greater detail the ground rules for Bill's seeking employment. If the direct, logical approach failed after carefully planning the implementation details, the hypothesis about disruption of homeostatic functioning would be supported, and a more indirect strategy might be used to solve the problem. The family was given explicit feedback about how their pessimistic, absolutistic statements polarized their interactions and became self-perpetuating prophecies of failure. They were encouraged to treat the solution as an experiment to be conducted, with the possibility that it might work. Mr. and Mrs. Millenson agreed to give Bill a second chance to look for jobs, to stop confiscating his cigarettes, and to consider permitting him to spend his earnings as he wished. Bill agreed to apply for several jobs. The session ended on a somber note.

Family interactions went from bad to worse between the fourth and fifth sessions. The smoking issue was eclipsed by a new crisis. The school called to inform the parents that Bill was skipping so many classes and arriving late so often that he was in danger of losing all his academic credits for the year. He was also loitering around the local shopping center after school and not coming home until just before dinner, contrary to a previous agreement to come home directly from school. At the beginning of the fifth session, family members were depressed, and trust was at an all-time low. Mr. and Mrs. Millenson felt that Bill was making no effort to follow the lawyer's suggestion to demonstrate increased responsibility at home and at school. A date had been set for an initial court hearing, heightening the tension. Bill felt that he was demonstrating responsibility and denied all wrongdoing. The parents and teenager argued bitterly even over facts such as what time he came home the previous night. Mrs. Millenson began dropping Bill off and picking him up at school with a threat to escort him from class to class if necessary. Bill was permanently grounded except for attending school. Mr. Millenson took little responsibility for this increased control, preferring as usual to have his wife deal with their son. Naturally, Bill's negative perception of his mother's overcontrolling behavior was aggravated. He decided that his privacy had been violated to the point where "I don't care about any rules." He openly defied the additional restrictions, sneaking out of the house when his mother wasn't watching. Even his father's intervention failed to bring Bill in line.

The therapist hypothesized that either Bill wanted to have "one last fling" before the court hearing or was trying to force his mother to expel him from the family. An individual interview with Bill confirmed the impression that he felt helpless, worthless, isolated, and deserving of severe punishment. He reported having nightmares about seeing a boy whom he had hit with the car lying on the street in pain as Bill pulled away from the scene of the accident. Although angry, Mrs. Millenson perceived the seriousness of her son's depression and self-derogation and was very worried about Bill. Her husband failed to see anything but Bill's rebellious behavior as a problem.

The therapist predicted an imminent, even more severe crisis if the cycle of reciprocal negative interactions escalated further. Despondent, hopeless, and impulsive, Bill could easily attempt suicide, run away, or commit another delinquent act. To conduct a problem-solving discussion would have been tantamount to placing the burden for finding solutions to avoid a crisis on an already overburdened family. Instead, the therapist intervened directly by negotiating a graduated reciprocal initiative in tension reduction (see Chapter 7). With this technique, one family member is convinced to announce a "spontaneous" de-escalation of a conflict, taking the others by surprise and compelling them to follow suit with further de-escalations. Meeting with the parents, the therapist emphasized the depths of their son's depression and self-derogation. They were told that as the responsible adults in charge of a minor, they needed to take the first step toward reducing tension. If they relaxed a restriction, Bill would be likely to reciprocate by increasing his level of compliance with rules, prompting restoration of trust. To circumvent their objections to giving in to a misbehaving youth, the therapist reframed relaxing a rule as a charitable gesture by wise parents who wished to use a sophisticated strategy to overcome their son's resistance to change. The Millensons agreed to permit Bill to stay out until 11 p.m. one weekend evening. In an individual meeting with Bill, the therapist then emphasized that while he didn't think it was possible for Bill's parents to make large concessions, he would stand up to them for Bill and fight for one small concession since he understood how "caged in" Bill felt. However, the therapist could only help Bill if Bill could absolutely assure him of compliance with the changed rule. Bill promised to comply.

Having preprogrammed the reciprocal de-escalation, the therapist brought the triad together. When the parents announced the change in weekend curfew, Bill was pleased and agreed to comply. They decided that failure to follow the agreement would be handled by the therapist at the next session, not by the family at home.

Sessions Six through Eight: Calm and Storm

At the sixth session the family reported that everyone had complied with the curfew agreement and was pleased at the outcome. Family relations had been relatively peaceful throughout the week. The agreement was extended for another week, despite the father's concern that Bill was "getting something for nothing." The graduated reciprocal initiative in tension reduction had temporarily interrupted the escalating cycle of negative reciprocity, giving the therapist room to maneuver.

Most of the session was devoted to an individual meeting with Bill, since the therapist believed his continued positive response to the parents' peace offering was essential to restore enough trust to permit successful implementation of solutions to any future problem-solving discussions. Bill revealed that he had recently had suicidal thoughts but no specific plan to hurt himself. He continued to obsess over the car theft and injury to the child in a self-blaming fashion. He also revealed that he currently felt that he had no close friends and that he perceived himself to be an outsider at school as well as at home. The seriousness of this youth's distress, especially his isolation from any close interpersonal relationships and his deep fears about the court case, became increasingly clear at this time. However, the therapist did not judge Bill in immediate danger of suicide since the recent curfew agreement with his parents had reduced the crisis atmosphere and relaxed tension at home considerably. The therapist decided to try to increase positive interactions between Bill and his father by assigning joint father–son tasks in the near future, with the goal of interrupting negative functional patterns by giving the father a nonthreatening alternative to his peacemaker role and providing Bill with paternal attention not contingent on negative behavior.

During the seventh session the family reported that Bill had again been permitted to go out on the weekend, but had returned home 1 hour late. Bill claimed his friend got a flat tire, delaying his return. This infraction was handled without an argument, a real accomplishment for the Millensons. The parents postponed disciplinary action until the therapy session in accordance with the therapist's request. The therapist briefly informed Bill that the agreement would be suspended for 1 week, a consequence accepted by everyone. Mr. and Mrs. Millenson reported attempting to use positive communication skills with their son and to overlook minor rule infractions. Mrs. Millenson had become much more attuned to her style of interacting with her son. For the first time since therapy began, Bill complimented his mother for talking nicely to him throughout the week. He had reciprocated by spontaneously accelerating his assistance with household chores. Mother and son appeared less depressed than the previous week. The therapist was guardedly optimistic. Building upon the recent positive interactions, the therapist coached Bill and his mother to exchange compliments and carry on a nonconflictual conversation during the session. As homework, Bill and his father were assigned the task of going someplace without his mother.

The eighth session took place the evening before Bill's court appearance. Two nights before, Bill had ingested a bottle of aspirin in a suicide attempt and was rushed to a local hospital, where vomiting was induced before physical damage was done. He was quickly released. Bill had been very frightened about the court hearing and had not wanted to face it. He claimed the suicide attempt was "stupid" and that he would never again try it, but the therapist considered whether Bill should be hospitalized to avoid another suicide attempt. A careful review of the incident revealed that Mr. and Mrs. Millenson had both reacted strongly and swiftly with appropriate concern, strengthening Bill's perception that they cared about him and did not want to expel him from the family, and actually drawing the family closer together. The therapist suspected that Bill's suicide attempt was in part designed to obtain a sympathetic response from his parents and test the hypothesis, "They hate me." The therapist judged Bill not to be in immediate danger of another attempt, and after warning his parents to watch him carefully prior to future court hearings, dropped the idea of hospitalization. The therapist then returned to the original agenda of treatment— helping the family improve problem-solving communication and resolve basic conflicts.

Framing Bill's suicide attempt as his way of testing his parents' concern for him, the therapist suggested that Bill might learn to ask important questions about his relationship with his parents in a more direct, less harmful manner. Mrs. Millenson began to cry, and Bill revealed that her tears inhibited him from asking her questions because he felt terribly guilty when she cried. This comment set the stage for a communication training session designed to teach the dyad to exchange affectual messages. The therapist prompted the parents to encourage Bill to ask questions or express any feeling he wished. Bill asked to be told the circumstances surrounding his adoption and whatever was known about his natural parents. For the first time, his parents presented the small amount of factual information they had about Bill's natural parents and the adoption. He was genuinely appreciative. This discussion transpired with minimal accusation, defensive comments, or other negative communication habits, to stark contrast to earlier discussions.

The therapist also asked the family to reach a revised agreement to reinstate Bill's late curfew on weekends. After a circumscribed problem-solving discussion, again characterized by minimal interference from negative communication habits, they agreed to permit Bill an 11 p.m. curfew one weekend night if he came home from school by 3:30 p.m. Tardiness and skipping classes were no longer reported by school authorities, representing improvement in these areas. During the previous week, Bill and his father had gone out to lunch together. Homework assignments were for Bill and his father to engage in another joint activity and for the family to implement the revised curfew agreement. The session ended on an upbeat note.

Session Nine: Interlude

On the way to the ninth session, Mrs. Millenson accused her son of taking money from his sister and father, provoking an argument in the car. The family entered the session angry and hostile. The therapist devoted considerable time to modeling, rehearsing, and giving feedback concerning nonaccusatory problem definition statements about stealing, preparing the family to generalize the use of such statements to crises at home. After several attempts, Mrs. Millenson was able to say, "I get upset when money disappears from our home, and Bill's past behavior leads me to believe he took it." Bill defined the problem as "I get angry when my mom falsely accuses me of taking money." The family became bogged down during the solution-listing phase of the discussion, unable to generate more than a few highly punitive options.

Remembering the resistance to implementation of the smoking solution, the therapist decided to prescribe an indirect, paradoxical solution to the problem. The family was asked to conduct a 1-week "experiment" designed to test the hypothesis, "Bill is dishonest and steals his family's money." The parents were convinced Bill had stolen the money and were concerned that he might repeat such thefts. Bill vehemently denied stealing. Aware of Bill's previously documented thefts and his impulsive tendency to act without considering consequences, the therapist doubted (but did not express aloud) the veracity of Bill's denials. The therapist instructed the parents to designate a sum of money for the experiment and purposely leave it scattered in several locations throughout the house. If the money disappeared within the week, they were to conclude that Bill was dishonest. If the money remained, they were to conclude that he was honest. Bill agreed to participate in this experiment. By making explicit the rules for evaluating Bill's honesty and challenging him to refrain from stealing money, the therapist hoped to induce Bill to consider the consequences of his actions and stop taking money. Since Bill was claiming to be honest, he couldn't easily refuse to participate in the experiment without appearing guilty. If successful, the "experiment" was to be continued over a number of weeks.

Aside from the argument over stealing, family relations had been moderately positive throughout the past week. The weekend curfew agreement had been successfully implemented, and the father and son had spent time together for a second week. Bill had shown no additional suicidal tendencies. His court hearing had been preliminary and procedural, with a substantive hearing scheduled for the next week. The therapist instructed the parents to call if they noticed severe depression and/or recurring suicidal tendencies before the second court hearing.

Session Ten: Premature Finale

At this time the reality of Bill's criminal offense overtook the pace of treatment. At the second court hearing, the judge made Bill a ward of the court until age 19, and remanded him for an indefinite period to a local therapeutic facility for juvenile offenders. Until an opening was available at the juvenile facility, the judge gave the family a choice of placing Bill in a psychiatric hospital or a juvenile detention center. The family was shocked, believing the court had acted harshly for a youth of Bill's age. The family's lawyer indicated that they had been lucky Bill had not been tried as an adult. Bill was extremely frightened and agitated but not suicidal. He reportedly handled himself in a polite, adultlike manner in court. Distraught and tearful, Mrs. Millenson called the therapist to seek recommendations. The therapist was supportive and advised that psychiatric hospitalization was preferable to juvenile detention. He made arrangements for Bill to enter an adolescent inpatient program as soon as possible.

The tenth and final session, conducted the night before Bill was to enter the hospital, was a somber occasion. Bill refused to leave the car and enter the clinic. The therapist talked with him alone in the car, taking a supportive stance. Bill was clearly agitated, trembling with fear, in touch with reality but near panic. He felt extremely guilty about his actions, worthless, and depressed.

The parents also felt depressed and guilty. They blamed themselves for their son's misdeeds and reported feeling helpless. For the first time, Mr. Millenson cried. The therapist reframed inpatient treatment as the intensive help Bill needed to get started in the right direction.

Bill went into the hospital the next morning, with trepidation but without resistance. The therapist had several phone conversations with Mrs. Millenson afterwards but no further sessions. The psychiatrist at the hospital convinced the court to permit Bill to remain in an inpatient psychiatric hospital rather than be transferred to a juvenile facility. Bill was hospitalized for 4 months. He reportedly participated actively in ward activities, individual therapy, and family sessions at the hospital. The staff felt he was beginning to overcome his depression and gain increased self-confidence. While Bill was in the hospital, his father sought and obtained a new job with fewer time demands in another part of the country and arranged for the family to move. With encouragement from the psychiatrist, the court agreed to transfer the case to the juvenile authorities in the new location and release Bill on probation if he continued in therapy there. Mrs. Millenson called the therapist to provide details of the impending move and thank him for his help. She was excited about the possibility of a fresh start in a new environment. The fact that her husband had taken steps to relocate the family reaffirmed his genuine commitment to them and strengthened the marriage. Mrs. Millenson thanked the therapist for the two things she felt helped her the most: (1) support and empathy during times of real family crisis; and (2) help getting her son into a psychiatric hospital rather than a juvenile facility. It was interesting that the skill-training component of treatment was not a feature she recalled as helpful. After the family moved, there were no further contacts with the therapist.

In retrospect, behavioral family therapy was, at best, marginally successful with the Millensons. At intake the family had been severely distressed, with skill deficits, cognitive distortions, intrapersonal problems, and marital conflict. To treat them with problem-solving communication training alone would have been akin to putting a Band-Aid on a gunshot wound. A broader approach was undertaken, with skill training as one component. On the positive side, some progress was made in interrupting reciprocally negative parent–adolescent interactions, and several specific agreements were successfully implemented at home. The sequence of interlocking contingencies depicted in Figure 13-1 was partially interrupted. By termination, the mother–father coalition had become stronger, as indicated by their joint disciplinary decision making; the father had also become less disengaged from his family, and Bill no longer needed to rebel to make contact with his father and avoid an overprotective, enmeshed relationship with his mother. But time ran out before Bill's impulsive behavior could be modified, the factors promoting the car theft could be addressed, the parents' basic marital conflicts could be resolved, or positive problem-solving communication skills could be overlearned to the point where generalization across time and settings was highly probable.

Apparently the disruption of homeostatic functioning caused by the court action and Bill's hospitalization had a positive impact on the system. Mr. Millenson finally responded to his wife's cry for more involvement in the family and marriage and arranged for a complete change of environment for the family. To the extent that Bill's rebellious behavior functioned to coerce his father to attend to his mother and the family, Bill achieved the ultimate "success" with his conviction and hospitalization, but at great emotional cost to the family. Ironically, the original therapeutic contract for 10 sessions was strictly followed.

NOTE

1. An abbreviated version of this case was reviewed in Robin (1979). Names and details of both cases have been altered to protect confidentiality.

CHAPTER FOURTEEN

Treatment Outcome Research

The ultimate determinant of the lifespan of any treatment is its effectiveness. Ineffective therapeutic approaches are ultimately doomed, regardless of their conceptual elegance and intellectual or personal appeal. Data-based investigations have replaced unsubstantiated testimonials over the past three decades as methods of evaluating treatment outcome. This chapter explores how problem-solving communication training has fared empirically in changing disturbed parent–adolescent relations. We then turn to a summary of comparable approaches in a search for shared outcome-enhancing components of effective but differently focused family treatments.

RESEARCH QUESTIONS IN FAMILY THERAPY

Documentation of therapy effectiveness can take many forms, depending upon the research question the investigator poses. Among the more important of these questions are those listed below, each accompanied by an overview of associated methodological concerns. Because evaluation of problem-solving communication training has used group designs, we will not consider issues involved in single-subject treatment evaluation (see Hersen & Barlow, 1976, and Kazdin, 1982, for detailed coverage of single-subject strategies).

Is Treatment Actually Necessary? Will the problem resolve itself in the absence of treatment? This issue is particularly relevant in child and family outcome research, where a child's maturation may set processes in motion that produce "spontaneous" cures. To control for maturation, a treated group may be compared with untreated controls. When a "pure" no-treatment control group is unfeasible or unethical, a wait-list control group is often employed.

Neither of these strategies is completely problem-free. It can be argued that a wait-list group is not a true control for mere passage of time, as the expectation of imminent treatment may alter families' behavior at home during the waiting period and/or responses to assessment instruments at the end of the waiting interval. In addition, studying control groups over a period of only a few weeks may be insufficient. This may be particularly true for parent–adolescent relations, which are popularly believed to be fluid, with heightened conflict disappearing and reemerging throughout adolescence. Two studies Kent and O'Leary (1976, 1977) conducted with preadolescent children illustrate how maturation can wipe out treatment effects. They compared the classroom behavior of children receiving behavior therapy with that of no-treatment control children immediately before and after treatment and at 1-year follow-up. While the treated group was superior to the control group at postassessment, the control group improved considerably over the follow-up interval. By follow-up, there were no differences between the groups.

What Is the Long-Term Impact of Treatment?   The long-term impact of treatment refers to maintenance of treatment effects, typically assessed after some follow-up interval. As just mentioned, following an untreated control group as well as treated families is extremely desirable, although not always practically or ethically feasible.

Drop-out is a particular problem in follow-up assessment—families are unavailable or refuse to complete follow-up data collection procedures (O'Leary & Turkewitz, 1978). If the initial number of families is small, drop-out can reduce the number of subjects to the point where inferential statistics lose power and meaning. On the other hand, including the data of the families that later dropped out in statistical comparisons and estimating follow-up scores can produce misleading results and conclusions (Kent, 1976). In addition, Oltmanns, Broderick, and O'Leary (1977) found that follow-up data were most difficult to obtain from families who appeared to have benefited least from treatment. If this finding represents a widespread phenomenon, follow-up data from subjects who agree to participate should be analyzed separately from subjects who drop out and interpreted in light of the potentially biased subsample of the treated population that they represent.

What Is the Locus of Treatment Effects?   A variety of domains can be examined in search of the consequences of treatment. Rosen and Proctor (1981) point out that therapy evaluation should address at least two types of outcomes. The first are what they term ultimate outcomes; these usually involve clients' presenting problems, and their achievement is sufficient for termination and leads to the conclusion that therapy has been successful. The second type of outcomes they call instrumental; these are defined more by the theory the therapist holds than by the problems the client brings in. These are the outcomes that a theoretical framework postulates are sufficient, when taken together, to produce ultimate outcomes—that is, resolution of presenting problems. Instrumental outcomes of effective problem-solving communication training for all families should be enhanced verbal problem-solving and communication behaviors, generalized use of those behaviors at home, altered systemic interaction patterns, and decreased conflict about problems resolved during therapy. When cognitive distortions and misattributions have also been targeted for treatment, changes in cognition would also become instrumental outcomes. Ultimate outcomes would depend on the family, but might include increased relationship satisfaction, decreased feelings of anger, resentment, and hostility among family members, and reduced conflict around various issues.

Failure to measure directly the predicted locus of treatment effects confuses interpretations of treatment outcome research. If the treatment produces improvements on measures of ultimate outcomes, is this because of changes in targeted behaviors, skills, and so forth, or is it a function of some unrecognized but important alternate aspects of treatment? Conversely, if treatment fails to produce desired ultimate outcomes, it could be due to an ineffective therapy *or* to therapists' poor implementation of a valid treatment, achieving no instrumental outcomes. The correlated presence of instrumental and ultimate outcomes does not prove that the former produce the latter. However, the absence of instrumental effects when ultimate effects are present does indicate that the aspects of therapy reflected in measures of instrumental outcomes were not essential for producing changes in the clients' presenting problems.

This is not to deny the importance of measuring ultimate outcomes. Evaluation of ultimate outcomes is particularly important when therapy focuses almost exclusively on behavior change, and is susceptible to the criticism that statistically significant behavior changes can be personally meaningless to family members. Kazdin (1977) and Wolf (1978) have convincingly argued that changes in behavior must be shown to have social significance or "validity" for the consumers of these changes and recommend assessment of subjective judgments as one method of documenting important ultimate outcomes. An alternate way is to establish and monitor progress toward family members' goals, which presumably are quite meaningful to the individuals who provided them. From alternate theoretical orientations, Gurman and Kniskern (1978) and Olson (1977) have argued for including multiple perspectives in outcome assessment, some of which represent measures of ultimate outcomes.

How Does the Treatment Compare with Alternative Therapies?   Does problem-solving communication training produce greater improvement in family functioning than do available alternatives, such as strategic family therapy? The usual approach to this question employs comparative group outcome studies in which two or more treatment methods are pitted against each other as well as a control group.

Appropriately executed comparative group outcome studies require attention to several methodological factors that do not arise in simpler treatment-versus-control outcome investigations (Gurman & Kniskern, 1978; O'Leary & Turkewitz, 1978). First, treatments should be equally valued by clients and therapists. Second, therapists should be selected carefully. When different individuals conduct the alternative treatments, they should be matched on experience level, number of therapists per condition, and experience with the approach they are using. A sufficient number of therapists should be used to ensure generalizability to the broader population of therapists. This is particularly important if the investigators are also therapists, which should be avoided because of the possibility that investigators' investment in treatment outcome will influence their behavior as therapists in unreported and unreplicable ways (Gurman & Kniskern, 1978; O'Leary & Turkewitz, 1978). Using the same therapists to conduct different interventions does control for some of the matching factors described above, but therapists may also have stronger theoretical orientations, more experience, and greater personal biases toward one of the treatments than toward the others, thus producing confounding variables. To mitigate this problem, O'Leary and Turkewitz suggest using several therapists with different orientations and providing intensive training in the alternative approaches. Gurman and Kniskern also recommend that the length and duration of treatment be equated. This is difficult, however, when a brief therapy is compared with a therapy that posits, as a crucial assumption, that treatment requires many hours over a long time period.

Additional issues concern dependent variables chosen for the study. Measures should be "fair" to all treatment approaches, providing adequate tests relevant to each treatment's presumed instrumental goals. Changes in projective test responses, for example, might be a good instrumental measure for psychoanalysis but a poor way of assessing behavioral methods. Ideally, measures of ultimate outcomes should be the same for all treatments, and assessments of instrumental outcomes should include measures relevant to the theoretical mechanisms by which each treatment is presumed to operate.

Finally, a check on the manipulation of the independent variables documents that the treatments were actually conducted as prescribed (O'Leary & Turkewitz, 1978). This is especially important when treatments are quite similar and the investigator must insure that therapists did not inadvertently include elements of one treatment in the other approach.

Which Aspects of Treatment Account for Its Effects? Investigations addressing this issue attempt to identify necessary and sufficient conditions for family change. Factorial designs test all different combinations of relevant treatment components and allow estimates of the effects of various aspects of treatment when offered both individually and with other components. An example of a factorial design might be to compare problem-solving communication training, cognitive restructuring, problem-solving communication training with cognitive restructuring, and no treatment.

A less informative but also less demanding alternative to a factorial design involves comparing only two treatments, one of which adds a new component to the other. Problem-solving communication training, for example, could be compared to problem-solving communication training with cognitive restructuring added. This allows an estimate of the additive effects of cognitive restructuring when combined with PSCT, but does not permit an evaluation of the effects of cognitive restructuring per se.

Factorial designs share many of the methodological requirements of comparative group outcome studies. An additional concern lies in time allocated to combined treatments versus single-component treatments. In the example just given, it would be important to avoid enriching the problem-solving communication training treatment received by the families not receiving cognitive restructuring, as the problem-solving communication training component of the two groups' intervention would not be comparable. On the other hand, it is also important to equate the amount of therapist contact for the groups. There is no perfect solution to this problem, but a partial resolution can be achieved by using identical treatment components in different groups, and equating the amount of therapist contact by including a certain amount of nonspecific conversation in the less complex intervention to fill the extra time required to make it comparable to the treatments with more components.

Which Families Benefit Most from Treatment? Underlying this question is the assumption that families do not all derive equal benefits from a given therapy. Different treatments may be appropriate for different families, depending on factors such as the nature of the presenting problem, family structure, and socioeconomic status.

Several methods can be used to explore this issue empirically. Statistical analyses can be conducted after an outcome study is completed. Families can be sorted into groups based on the variable of interest (e.g., single-parent vs. dual-parent household) and the amount of change from pre- to postassessment can be examined to see if any of the different groups improved more than others. Alternatively, correlations between change scores and family variables can be computed.

More complex research explorations build in family type as an independent variable in the design of the outcome study. For example, families might be categorized based on the age of the adolescent (junior high vs. high school age), then randomly assigned within each group to the treatment(s) under investigation. Subsequent analyses would explore whether treatment was more (or less) effective with families with younger adolescents than with families with older teens. Of course, it is important in this type of design to ensure that different subgroups of families are equivalent prior to treatment on family variables other than those under investigation, in order to ensure that differences in extraneous characteristics could not account for any differences found in the groups' responses to treatment.

Ideal Evaluation Criteria

The review of research questions in family therapy suggests a number of "ideal" criteria against which to evaluate existing research on problem-solving communication training and related approaches:

1. To determine whether treatment is actually necessary, investigators should at minimum compare intervention to wait-list or no-treatment controls using random assignment of participants to conditions.

2. To determine the long-term impact of treatment, investigators should conduct follow-ups of treated and, wherever possible, untreated groups over

follow-up intervals at least 6–12 months. When there is a significant dropout problem, analyses should be conducted separately for families who remain and who drop out.

3. The ultimate and instrumental goals of treatment should be clearly operationalized, and multidimensional, psychometrically sound measures of each type of effect should be collected.

4. Checks should be made to ensure that the treatment is implemented as prescribed.

5. In comparative outcome studies, therapists should be comparable, dependent measures should be fair to different treatments, and length of treatment should be equated as much as possible.

6. In component analyses, factorial designs should be employed whenever feasible, following guidelines for comparative outcome studies.

7. Treating family characteristics as independent variables in the design of studies is the most appropriate way to determine which families benefit most from which treatment.

RESEARCH ON PROBLEM-SOLVING COMMUNICATION TRAINING

Having discussed general considerations related to family outcome research, we now turn to specific studies designed to answer some of these questions with regard to problem-solving communication training. Robin (1975) conducted an initial study as a doctoral dissertation; Robin et al. (1977) later published this in abbreviated form. This investigation evaluated whether a basic problem-solving communication training package was more effective than no treatment in reducing mother–adolescent conflict. Twenty-two mother–adolescent dyads were recruited by newspaper and radio announcements describing a program to help mothers and adolescents improve their communication. Participants were blocked according to severity of arguments and socioeconomic status, then randomly assigned to either a wait-list control group or problem-solving communication training. Children ranged in age from 11 to 14, and half were female.

Three graduate students in clinical psychology provided treatment for five sessions. The first three sessions included modeling, coaching, behavior rehearsal, and social reinforcement to teach the dyads the basic skills of problem solving with hypothetical problems of gradually increasing difficulty. During the last two sessions, mother–adolescent dyads practiced the skills using real problems they identified in their own relationship. Therapists also targeted and corrected communication styles as they interfered with the problem-solving sequence.

Measures were administered before and after training, to assess acquisition of problem-solving skills. Mother–adolescent dyads were audiotaped discussing both a hypothetical and a real problem, and these tapes were later coded by trained observers who counted the frequencies of each component behavior in the problem-solving process. Treated mothers and teenagers showed large, significant gains in problem-solving behaviors on both hypothetical and real problems; control dyads did not.

Questionnaire measures tapped mother and adolescent perceptions of changes in communication and conflict. The Communication Checklist assessed perceptions of the audiotaped discussion, while two Communication Habits Surveys surveyed perceptions of communication–conflict behavior (i.e., blaming, lying, interrupting) and frequency and intensity of discussion of specific issues at home (the second of these surveys was a forerunner of the IC). Analyses revealed in general that families perceived little change in their behavior at home, although treated mothers' data showed a trend toward decreases in specific disputes following treatment. However, when individual items were analyzed using sign tests to assess the direction of reported changes, the treated group (particularly mothers) showed significantly more change in positive directions than did the control group on most measures.

The preassessment measures also included a measure of perceived level of parental authoritarianism in child rearing—Elder's (1962) 7-point scale of decision making, including autocratic, authoritarian, democratic, egalitarian, permissive, laissez faire, and ignoring. Adolescents rated mothers' and fathers' decision-making style, while mothers provided self-ratings. When level of parental authoritarianism was correlated with problem-solving behavior, an interesting pattern emerged. There were no significant relationships between problem-solving behavior and adolescent ratings of parental authoritarianism at preassessment, but there were moderate correlations between these adolescent evaluations of mothers prior to treatment and problem-solving behavior after treatment ended ($rs = .51–.54$). These findings suggest that adolescent perceptions of mothers as democratically oriented in decision making predicted more positive outcomes following problem-solving training.

This preliminary investigation indicated that problem-solving communication training procedures led to acquisition of component steps of problem solving in an analogue clinic observation. However, mothers and teens reported little change in specific disputes or communication at home. Because the psychometric properties of the questionnaire measures were unknown and the treatment had been very circumscribed, it was impossible to ascertain whether the limited results were a function of inadequate measures or treatment methods (or both).

In a subsequent study, Foster (1978; also reported by Foster *et al.*, 1983) broadened the intervention, included measures with sounder psychometric backing, and replicated and extended Robin's work. Three questions were addressed: (1) What is the impact of problem-solving training, relative to no treatment? (2) Are treatment effects maintained over time? and (3) What are the additive effects of strategies designed to enhance generalization of basic problem-solving communication training?

To answer these questions, 28 families with an adolescent between the ages of 10 and 14 were recruited by newspaper notices announcing a communication training program. These families were blocked according to severity of conflict based on CBQ scores and randomly assigned to either a wait-list control or to one of two treatment groups. One treatment (skill training) consisted of seven sessions of problem-solving communication training, emphasizing skill building but not skill use at home. The second group (skill training plus generalization) received the same training and, in addition, a generalization program. The generalization program consisted of weekly homework assignments of graduated difficulty and discussions in sessions about homework and about how to use communication and problem-solving skills at home. To equate the treatment groups for the amount of skill building, the skill-training group spent the first and last 10 minutes of each session in nonspecific discussion, while the generalization group discussed issues related to home use of their skills. Coding of audiotapes of the first and last 10 minutes of each therapy session verified that significantly more discussion of both communication and problem solving at home occurred during sessions with the generalization families than with the skill-training families.

The skill-training component of treatment differed in several important respects from that employed by Robin. Fathers (in two-parent families) were included. Treatment was lengthened to seven sessions, and families worked only with real problems, starting with simpler, less anger-provoking topics, then gradually advancing to more difficult issues. Therapists also had the option of spending one session on crisis intervention, working on a specific communication skill or some topic other than problem solving, if needed. As in the Robin study, therapists were graduate students in clinical psychology (two of the same therapists participated in both studies).

Measures included the IC, CBQ, and Daily Home Reports. Audiotapes of 10-minute mother–child discussions of a currently troublesome, real problem were rated using two observation codes: the IBC and a problem-solving verbal behavior code similar to that employed by Robin. In addition, during the pretreatment assessment session, each family member set specific goals for what s/he would like to accomplish during the training program and later rated achievement of these goals. IC, CBQ, and observational measures were collected before and after treatment for all three groups; the two treated groups were assessed again at a 6–8-week short-term follow-up. Goal ratings were collected at postassessment and at follow-up.

At postassessment and at follow-up, each family in the two treated groups was given a list of family members' communication targets and asked to rate each member's improvement in the sessions and at home. They also rated how problematic each of the issues discussed in sessions was to them currently. Finally, each family was asked to estimate the number of times they had used the problem-solving strategy at home (excluding homework for the generalization group).

Analysis of pre- and posttreatment audiotapes provided evidence for change in only negative maternal behavior, with the generalization group superior to the wait-list dyads. Problem-solving behavior showed minimal change, although these results were limited by low interobserver agreement on many of the problem-solving code categories. In contrast with Robin's findings, families showed considerable variability in problem-solving and communication skills prior to intervention, although it is unclear whether population differences or less restrictive definitions of problem-solving code categories accounted for the discrepancies. By follow-up, the negative behavior of the generalization group mothers no longer differed significantly from pretreatment levels.

By contrast, questionnaire data reflected several gains as a function of treatment. Mothers in both treatment groups reported significantly lower anger-intensity levels of specific disputes on the IC than did wait-list mothers; fathers in the generalization group indicated lower anger-intensity levels than fathers in the skill-training group. Adolescents in the skill-training group improved more in their relationships with their mothers as reported on the CBQ than adolescents in either the wait-list or generalization groups. Ratings of attainment of goal-related behavior were higher for the two treated groups than the control group. Most of the questionnaire variables also indicated that the wait-list group improved significantly from pre- to postassessment. The reasons for this improvement were not clear, but posttreatment assessments were conducted as the school year ended, and seasonal changes may have ameliorated child-related behavior problems.

Most of the treated groups' gains were maintained at follow-up. However, a small number of measures showed continued improvement for the skill-training group but some deterioration for the generalization group. These included mother anger-intensity levels on the IC, dyadic conflict scores for both mother and adolescent CBQs, adolescent report of severity of problems discussed in training, and maternal rating of communication skill use at home. Contrary to predictions, the generalization strategies seemed to impede maintenance of family gains, at least in some domains.

Furthermore, there was no evidence that the generalization strategies employed in the study actually enhanced generalization. A majority of families in both treatments reported using problem-solving strategies at home, and their frequency of reported use did not differ. At postassessment mothers and adolescents in both groups reported superior communication in sessions than at home: The two groups were equivalent on these ratings. Of course, as self-report data, these results may not correspond to actual behavior. Clearly, though, families' perceptions of generalized skill use did not differ for the two treatment groups.

Unfortunately, several methodological decisions made early in the design of the study limited its conclusions. Only mother–adolescent dyads were included in the communication task, to provide data comparable to those of an earlier validity study (Prinz *et al.*, 1979). This, however, meant that the family unit assessed was frequently not the unit treated (i.e., mother, adolescent, and father). Thus, the lack of change evident in communication measures may have represented either (1) little or no family change or (2) failure to generalize skills performed by a parent–adolescent triad to a parent–adolescent dyad.

Another unexpected complication arose from the improvement of the wait-list control group at postassessment, coupled with the unavailability of controls at follow-up. Thus, although the treatment groups maintained their improvements (for the most part) at follow-up, it was difficult to interpret this finding. Would the families in the control group have sustained their gains too, or was their earlier improvement a temporary phenomenon? Both ethical and practical considerations had mandated that the control group be treated immediately following the postassessment. Nonetheless, the absence of a control group was unfortunate, given the questions raised by the data.

A third study conducted by Robin (1981) compared problem-solving communication training to a best-alternative-treatment group as well as to a wait-list group. Thirty-three families with reports of parent–adolescent conflict were recruited through announcements; matched according to number of parents participating in treatment, sex of adolescent, and severity of conflict on the CBQ; then randomly assigned to one of the three groups. Adolescents ranged in age from 11 to 16, and families were predominantly middle-class.

Problem-solving communication training and generalization strategies in the study were similar to those used by Foster (1978). In addition, for the first time cognitive restructuring was added to the treatment package. Training lasted seven sessions; therapists included PhD and master's-level psychologists.

Families treated with alternative family therapy received one of several different interventions available at the clinic where the study was conducted. The alternative therapies were employed instead of an attention-placebo group for ethical reasons. These interventions also lasted seven sessions and were conducted by a psychiatrist and master's-level psychologists who endorsed the notion of short-term intervention and characterized their orientations as either "family systems," "eclectic," or "psychodynamic." All alternative family therapists agreed that the dependent measures provided fair assessments of their treatments. Assessment of family members' expectations after the first session indicated that family members in the two treatments had equivalent expectations of treatment success.

Despite these facts, it is important to note that the alternative treatment group was not intended as a test of a specific type of family therapy, for several reasons. First, measures assessed instrumental outcomes only for problem-solving communication training; the instrumental effects hypothesized to result from the various forms of alternative family therapy were neither specified nor assessed. Secondly, therapists were not matched for number or experience. Finally, while problem-solving communication training interventions were fairly homogeneous in structure, alternative family therapy approaches were more diverse. Thus, this study is best viewed as a comparison of problem-solving communication training with alternative therapies that control for therapist attention and other nonspecific factors of treatment, rather than as a comparative outcome study.

Measures included the IC, CBQ, Daily Home Reports, and an attitude survey measuring consumer satisfaction with treatment. In addition, each family triad (or dyad, in single-parent families) discussed two problems selected based upon the highest weighted frequency by intensity ratings on the IC. Audiotapes of these discussions were later rated using the PAICS. Both treatment groups and the control groups were assessed immediately before and after treatment. The two treated groups also completed a follow-up evaluation consisting of the CBQ and IC by mail, 3 months after the postassessment.

Results at the postassessment revealed that parents and adolescents in both treatment groups improved significantly on the weighted frequency by anger-intensity index of the IC, on CBQ ratings of the dyadic relationship, and on a composite score of problem-solving communication behavior derived from the PAICS. Problem-solving communication training was superior to the alternative treatment on both the problem-solving and positive communication categories of the PAICS. Parents in problem-solving communication training also displayed greater consumer satisfaction with the program and its effects than did parents in alternative family therapy. Neither group improved on the Daily Home Report.

Follow-up data were collected from a reduced sample of families (approximately 60%). Respondents in both treatments indicated maintained improvement on quantity of issues and on both CBQ scales, but the weighted frequency by anger intensity of issues showed some deterioration from postassessment to follow-up. There were no differences between the two treatment groups on questionnaire results.

Despite similar training packages, the Foster *et al.* (1983) and Robin (1981) studies produced discrepant results. Robin's families demonstrated considerable improvement in communication and problem-solving skills as a function of treatment, while Foster *et al.*'s did not. Robin failed to find the maintenance decrement reported by Foster *et al.*, despite the use of similar generalization strategies. These divergent results could be due to any number of methodological factors, including inclusion of fathers in the audiotaped discussions, different observational systems, and the availability of only a partial sample at follow-up. Alternatively, the addition of cognitive restructuring to the treatment package may have boosted the impact of problem-solving communication training on skill acquisition and/or maintenance of treatment gains. Finally, families may have received better skill training in the Robin study, possibly resulting in superior maintenance.

A final study by Stern (1984) evaluated problem-solving communication training taught in groups with parent–teen dyads. Since the purpose of the study was to assess the additive effects of a component designed to enhance anger control, only two treatment groups were included: one received only problem-solving communication training over eight 2-hour weekly sessions; the second received problem-solving communication training plus strategies derived from stress control and anger management literatures. Mothers and teens in both groups improved significantly on the CBQ, and mothers in both groups reported fewer issues and less anger intensity on the IC after treatment. Only the adolescents who received the combined treatment reported similar changes on the IC.

Observations of videotaped communication about real problems showed significant gains in positive behavior for teens, decrements in negative behavior for parents, and reduced insultingness for parents and adolescents, regardless of treatment condition. Thus, problem-solving communication training was associated with positive change, but there was little evidence that the additional component enhanced the effectiveness of this training. Unfortunately, no follow-up data were reported.

Although the studies reviewed here demonstrate the statistical significance of the treatment effects obtained with problem-solving communication training, they do not address clinical significance. In order to examine the clinical significance of the changes, Koepke, Robin, Foster, and Nayar (1988) pooled outcome data on the IC and CBQ from two of the studies reviewed here (Foster *et al.*, 1983; Robin, 1981) and one additional unpublished study (Nayar, 1985) using standardized score transformations. Data from 45 problem-solving communication training families and 29 wait-list control families were analyzed. A one standard deviation decrease on the IC anger-intensity score and the CBQ total score was defined as "clinically significant." On the CBQ, 68% of the treated parents and 39% of the treated adolescents reported clinically significant improvements compared to 24% of the wait-listed parents and 24% of the wait-listed adolescents. These differences were significant, based on chi-square tests. On the IC, 54% of the treated parents and 27% of the treated adolescents reported clinically significant improvements compared to 24% of the wait-listed parents and 31% of the wait-listed adolescents; the differences were significant for parents but not for adolescents. Thus, problem-solving communication training was effective for one-half to two-thirds of the families in ameliorating self-reported conflict and specific disputes, with stronger effects for parents than for adolescents.

To what extent has problem-solving communication training answered the questions posed earlier in the chapter? How does it match up with our ideal research criteria? Answers to both questions are mixed. Three of four outcome studies employed wait-list control groups to assess whether problem-solving communication training was better than no treatment. In two out of three studies, it was superior to no treatment in (1) changing communication and problem-solving behavior in laboratory discussions of real-life problems (instrumental outcomes), and (2) reducing indices of family conflict in the home (ultimate outcomes for most families). The one study that most directly assessed ultimate outcomes (Foster *et al.*, 1983) also found improvements in family members' ratings of goals they had set for treatment. Although no control group was used in the Stern (1984) study, changes from pre- to posttreatment were comparable to those of the controlled investigations. Most gains following problem-solving communication training have maintained at 6–8-week follow-up; however, no control groups have been assessed at follow-ups, and longer term follow-ups are needed.

Problem-solving communication training measures assess both ultimate and instrumental effects of treatment, and considerable research on psychometric properties of these instruments has been conducted (see Chapter 5). However, development of measures to assess communication and problem solving at home using means other than self-report would be helpful, as would methods of assessing family members' cognitive patterns.

In comparison with alternative family therapy, problem-solving communication training produced greater changes in laboratory communication and in treatment satisfaction, and was equivalent in its effects on indices of family conflict. While therapists conducting the two interventions were not strictly comparable (the alternative family therapists had more experience), this difference should have worked against problem-solving communication training, and treatment durations were comparable. However, because instrumental effects of the alternative therapy were not assessed and because of the mélange of orientations of the alternative family therapists, comparisons of problem-solving communication training with more clearly specified alternative approaches remain to be done.

What contributes to the effectiveness of problem-solving communication training? What families benefit most from it? At present, our answers to these questions are scanty or contradictory. Addition of a "generalization package" to basic problem-solving communication training appeared to have little impact on measures of generalization and to impede maintenance in one study. Yet findings from a second investigation that included these components failed to replicate the maintenance decline. Further, problem-solving communication training outcome studies with similar components have not all yielded the same findings. Yet each outcome study, in attempting to improve on previous interventions, has added new components to the treatment. Process measures might assist in sorting out similarities and differences in how therapists implemented problem-solving communication training in the different studies. Unfortunately, though, only one investigation included process measures, and these were limited to checking for differences between problem-solving communication training with and without generalization treatments during the beginning and end of sessions (when the two treatments were supposed to differ). Without more in-depth measures of therapist–client interaction during sessions or factorial designs, the active ingredients of problem-solving communication training cannot be determined. Further, the types of families who respond best to this training have not been established, and certainly this important issue requires future attention.

ALTERNATIVE APPROACHES

Many approaches other than problem-solving communication training have been developed for parents and teenagers. Several have garnered programmatic outcome data to support their efficacy. Three of these, each bearing some similarity to problem-solving communication training, are reviewed here.

Functional Family Therapy

Functional family therapy has been described by its creators as "an integration and extension of two major conceptual models of human behavior: systems theory and behaviorism" (Barton & Alexander, 1981, p. 403). Functional family therapists view behaviors in families as serving interpersonal functions for family members, functions that are defined by the intimacy, distance, and regulation outcomes produced by behavior (see Chapter 6 for further discussion of these concepts). Functional family therapists see dysfunctional behavior of family members as serving legitimate intimacy or distance-producing functions, but in ways that simultaneously result in negative consequences for one or more family members. Treatment focuses first on identifying regular patterns of behavior and postulating the functions served by each member's responses. Then it moves to what Alexander and Parsons (1982) call "therapy," a phase "designed to modify the cognitive sets, attitudes, expectations, labels, affective reactions, and assumptions of the family" (p. 47). Various strategies can be employed toward these ends, including relabeling and making nonblaming statements; interrelating thoughts, feelings, and behavior; and highlighting different aspects of the sequences of behavior that comprise family interaction patterns. The "therapy" phase leads into an "education" phase of treatment, in which specific interventions are introduced to promote and maintain positive changes in the family. Communication and negotiation training, consequence delivery systems, charting and graphing methods, and setting up methods of exchanging information (e.g., bulletin boards, notes) are among the strategies employed. Homework assignments ("interpersonal tasks") are also used to restructure interactions in the family (Alexander & Parsons, 1982).

Empirical evaluations of functional family therapy have been conducted principally with delinquent youths and their families. In an initial study (Alexander & Barton, 1976), 40 families with teenagers on probation for status offenses were randomly assigned to family therapy alone, family therapy plus individual therapy, individual therapy, or no treatment. Family therapy consisted of teaching families communication and contracting skills in small groups. Individual therapy consisted of four 1-hour weekly meetings with the teenager and varied according to the therapist's usual method. Three of the five family therapists also served as individual therapists; three other therapists worked only with individuals. Outcome was evaluated in terms of changes in the ratio of supportiveness to defensiveness in family communication. These ratios improved only for the two conditions that received family treatment.

As Alexander and Barton note, these data are limited by several factors, including differing amounts of therapist contact across groups and possible nonequivalence of therapist enthusiasm across conditions. In addition, the measures only tapped factors related to the goals of family therapy, not individual therapy. Finally, the treatment evaluated was a precursor rather than a representative example of functional family therapy as currently practiced. Nonetheless, the study demonstrated that family communication could be altered as a function of communication training and contracting.

A more elaborate study was subsequently conducted (Alexander & Parsons, 1973; Parsons & Alexander, 1973). Families were referred from the courts based on behavior problems displayed by their 13- to 16-year-old sons or daughters (running away, ungovernability, possession of illegal substances, shoplifting, or truancy). Families were randomly assigned to family therapy, client-centered family treatment, a church-sponsored, psychodynamically oriented family counseling program, or no treatment.

Functional family therapy consisted of training in contingency contracting, first with minor issues, later with major issues. Therapists also taught communication skills and assisted some families in setting up token economy programs. Client-centered treatment consisted of group meetings focusing on attitudes and feelings about family relationships. Psychodynamically oriented counseling consisted of insight-oriented meetings with individual families. Functional family therapy and client-centered treatment each involved eight meetings with the therapist (twice weekly for 4 weeks); psychodynamic treatment averaged 12–15 sessions. Therapists differed across conditions, with the functional family therapists considerably less experienced than the others. However, the functional family therapists received extensive training and supervision (6 hours/ week) during the project.

Outcome was assessed using communication measures (administered after treatment only), which were collected on the functional family therapy families but only on a subsample of the client-centered and no-treatment families. Results showed that functional family therapy was associated with less variance in talk time, less silence, and more interruptions than were client-centered therapy or no treatment. In addition, recidivism rates 3–15 months after treatment averaged 26% for functional family therapy families, whereas it was 47%, 73%, and 50%, respectively, for client-centered, psychodynamic, and no-treatment groups. A replication sample of 45 families seen for functional family therapy with different therapists during subsequent years yielded a recidivism rate of 27% (Alexander & Barton, 1976). A subsequent study (Klein, Alexander, & Parsons, 1977) examined court records 2½–3 years after intervention to assess court contacts of the siblings of teens in the 1973 study. Sibling referrals were 20% for functional family therapy, 40% for no treatment, and 59% and 63% for the client-centered and dynamic treatments.

These results suggest that functional family therapy was superior to client-centered treatment and to no treatment in improving family communication, although the limited assessment of communication done only after treatment attenuates this conclusion. Functional family therapy has also proven superior to all of the alternative interventions examined in Alexander and Parsons's outcome studies in reducing immediate recidivism and later sibling court contact. This finding is particularly striking in light of the presumed importance of reduced recidivism as an ultimate goal for all of the treatments. Nonetheless, measures representing the instrumental goals of the alternate therapies were not used, nor were measures collected on areas of family functioning other than communication in analogue settings. Finally, therapists were not matched for experience level, nor for amount of supervision in their approaches. While the former should have biased the results against functional family therapy, extensive supervision may have produced different levels of therapist enthusiasm and commitment to producing change across treatment conditions.

Barton, Alexander, Waldron, Turner, and Warburton (1985) replicated some of the results of the above studies in three additional investigations. In the first, paraprofessional therapists (undergraduates with extensive training and supervision) saw families in which the adolescent had committed several status offenses; no control group was included. The recidivism rate for the sample 13 months after treatment was 26%, comparable to that produced in earlier studies. Therapists also rated family members' defensiveness in session, which declined from the first to fourth or fifth session. Unfortunately, no interrater agreement data were provided or these data, which are even more suspect given therapists' obvious personal involvement in the cases.

The second study resulted when two participants in a functional family therapy workshop systematically incorporated functional family therapy into their work and evaluated its effect by reviewing their case notes and those of "control" coworkers before and after beginning to use this therapy. The two therapists reduced the proportion of teenagers referred to foster care for unmanageable behavior from 48% to 11%; control coworkers' rates remained stable (43% pretreatment, 49% posttreatment). Implementing functional family therapy was also associated with increased efficiency in service delivery. As Barton *et al.* note, however, the high motivation level of the two workers may limit the generalizability of these findings.

The third study involved incarcerated delinquent youths who were eligible for return to the community. Thirty hours functional family therapy included standard therapy procedures plus "supportive social services such as remedial education, job training," and so forth (p. 23). An alternative comparison treatment group consisting of youths incarcerated for similar offenses at approximately the same time at another facility received a mélange of combined services, mostly in group homes, with supportive social services generally provided to these youths as well. After 15 months, functional family therapy produced fewer offenses and lower recidivism rates than the alternative treatment; however, recidivism was still 60% for functional family therapy youths (93% for the alternative group).

In terms of the questions and ideal research criteria posed earlier in the chapter, functional therapy has proven better than no treatment for changing selected aspects of family communication patterns assessed immediately after treatment. No follow-up studies have examined durability of these effects. However, recidivism rates 3–18 months after treatment and sibling court contacts 2½–3 years after treatment were half as frequent with functional family therapy than with no treatment. In addition, functional family therapy appears superior in reducing recidivism to the forms of client-centered and dynamic therapies examined by Alexander and Parsons (1973). Preliminary data imply that it may reduce foster home placements for unmanageable behavior, but these findings should be replicated.

Studies of functional family therapy have fallen short of the ideal, however, in operationalizing and assessing its instrumental effects and those of alternative treatments. No checks on treatment manipulations have been conducted, nor have comparison therapies been equated with functional family therapy for therapist characteristics, treatment duration, and the like. Further, the active ingredients and characteristics of families who benefit most from the treatment have not been explicated, although it has been shown that families seen by therapists receiving higher supervisor ratings of directiveness and supportiveness progress better in treatment (Alexander *et al.*, 1976), and it seems—not surprisingly—that families with status offenders benefit more than families with hard-core delinquent youths.

Functional family therapy and problem-solving communication training share many common features, including the use of directives, communication and negotiation skills training, and reframing and relabeling to modify maladaptive cognitive styles. Both focus on altering the structure of family interaction and emphasize the functions behavior serves for family members. Both emphasize directive yet supportive therapeutic intervention. Both punctuate interactions at molar levels when this approach promotes therapeutic conceptualization and intervention. Both define change in the presenting problem(s) as the goal of treatment.

Functional family therapy and problem-solving communication training differ in sequencing treatment components. The functional family therapist relabels and restructures attributions before skill building; in problem-solving communication training these activities are intertwined. The skill-training and cognitive restructuring components of problem-solving communication training appear more structured than similar interventions used by functional family therapists, although the extent to which this distinction holds in practice is not clear. Another difference lies in the programming of new interactions: Functional family therapists do not attempt to change the functions served by family members' behaviors—rather, they try to change the topography of the interactions to achieve the same functions with less pain and conflict. Problem-solving communication training, in contrast, may or may not attempt to alter the interpersonal functions of behavior. Further, we postulate that several sets of functions can maintain problematic behavior, and that these operate based on principles of learning. Functional family therapy considers only two functions—

intimacy and distance—and does not use behavioral principles to explain the process by which the behavior–function relationship is maintained, although explanations offered by functional family therapists are not incompatible with a behavioral framework.

Relationship Enhancement

Guerney and his colleagues (Guerney, 1977; Guerney, Coufal, & Vogelsong, 1981; Grando & Ginsberg, 1976) developed relationship enhancement programs for father–son and mother–daughter parent–adolescent dyads. These programs are described as basically preventive and educational in nature. Rogerian theory provides the philosophical underpinnings of relationship enhancement, which emphasizes openness and empathy in communication. Behavioral strategies such as behavior rehearsal and feedback are used to teach relationship enhancement skills.

With relationship enhancement, dyads attend small group sessions in which they are taught four kinds of communication skills. These skills were designed to promote verbal sharing and understanding, communicated in a democratic fashion (Grando & Ginsberg, 1976). *Expresser skills* involve clear, specific statements of views and feelings, emphasizing positive underlying feelings. *Responder skills* include appropriate listening and empathy. *Facilitator skills* are behaviors that assist an expressor or responder by redirecting the conversation, praising, and helping the other to clarify or improve a previous statement. *Mode switching skills* revolve around turn-taking in the conversation (Guerney, 1977). To teach these skills, the leader models the behavior, asks the participants to practice it, and then provides praise and/or corrective feedback contingent upon their performance. The leader takes an active role in structuring and directing the sessions. Because the emphasis is on skill building, the leader avoids interpretive statements, advice, and explanations about the relationship (Guerney, 1977).

Ginsberg (1971) explored the efficacy of relationship enhancement with father–son dyads (adolescent age averaged about 13). Dyads recruited from the community were randomly assigned to either relationship enhancement or wait-list control groups. Participants completed pre- and posttreatment questionnaires and were audiotaped during structured interactions and while waiting for experimenter instructions. Conversations were later rated using scales that measured speaker and listener behavior, representing assessment of instrumental outcomes of treatment. The treatment groups improved on most behavioral and questionnaire measures relative to the controls, indicating that they had acquired communication skills and perceived their relationships to have improved.

In a second study, Guerney *et al.* (1981) examined a similar relationship enhancement program with 54 mother–daughter dyads (mean age of daughter, 13), comparing it to a discussion group and a wait-list control group. Participants were recruited from the community and completed questionnaire and audiotaped behavior-sample measures before and after treatment. Audiotaped samples consisted of structured discussions in which each member of a dyad discussed things she would like to change about herself or her partner.

Relationship enhancement followed the general procedures described earlier and was implemented with small groups (2–3 dyads) meeting for 12–15 2-hour weekly sessions. Discussion groups met an equivalent number of times, focusing on mutual support and participant-selected topics rather than systematic skill building. The same leaders conducted both treatments, and client evaluations of their leaders after treatment showed no significant differences across the two interventions.

Results revealed that, relative to control and discussion groups, the relationship enhancement group showed significantly greater gains in ratings of listener and speaker skills in the audiotaped conversations. Most questionnaire measures showed identical results; in only one case were the responses of discussion group dyads superior to those of control dyads.

Vogelsong (1975) collected 54-month follow-up data from participants in both treatments and in the control group. In addition, half the participants in each treatment group received "booster" weekly phone calls and meetings every 6 weeks. Results based on pretreatment to follow-up behavioral and questionnaire measures were virtually identical to those obtained immediately following treatment: Relationship enhancement was superior to the other two groups, which did not differ from each other. Booster sessions produced greater gains than no booster sessions on questionnaire (but not behavioral) measures, and only for the relationship enhancement condition. Together, these studies suggest that relationship enhancement training can produce significant gains in laboratory-based measures of the skills targeted by the program. These changes were accompanied by improved reports of the quality of parent–teen relations at home, which were maintained over a 6-month follow-up interval. The failure of an alternative treatment, in which dyads discussed problems without skill training, to yield similar gains implies that the specific structure of relationship enhancement training accounted for its therapeutic impact.

With respect to the research questions and criteria offered earlier, relationship enhancement is more effective than no treatment in improving speaker and listener skills (instrumental outcomes) and perceptions of parent–adolescent relationships at home (ultimate outcomes). However, participants have been assessed using Guerney's own assessment instruments, and without comparative data it is difficult to determine to what extent these samples differed from clinic populations in other studies. In fact, it appears that the research samples were primarily mildly distressed families interested in an enrichment program. Gains in behavior and verbal report maintained for as long as 6 months and were enhanced with "booster" phone calls and meetings. Relationship enhancement appears to be superior to parent–teen discussion groups, suggesting that its structure might be an active ingredient responsible for treatment gains. In this comparison, treatment lengths were equated and leader characteristics assessed to ensure comparability. However, checks that treatment was implemented as prescribed have not been conducted. In addition, further specification of active ingredients of relationship enhancement is needed, and comparison with other forms of intervention with clinical populations would be worthwhile.

The kinds of families that benefit most from relationship enhancement have not been systematically studied. However, Grando (1972) examined pretraining and process variables related to father–son relationship improvement in the Ginsberg (1971) study, identifying several predictors of therapeutic improvement. Self-reported communication was most likely to improve for fathers and sons who had better relationships and were more empathic with each other prior to training. Greatest gains in self-reported relationship satisfaction occurred for fathers with greater openness before training and with sons who were more impulsive. From these findings, it would seem that dyads (at least fathers and sons) with the least disturbed relationships respond best to relationship enhancement, although this conclusion is tentative because pretreatment variables predicted treatment outcome only weakly in the Grando study.

Relationship enhancement, like problem-solving communication training, emphasizes structured communication training for discussing important relationship issues. Both employ modeling, feedback, behavior rehearsal, and home assignments to teach selected skills. Therapists play directive yet supportive roles in skill building. Components of "listener" and "speaker" skills described by Guerney (1977) are frequently chosen in problem-solving communication training as family communication targets. The interventions differ in their focus on clinic versus nonreferred populations, dyads versus triads, use of group versus individual family sessions, and preset versus family-tailored curricula. Unlike relationship enhancement, problem-solving communication training includes training in problem solving, attempts to restructure interlocking interaction patterns, and contains cognitive restructuring components. Finally, problem-solving communication training is founded on thorough assessment of interaction patterns and skill repertoires; relationship enhancement is based on an educational model and does not utilize this kind of detailed assessment.

Behavioral Contracting

Behavioral contracting involves designing a specific written agreement between parents and adolescents, specifying the relationship between particular target behaviors (usually the child's) and their contingent consequences (usually provided by the parents). In theory, the purpose of the contract is to restructure the environment to provide sufficiently consistent reinforcers to establish and maintain adaptive teen behavior. While behavioral contracting has been associated with positive results when used as a prominent component of marital therapy (see Jacobson & Margolin, 1979), contracting results with parents and teenagers have been more equivocal, in part due to methodological problems of studies exploring the efficacy of contracting.

Early evaluations of contracting conducted by Stuart and his colleagues focused on the school behavior of adolescents labeled "predelinquent" and "delinquent" (Stuart & Tripodi, 1973; Stuart, Jayaratne & Tripodi, 1976). Stuart and Tripodi varied the treatment durations (15, 45, or 90 days) of a contingency contracting intervention and compared these groups with a defector control group composed of families who refused treatment. The experimental groups displayed less deterioration in school attendance and grades relative to the control group but no differences in tardiness or number of court contacts. While parent and teacher reports of teenagers' behavior showed some improvement following intervention, comparable data were not available for the control group. Furthermore, no statistical tests were reported to evaluate pre- to posttreatment changes for the treated families. Finally, minimal descriptions of the types and severity of adolescent referral problems were provided. The nonequivalence of treatment and control groups, lack of control data for many dependent measures, and poor definition of population parameters render Stuart and Tripodi's tenuous measures of success largely uninterpretable.

Some of these difficulties were corrected in a second study (Stuart *et al.*, 1976). Sixty students referred from five junior high schools were randomly assigned to either a contracting or a placebo control group. Placebo treatment consisted of activity periods with therapists. Contracting included use of daily reports from the teachers to the parents, with parent consequences for school behavior delivered according to contracts established and refined by the therapist, teenager, teacher, and teen's parents. Therapists spent an average of about 15 hours with adolescents, teachers, and families in the contracting condition, but only 2¼ hours in the placebo treatment.

Dependent measures included grades, frequency of absences, court contacts, and evaluations of behavior made by parents, teachers, and counselors. Teacher and counselor evaluations of school behavior improved for both treatment groups but significantly more for contract group adolescents. Maternal evaluations of marital adjustment and of the mother–son relationship also showed significant gains relative to the control group, which deteriorated on both of these measures. The authors argue that these data represent a conservative estimate of differential treatment effects, since several more severely disturbed adolescents had to be dropped from the placebo group to receive more intensive treatment, while other control subjects sought and received interventions similar to behavioral contracting on a private basis.

Despite these arguments, the small amount of contact between therapists and control subjects indicates that the placebo treatment did not control adequately for amount of therapist attention and/or other nonspecific factors. Thus, contracting per se may not have accounted for the differential treatment gains. In addition, gains were obtained only on paper-and-pencil measures; psychometric and normative data were not available for these instruments. Finally, as in the Stuart and Tripodi (1973) study, referral problems of adolescent subjects were not specified.

In a third study, Stuart, Tripodi, Jayaratne, and Camburn (1976) compared contracting with no treatment, using a large sample of predelinquents with unspecified referral problems in grades 6–10. Contracting focused first on school behavior, and involved counselor intervention with teachers, students, and parents. Later contracts addressed behavior changes at home. Relative to the controls, adolescents in the contracting group showed superior improvement in parent and teacher questionnaire measures of school behavior and in mother reports of parent–child interaction. However, absolute gains on these measures (although significant) were quite small. The groups did not differ in grades, attendance, or reports of home behavior. Unfortunately, this study suffered from some of the same problems as previous investigations, including unspecified presenting problems and measures with unknown psychometric properties.

Evaluating contracting with an older adolescent hard-core delinquent population (ages 14–17), Weathers and Liberman (1975) employed a multiple baseline design in which families began contracting after varying baseline durations. Intervention consisted of one session of contract negotiation and two sessions of training in negotiation and communication skills. Only 6 of 28 families completed the study. Parent-collected data revealed minimal changes in home behavior. School grades, school attendance, and recidivism also did not change. The authors concluded that contracting may not be a viable approach for this population (juveniles with several court contacts).

Blechman (1977) speculates that the brief duration (three sessions) as well as the structure of Weathers and Liberman's approach (which did not include the opportunity to renegotiate failing contracts) may have prevented accomplishment of these steps, thus limiting their success. Blechman specifies four conditions she believes necessary for establishing successful contracts: (1) the therapist and family must have established a positive relationship so that therapist opinions are valued, (2) contracts must enable teenagers to increase their influence over parent behavior, (3) family members must value contract success, and (4) strategies applicable to new problems should be taught as part of contracting.

While Blechman's prerequisites for successful contracting remain to be verified with empirical tests, research involving a "family contract game" she developed has been promising. The contract game helps a family arrive at a negotiated agreement to a dispute (Blechman, 1974; Blechman & Olson, 1976) by prompting problem definitions, specifications of desirable alternative behaviors, reward systems for performance of the alternative behaviors, and data collection systems. Single-subject ABA designs with four single-parent families indicated that using the game produced significantly more on-task and fewer off-task verbalizations than not using it when discussing a problem. Unstructured discussions of problems showed significant gains in on-task behavior from pre- to posttesting, with no decrease in off-task behavior. Ratings on the Devereux problem scale also changed significantly.

This research unfortunately has several shortcomings. First, there were no reports of whether agreements from the contract game were implemented or whether the game was utilized at home. Second, a second implementation of the game condition would be necessary for definitive statements that the game controlled verbal behavior. Third, it is not clear whether the game format or its contracting component was responsible for the changes in interaction: that is, would playing Monopoly produce the same changes as playing the contract game? Fourth, the authors relied upon use of the game to control verbal behavior and did not specifically teach communication skills that could be used cross-situationally without the game. Thus, although outcomes are more promising than those produced by alternative contracting approaches, definitive conclusions regarding the contract game must await more carefully controlled evaluations.

A final study by Besalel and Azrin (1981) examined a combined contracting-communication approach with 29 youths ranging in age from 6 to 16 (average age, 12) referred by public and school agencies. Youths were randomly assigned to either a wait-list control group or to a four-session intervention consisting of family communication training, written contracts, and overcorrection. Treatment was evaluated using a checklist assessing severity of problems in the family. Treated families reported significant decreases in problem severity relative to controls. The wait-list group was then treated, replicating the results of the original treatment group. Gains were maintained at a 6-month follow-up. While the results of this study were quite positive, the authors unfortunately relied upon a single unvalidated questionnaire to evaluate treatment outcome. In addition, a breakdown of the results for adolescents versus preadolescents would have been useful to examine the generality of results across the wide age range included in the study.

Because many behavioral contracting studies include other techniques, it is difficult to reach definitive conclusions concerning the impact of contracting. In addition, the few studies relying exclusively upon contracting have not been promising. Whether contracting produces changes relative to no treatment or to alternate treatments cannot be answered definitively at present, given the designs and limitations of existing studies. Nonetheless, the Blechman studies imply that a structured contract game can improve family interactions when the game is in use, and a blend of contracting and communication training appears to reduce families' reports of problems compared to a wait-list control (Besalel & Azrin, 1981).

Long-term effects of contracting without communication training have not been explored. Short-term effects may include changes in parent, teacher, and child reports of behavior and family interactions; some of these may be associated with ultimate outcomes desired by families, but this is hard to ascertain. Only Weathers and Liberman directly evaluated instrumental effects of treatment (i.e., results of contracting on behaviors specified in the contract), and their results indicated minimal changes. On the other hand, Stuart et al. (1976) measured improvement in school behavior as a function of contracting and these measures presumably represented instrumental effects of contracting for at least some of their subjects. Treatment components and families benefiting most from contracting have not been evaluated, although Blechman (1977) speculated on these factors.

Both behavioral contracting and problem-solving communication training focus on reaching specific negotiated agreements between parents and adolescents. Problem-solving communication training constrains the process by employing the problem-solving format; only the contracting game provides similar constraints. Problem-solving communication training's focus on specific communication skills and family interaction process has been deemphasized in contracting, which appears to stress changes in contingency systems rather than in verbal interaction processes as a central goal. Finally, considerations of structural and cognitive variables as well as functional analysis of family negotiation patterns do not appear in written discussions of contracting.

SUMMARY

The results of the evaluations of problem-solving communication training, functional family therapy, relationship enhancement, and behavioral contracting suggest that a variety of interventions have proven effective in ameliorating parent–adolescent conflict and family problems. Most treatments that have demonstrated short-term effectiveness have also documented maintenance of treatment gains over intervals ranging from 6–15 months.

The populations that have been successfully treated have varied widely, including juvenile offenders, clinic-referred and self-referred families with independence-related conflicts, adolescents with school difficulties, and dyads seeking an educationally oriented enrichment program. While the lack of treatment method by family type factorial studies precludes definitive conclusions concerning which approach works best for which families, some tentative recommendations for practicing clinicians can be made based upon examination of characteristics of interventions that individual investigations selected to use for specific populations.

It appears that the more seriously distressed the family, the more important it is to include treatment components that address both communication skills and interactional process variables such as family structure and the function of interactants' behavior within the family system. Interventions limited to direct behavioral contracting and communication skill training appear sufficient to achieve gains only with mild-to-moderately distressed parents and adolescents.

This conclusion is based upon a rank ordering of the level of distress of the families who participated in the research evaluating functional family therapy, problem-solving communication training, behavioral contracting, and relationship enhancement, and a comparative analysis of the outcomes of this research. Judging from authors' descriptions of their samples, Weathers and Liberman worked with older adolescents with multiple delinquent offenses, the most distressed group. Alexander and his colleagues worked for the most part with court-referred juvenile status offenders, also seemingly seriously distressed families. Stuart and his colleagues worked with youths and families with multiple school, home, and community problems, while Robin, Foster, and Stern worked with less seriously distressed clinic or self-referred families with few juvenile offenses. Guerney and his colleagues worked with the least seriously distressed population, a group self-referred for an enrichment experience. Blechman also appears to have worked with mildly distressed families.

While functional family therapy, which addresses interactional process variables, proved successful with juvenile offenders, behavioral contracting was not successful with seriously disturbed families (Weathers & Liberman, 1975). It was, however, successful with the more mildly distressed group recruited by Blechman. Relationship enhancement proved successful with the mildly distressed enrichment group. Families from a moderately distressed population referred primarily for difficulties in conflict management responded well to problem-solving communication training, which includes some emphasis on structure and function but not as great an emphasis on these variables as functional family therapy has. As we noted in earlier chapters of this book, clinical experiences have indicated the importance of adding functional/structural components to problem-solving communication training when the level of distress is severe, multiple problems warrant treatment, and the adolescent is inappropriately involved in cross-generational alliances, triangulated or enmeshed patterns, or marital conflict.

Many treatment-related questions remain to be answered. Ultimate and instrumental effects of treatment have rarely been examined simultaneously in investigations. It is therefore often difficult to know whether processes hypothesized to occur during treatment actually happen. This relationship is crucial for determining whether a treatment impacts relationships in the ways its proponents speculate. In a related vein, parametric investigations to determine the active ingredients of effective interventions have not yet been conducted, nor have comparisons between approaches (e.g., problem-solving communication training vs. relationship enhancement) been attempted. Thus, we cannot at this point offer an empirically grounded framework for matching clients to treatment procedures and specifying how to help families who fail to benefit from the treatments described in this chapter.

Another set of treatment questions concern process variables, particularly therapist skills that are important during particular phases of behavioral family therapy. Alexander *et al.* (1976) provide data supporting the importance of relationship and structuring skills for propelling a family toward meaningful improvement with functional family therapy. Blechman (1977) also noted the importance of a strong, positive therapist–family relationship in the success of behavioral contracting. What is the appropriate balance of structure and flexibility for a behavioral family therapist to maintain during the early, middle, and later stages of treatment? Failure to deviate from a preplanned agenda when a family is in crisis can undermine a therapist's effectiveness, but repeated deviations whenever interesting material arises can lead to chaotic sessions where skills are not acquired, goals are not achieved, and the therapist becomes a part of the system maintaining the presenting problem (Haley, 1976, 1980). To complicate matters further, variables such as the therapist's age, sex, marital status, child-rearing experiences, and family-of-origin experiences are likely to influence his/her reactions to particular constellations of parent–adolescent interactions.

Numerous investigators have begun to accumulate empirical knowledge about the kinds of skill-oriented interventions that can be effective with parents and adolescents with relationship problems. Nonetheless, much remains to be done. The predominant direction of the approaches reviewed here has been towards an integration of traditional behavioral procedures with selected aspects of other therapies, notably family systems and Rogerian approaches. Behavior therapy has reached a stage in its development where it has established a sense of identity, achieved a sense of self-acceptance, and can be self-critical and self-evaluative, looking to other specialties for innovative ideas and mutual sharing (Kendall, 1982). In the area of individual problems, integrationists have moved in the direction of dynamic therapies (Goldfried, 1982; Wachtel, 1982). In the area of family and parent–adolescent problems, the natural comrade is family systems therapy (Foster & Hoier, 1982). Yet integrationism, like any therapy, must involve an internally consistent theoretical framework that produces treatment procedures able to pass the ultimate tests—methodologically sound and comprehensive evaluations of long-term effectiveness.

CHAPTER FIFTEEN

Future Directions

It should be abundantly clear from previous chapters that the knowledge base for theory, assessment, and treatment of distressed parents and adolescents is far from complete. While on the one hand it is frustrating to build much of our theoretical and practical framework on hypotheses rather than established facts, on the other hand this state of affairs opens the possibility of laying the empirical and conceptual groundwork that will establish these facts.

Throughout this volume we have attempted to adopt an appropriately self-critical stance, stressing the need to verify or disconfirm the hypotheses we offer. We pointed out many areas in need of further development and research as the book progressed. This chapter overviews additional issues that we believe should be addressed to advance our understanding of parent–adolescent dysfunction, assessment, and treatment.

THEORY

The behavioral–family systems theoretical framework offered in this book proposes behavioral, cognitive, structural, and functional patterns believed to promote the *development* and *maintenance* of intense parent–adolescent conflict. As clinicians and researchers develop and further test this model, it will be important to consider the relevance of findings emerging from developmental psychology research on adolescence and the family (Grotevant & Cooper, 1983; Montemayor, 1983).

In a review of the developmental literature on parent–adolescent conflict, Montemayor (1986) found that while parent–adolescent relations vary widely in degree of discord, survey research suggests that most families have generally harmonious relations, with only a minority experiencing frequent, bitter acrimony. Montemayor reaffirmed the contribution of interactional and parenting skill variables to parent–teen discord and suggested the importance of three additional factors: family social context, family composition, and characteristics of individual family members. The social context of a family includes historical period, cultural and ethnic traditions, and socioeconomic status. Family composition refers to family size, intact or divorced family, or stepfamily; parental divorce and remarriage are both associated with increased mother–adolescent conflict. The characteristics of family members include the sex of the adolescent, the biological changes of puberty and the stage of adolescent development, and organismic variables such as temperament, self-esteem, depression, and so forth. A variety of specific findings, too numerous to summarize here, have been noted concerning these variables. To these variables we would add a need for considering the parents' experiences in their families of origin, since these provide much of their learning history for parenting behavior. This is often discussed but rarely researched by other schools of family therapy (Gurman & Kniskern, 1981).

Research comparing distressed and nondistressed families supports the behavioral–family systems model. But findings that distressed families show poorer communication, more rigid beliefs, and more structural problems than their nondistressed counterparts do not address the role of these behaviors in the etiology or maintenance of conflict, since these studies are correlational in nature. It is possible, for example, that intense disagreements produce poor problem solving, rather than the reverse. Similarly, these findings say nothing about how negative interaction patterns came into existence. Longitudinal studies examining the evolution of parent–adolescent difficulties by assessing the relative contributions of problem solving, communication, cognitive distortions, and structural and functional patterns of interaction would be a first step in determining why clinically significant family conflict develops. In so doing, it will be important to consider the wealth of research on behavior problems with preadolescent children; the growing literature relating marital and child problems, reviewed in Chapter 3; and the factors involved in adolescent development (including those outlined above), which presumably set the stage for changes in family relations during the teenage years.

Patterson (1982; Patterson & Bank, 1986) provided a model for theory development and testing which is highly applicable to parent–adolescent relationship problems. In attempting to explain the etiology and maintenance of aggressive behavior in preadolescent conduct-disordered boys, he developed a performance model that relates poor parental discipline and inept parental monitoring of children's behavior to coercive parent–child interactions in the home and antisocial child behavior in the community (Patterson & Bank, 1986). In an elegant series of validation and theory testing studies, Patterson used the multitrait–multimethod matrix approach to develop composite scores of the constructs of discipline, monitoring, coercive child behavior, and antisocial child behavior, operationalizing each construct in a series of multidimensional measures provided by multiple informants. Then Patterson tested the model based on data from a new sample of families using structural modeling, deriving path coefficients indicating the strength of each direct and indirect relationship between the variables. A similar approach might be used to test the behavioral–family systems model of parent–adolescent conflict, employing multiple operationalizations of the basic constructs of skill deficits, cognitive distortions, problems in family structure, parent–adolescent arguments, and additional variables such as characteristics of the family members and family-of-origin factors.

Structural patterns that promote excessive conflict also warrant further examination from a behavioral vantage point. This in turn requires more precise operationalization of structural patterns in terms of specific response classes or interaction sequences (Foster & Hoier, 1982). Robin *et al.* (1986) found minimal differences between clinic-referred, acting-out adolescents and their parents, compared to their non-clinic-referred counterparts, on the Coalitions and Triangulation scales of the Parent Adolescent Relationship Questionnaire (PARQ), raising questions about the veracity of clinically derived family systems hypotheses about coalitional and triangulated interaction patterns. Examining structural patterns from a social-learning perspective to postulate how positive and negative reinforcement, punishment, and avoidance operate to maintain structural patterns is an additional step in understanding the interplay among behavior, affect, and cognitions at molecular and molar levels. Ultimately this process of refining an integrated picture of the parameters that produce and sustain family distress should also lead to a taxonomy of structural and functional patterns common to interactions of parents and teenagers presenting with various types of distress.

Behavior therapists generally have neglected the role of affect in dysfunctional interpersonal patterns, and research with families is no exception. Yet conflict is often typified by intense negative emotion. Is that emotion best thought of as a byproduct of poor communication skills and irrational thinking, as our model implies? Gottman and Levenson (1985) found that distressed couples showed more pronounced patterns of physiological linkage during conflictual exchanges than happier couples, suggesting that the physiological component of affect may be a more critical component of interpersonal exchange than previously thought. The experiences of positive and negative feelings during family interactions and the relationship of these experiences to dysfunctional thought and communication are also important to examine in further depth. Clinically speaking, we often find that a key to assessing the reinforcing or punishing value of a behavior is to ask how the parties involved felt before and after the behavior occurred. Whether these statements of feeling are epiphenomena and have little to do with the actual functions of behavior, or whether they accurately mirror physiological states underlying reinforcement processes, would be important to know for both practical and theoretical reasons. Interestingly, Robin *et al.* (1986) found that when they asked family members to report perceived warmth/hostility along with perceived communication and problem solving on a standardized inventory, affective self-reports correlated over .80 with self-reports of communication and problem solving; perceived warmth/hostility was also one of the strongest discriminators of clinic from non-clinic-referred families. Clearly, affect is closely associated with other dimensions of parent–adolescent discord, but further research is needed to determine its specific role.

ASSESSMENT

Although numerous assessment options are available for assessing family interaction, surprisingly few assess structural and functional patterns in the family systematically. Initial developments in these areas should benefit from direct observation of family process, to avoid problems inherent in interpreting self-reports. Gilbert *et al.* (1984) provide a model for how this might be done in describing a behavioral observation code designed to assess family alliances based on coding taped samples of family discussion.

As assessment approaches for describing more molar interaction patterns are developed, content and construct validity issues must be addressed. This is particularly important in operationalizing response classes presumed to index structural patterns, to ensure that global categories such as "triangulation" are comprised of relevant molecular subcategories. Russell's (1980) findings underscore the danger of neglecting this process: She compared three different indices of cohesion (the Family Environment Scale, the Family Adaptability and Cohesion Scale, and a family sculpture task), finding little relationship among them. However, the measures assessed very different behaviors, although each purported to assess the same general construct.

Recent validation research with the PARQ, a multidimensional self-report measure of skills, cognitions, affect, structure, and specific disputes, illustrates one approach to the problem of operationalizing nebulous concepts and investigating construct validity (Koepke, 1986). Twelve "constructs" were operationalized via behaviorally anchored scales consisting of self-report items: global distress, communication, problem solving, warmth/hostility, unreasonable beliefs, coalitions, triangulation, cohesion, school conflict, sibling conflict, somatic concern, and conventionalization. A structured family interview was also developed, after which the interviewer rated the family members on global-inferential rating scales covering the same 12 constructs. Fifty-one distressed families completed the PARQ and participated in the structured family interview. Interview ratings were correlated with PARQ scores across the 12 dimensions. For parents, the convergent validity correlations between the same dimensions across methods were higher than all of the across-method-within-content or across-content-within-method correlations on half of the scales; for adolescents the convergent validity correlations were highest for a third of the scales. In those cases where the within-content correlations were not highest, the scales were most highly correlated with closely related constructs (e.g., communication with problem solving or cohesion with triangulation). These results provided strong evidence for the construct validity of the PARQ scales as operationalizations of dimensions of the behavioral–family systems model.

Just as affect has received little attention from a theoretical perspective, its assessment has been relatively ignored. Marital therapists have developed several methods of assessing different aspects of affect, which could be adapted for parent–teen interaction. Behavioral expressions of emotion can be assessed with Gottman's Couples Interaction Scoring System (Gottman, 1979), or with more in-depth coding schemes (e.g., Gottman & Levenson, 1985). Gottman and Levenson (1985; Levenson & Gottman, 1983) also describe sophisticated physiological equipment for examining the physical substrate of emotion. Assessing the subjective experience of emotion has been accomplished via questionnaires (O'Leary, Fincham, & Turkewitz, 1983) and ratings of one's feelings during an interaction (e.g., Gottman, Notarius, Markman, Bank, Yoppi, & Rubin, 1976). The latter method has particular promise, as information on affective events could be correlated with observations of communication patterns to examine functional relations between the two. By adding a cognitive reconstruction session (in which the person views a videotape of an interaction and indicates what s/he was thinking as the interaction went along), cognitive events could be integrated into the analysis. Illuminating common sequences of thought–affect–behavior patterns that occur in actual interactions of distressed families could be enormously helpful both to practitioners and to researchers.

Also important is further exploration of the level of analysis at which functional patterns should be described. At a molecular level, we suspect that analyzing the functions of specific communication behaviors during discussion is particularly valuable as a precursor to communication and problem-solving training, which focuses on these molecular patterns. Yet molecular behaviors may be components of more molar sequences, too. For example, persistent interrupting may represent either a negative communication skill or an example of overinvolved, enmeshed interactions. Developing reliable, valid methods of differentiating between these two possibilities would be helpful to clinicians.

More molar analyses examining the functions of arguments, withdrawal, and problem behaviors over broader time frames seem especially useful when considering more general patterns that maintain problem behaviors. Rethinking these hypotheses often appears to help the therapist come up with new directions with families who have made limited progress in therapy. Yet whether in fact these speculations are accurate is an open question; Nelson and Hayes (1979) even raise the question of whether systematic functional analysis enhances therapy outcome, asking whether individuals or families should be treated with "treatment packages" matching their presenting problems, regardless of the functions their behaviors serve.

While functional analysis at molecular and molar levels may seem a fairly straightforward process, Felton and Nelson (1984) indicate that clinicians' agreement on antecedents and consequences of behavior problems described by individual clients may in fact be quite low. This is probably further compounded when dealing with family interaction, which involves several members and can be "chunked" in varying ways. The process of functional analysis is influenced by the questions clinicians ask, the responses family members provide, and the judgments therapists make about which patterns, grouped into which themes, are most salient and important in the interaction process. The last of these factors may be crucial to examine, not by looking for the "truth" of clinicians' judgments, but rather by examining their utility. In other words, which analyses lead to better outcomes in therapy? How should these be framed, and what assessment information is particularly important in guiding their formulation?

The reliability of clinicians' functional analyses of family interactions could

be improved through creating standard assessment protocols. Structured interview questions, informal observational probes, and self-report questionnaire
profiles yielding information concerning the common functional patterns discussed in Chapter 10 (weak parental coalitions, the overprotection–rebellion
escalator, triangulation, etc.) could be derived through empirical analysis. Clinicians might then be trained to use these protocols reliably, and the information
derived could be evaluated for its utility.

On a practical level, the assessment process relies heavily on family members' reports of their own and others' behavior, particularly during the interview.
But, as has been repeatedly emphasized, self-report may be inaccurate for a
variety of reasons. Nonetheless, the widespread use and convenience of client
report, coupled with practical difficulties arranging more direct methods of
collecting ongoing information (i.e., direct and self-observation), undoubtedly
assures its continued prominence in the assessment process. For these reasons, it
would be useful to be able to predict which clients are likely to be more (and less)
accurate in their reports. Similarly, it may be that certain types of problems or
behaviors are more likely than others to be reported inaccurately. For example,
Christensen, Sullaway, and King (1983), examining the daily reports couples
provided about their interactions, found higher levels of agreement for more
objective and specific items. This kind of research could produce guidelines
about which information from which clients can and cannot be taken at face
value.

Another approach to the problems of self-report data in clinical interviews is
to treat the interview as a psychometric measure and apply the same validation
standards used with other instruments. Chapter 4 reviewed research taking this
direction, noting many gaps in our knowledge. Standardizing the interview
format, separating information provided verbatim by family members from
interviewer judgments, and developing quantitative methods of recording both
types of information may help to improve the reliability and validity of the
interview.

Although we stress the need for accurate information about parent–
adolescent interaction, it can be legitimately argued that when family members'
perceptions are discordant with reality, the perceptions may represent more
important phenomena than the stark reality of the events. In fact, the therapist
may never determine "true reality." Following this line of reasoning and taking
into account the distorted information-processing styles hypothesized to
characterize parents and adolescents in conflict, it is only natural to expect
clinic-referred families to have more discrepant perceptions of their interactions
than non-clinic-referred families (see Chapter 5).

Finally, we emphasize that the initial assessment phase of treatment has
therapeutic as well as information-gathering objectives. Establishing rapport,
engaging reluctant participants, and framing problems within interactional
frameworks are assumed to enhance the success of and decrease resistance to
later treatment. While aspects of therapist behavior has been associated with

successful outcome (e.g., Alexander *et al.*, 1976), exactly how these behaviors influence the therapy process to enhance treatment remains to be examined. Similarly, guidelines for handling the kinds of problematic situations that commonly occur during family assessment should ultimately have empirical rather than intuitive bases.

TREATMENT OF FAMILY CONFLICT

Improvements in the treatment of parent–adolescent problems should come from (1) improvements in treatment procedures per se, and (2) improvements in treatment outcome research.

Improvements in treatment procedures are needed because both outcome research and our clinical impressions indicate that problem-solving communication training—while often helpful—does not always produce significant, long-lived changes in family functioning. Initial attempts to enhance the effectiveness of the treatment program led to the development of the cognitive restructuring component of therapy. Later attempts produced expanded consideration of functional/structural elements of family interaction. Whether these later additions to the skill-training components of treatment produce quantitatively demonstrable changes in families not helped by our initial treatment packages remains to be established, however, through a series of dismantling and/or factorial component analyses. Nayar (1985) compared problem-solving communication training with cognitive restructuring, to skill training alone and a wait-list control, finding marginal superiority in the combined condition compared to the skill-training-alone condition. Additional component research of this kind is needed.

Interventions designed to integrate problem-solving communication training and cognitive restructuring into a total treatment approach based on structural and functional considerations particularly need elaboration and systematization. While we provide preliminary suggestions and examples of how these concepts might be used, the kinds of practice-based guidelines that come from years of using these strategies remain to be developed. More systematic evaluation of when, what, and how intervention strategies borrowed from other schools of family therapy work would lay the groundwork for explaining why these techniques work under certain conditions—a *why* that should hopefully be conceptually consistent with the theoretical framework advanced in this book.

All of the preceding discussion points to examining our failures, with the ultimate goal of expanding or modifying the treatment program to help therapists deal more effectively with families who fail to acquire or to implement consistently problem-solving and communication skills during treatment. While some adaptations will undoubtedly arise from altering the content of treatment, it is also important to specify more fully those characteristics of therapists and therapy process that enhance treatment outcome. The detailed discussion of resistant behavior in Chapter 12 was designed both to provide practical guidance and to spur investigation specifying the form and functions of resistant behavior as well as methods of coping with it. Observation systems to code therapy process data would facilitate these investigations.

Just as failure challenges us to revise our theories and methods of approaching family conflict, success too raises the challenge of specifying how and why therapy worked. It is particularly important to establish the conditions under which problem-solving communication training is most likely to be successful without additional treatment components. Our hunch is that the skill-training modules of the approach are most useful for mild to moderately distressed families with few structural problems, and that protracted treatment heavily emphasizing structure and cognitions is not necessary for these families. But this is at present only a hunch, not an empirically established rule of thumb.

Therapy outcome research will be a key element in answering many of these questions. Chapter 14 highlighted critical elements in the methodology of outcome research with families. Most of these dealt with group design approaches. Single-subject strategies, too, could provide useful contributions, particularly if these studies were aimed at documenting effective strategies for coping with impasses or process problems in treatment. For example, a therapist who encounters a resistant adolescent could audiotape sessions and use particular strategies systematically to attempt to increase the teen's participation, using either an ABAB design, if a reversal would not jeopardize therapy outcome, or a multiple baseline across subjects. Mini-ABAB designs within sessions, such as those described in earlier chapters, could also be conducted and evaluated systematically.

As therapy outcome research increases in both scope and sophistication, assessment of different types of effects of therapy will be required. These include both consumer satisfaction and ultimate outcomes. Mittl and Robin (1987) assessed the social acceptability and consumer satisfaction of problem-solving communication training; they asked college students and their mothers to read vignettes describing typical cases of parent–adolescent conflict and rate the social acceptability of problem-solving communication training compared to three alternative interventions—behavioral contracting, paradoxical family therapy, and medication. Problem-solving communication training received the highest social acceptability ratings, followed in rank order by behavioral contracting, medication, and paradox. Further social acceptability research with clinical populations is in progress.

Assessment of ultimate outcomes is crucial for social validity reasons. It is important to address this issue by assessing and reporting clients' presenting concerns, rather than assuming that their ultimate goals are reduced conflict, no further contact with the juvenile court, and improved relationship satisfaction. In group design research, this will require that investigators either select subjects who share similar goals for treatment or individualize measures of presenting problems and therapy goals for each family. Instrumental outcomes are also crucial to assess, for these data can be of invaluable assistance in explaining why ultimate goals were or were not attained. When different therapies are compared, measures of instrumental outcomes appropriate to each type of treatment should be included.

In addition, it will be increasingly important to demonstrate the degree and variability of change produced by different family therapies. Jacobson, Follette, and Revensdorf (1984) appropriately criticize the practice of equating statistical significance and clinically significant change, noting that stable mean differences between pre- and posttreatment do not necessarily indicate either the percentage of families that have improved or whether the improvement was important to their lives. They propose a sophisticated strategy for evaluating the clinical significance of change based on normative means and test–retest reliability of the measure used to assess change, and apply their proposal in a reanalysis of outcome data from studies evaluating behavioral marital therapy (Jacobson, Follette, Revensdorf, Baucom, Hahlweg, & Margolin, 1984). As studies accumulate assessing the impact of problem-solving communication training and alternative therapies, these sorts of analyses will provide useful supplements to standard statistical tests of family change.

Further questions arise about the ultimate limitations of a problem-solving communication training approach. When conflict is part of psychiatric conditions such as affective disorders, personality disturbances, attention deficit disorders, psychosis, or eating disorders, can a problem-solving communication training approach contribute to an overall therapeutic regimen? Or is the effectiveness of our approach limited to milder forms of conflict occurring in the absence of serious psychiatric disorders, defined in traditional diagnostic terms?

Readers may mistakenly assume that our approach is limited to the milder forms of conflict because we have refrained from discussing traditional psychiatric syndromes. This is more a function of our behavioral orientation than a consequence of the fact that we have not worked with seriously disturbed families. Many of the youths who have participated in our programs have been diagnosed as conduct disordered, psychopathic, ADHD, depressed, or suicidal. Naturally, our clinical success rate is higher with milder disturbances, but adolescents with serious psychiatric problems and their families have benefited from our interventions. In such cases, problem-solving communication training often becomes part of a broader treatment approach.

Two important points must be emphasized about treating seriously disturbed families: (1) problem-solving communication training is rarely the only intervention needed, and it must be used as part of a broader approach; and (2) families must be willing to acknowledge the presence of overt conflict to benefit from an intervention that teaches conflict-resolution skills. When conflict is apparent to the therapist but not to the family, problem-solving communication training is not very useful.

The recent work of one of us (A. R.) with eating-disordered adolescents provides an example of an unusual application of problem-solving communication training within a broader therapeutic context. Families with adolescents diagnosed with anorexia nervosa often present with conflicts about eating but claim to have few conflicts in other areas. They report close relationships, few arguments over independence-related teenage issues, and little or no marital discord, and they generally cannot understand why their adolescent is starving herself. Further assessment often suggests that family members actively avoid conflicts by changing the topic or becoming distracted when difficult issues arise. Refusal to eat is one of the few oppositional behaviors the teenager exhibits, but the family does not perceive self-starvation as rebellious. The little overt conflict results because the adolescent is not demanding age-appropriate autonomy.

Restoring weight is clearly a primary goal of any treatment program for anorexia nervosa. Helping the anorectic begin to accomplish the stymied developmental tasks of adolescence—including seeking independence from her parents—and to increase her peer involvement is a major secondary goal. Accomplishing this goal usually involves teaching the adolescent to seek additional freedom and preparing the family to face rather than avoid or punish adolescent independence seeking and the normal conflicts that result. Problem-solving communication training can play an important role at this stage of treatment.

Robin and Siegel (1988) outline a broad-based behavioral–family systems approach to anorexia nervosa in adolescence. During the active weight-gain phase of the treatment, a pediatrician establishes a required target weight and rate of weekly weight gain, a dietitian establishes and adjusts as necessary a required daily caloric intake, and the therapists then give the parents complete control over their daughter's eating. Strategically, the parents are required to learn to work as a team to develop and implement a comprehensive behavioral plan for monitoring and consequating all daily eating behavior, in order to insure that the teenager eats and gains weight. The structural techniques for building a strong parental coalition outlined in Chapter 10 of this volume are used to help the parents assume control of their daughter's eating. As the teenager gains weight and eats regularly, the therapist shifts gears, focusing on adolescent autonomy, family communication, and extreme belief systems. The therapist may reframe refusal to eat as rebellious behavior, target negative communication patterns related to discussions of eating, and eventually encourage the adolescent to become involved in age-appropriate peer activities. Often we prescribe mildly rebellious adolescent behavior and block the family's attempts to avoid resulting conflict, then teach them to use problem solving to reach reasonable agreements. For example, one teenager was asked to commit a secret rebellious act, and her parents were instructed to try to guess what their daughter did. Her "rebellious behavior" consisted of changing the channel on the television when her father stepped out of the room during a football game. Her parents worried that their daughter would commit some ruinous rebellious act and did not guess accurately what she did. The therapist addressed their exaggerated, ruinous concerns through cognitive restructuring and taught the family to use problem solving to help their teenager generate a list of rebellious behavior more extreme than changing the television channel.

During the weight-maintenance phase of treatment, many normal conflicts of adolescence begin to arise. In our experience many anorectic adolescents and their families are absolutistic, "all-or-none" thinkers. With perfectionistic tendencies, when the adolescent emerges from starvation and begins to seek increased peer contact, she often goes to extremes, just as she did during self-starvation. One 16-year-old girl who had lost all interest in boys during her weight-loss phase rapidly had five relationships within 2 months of achieving her target weight. Her heterosexual relationships were tumultuous, impetuous, and characterized by sudden bursts of defiance towards her parents. A combination of cognitive restructuring and problem-solving skill training proved useful to help her modulate her intense approach to dating and to help the family establish new limits on her behavior.

In summary, problem-solving communication training can serve as one part of a more comprehensive behavioral–family systems therapy for eating disordered and other severely distressed adolescents and their parents. Individual components of the intervention are called upon flexibly as needed. Additional investigations are needed to determine how problem-solving communication training might be integrated into interventions for other adolescent behavior disorders.

CONCLUDING COMMENTS

Conducting family therapy provides challenges on many levels. Intellectual challenges abound, as the therapist must conceptualize interaction rather than individual patterns in ways that explain the behavior of involved family members. Observations of family process require that the therapist be simultaneously a participant and an observer in sessions, processing family members' behavior in both roles while guiding the session. Practical challenges require the therapist to balance rapport, direction, support, and feedback to engage family members with different points of view and goals in the therapeutic process. Furthermore, the therapist must maintain a goal-directed stance while at the same time responding to the inevitable crises and backsliding that often punctuate real change in family interactions.

The excitement of these complexities can easily turn to discouragement, particularly when the therapist is confronted with a difficult, resistant family with very real problems, when the therapist's efforts seem pointless, when fresh ideas seem as rare and unlikely as winning a daily lottery. It is for these occasions that this book was written. We hope that it will stand as a reminder of how much we have yet to learn. At the same time, we hope it will provide new ideas to help therapists expand their knowledge and their skills in dealing with parent–adolescent conflict. Even more important, we hope this volume will encourage therapists and researchers alike to evaluate both practical and theoretical ideas systematically, using their results to build our understanding of family process and dysfunction.

APPENDIX A

Self-Report Measures

Instructions for administration and scoring of the Issues Checklist (IC) and Conflict Behavior Questionnaire (CBQ) are included in this appendix. These measures have been discussed in Chapter 5.

Parent and adolescents independently complete each questionnaire. When mother and father are both available, each parent completes the questionnaires, and the adolescent completes the questionnaires separately for relations with each parent. (There are slight differences in wording for adolescent–mother and adolescent–father versions of the CBQ.)

The assessor should review the questionnaires with the family prior to their administration and check them over carefully for omitted items following their administration.

ISSUES CHECKLIST

Administration Instructions

When we administer the IC, we staple a blank cover sheet over the frequency and intensity columns of each page (right half) until the family has completed all of the quantity ratings. Then we ask them to remove the cover sheets. The IC is introduced as follows:

On these pages is a list of issues that sometimes get talked about at home. First, we would like you to look carefully at each topic on the left-hand side of the page and decide whether the two of you together have talked about that topic at all during the last 4 weeks. The talks may have been long or short, pleasant or unpleasant; it doesn't matter right now. If the two of you have discussed the topic together during the past 4 weeks, circle *yes* to the right of the topic. If the two of you together have not discussed it during the past 4 weeks, circle *no* to the right of the topic. Go down this column for all four pages and let me know when you have finished. Please do not remove the cover sheets until I instruct you to do so. Any questions?

(In the case of a triad, specify that each parent is to rate dyadic discussions with the adolescent, and that the adolescent is to rate dyadic discussions with the mother and father on separate ICs.)

When the family has completed the yes/no ratings, continue as follows:

Now tear off all of the cover sheets. Good. Now we would like you to go back over the list of topics. For those topics for which you circled yes, please answer the two questions on the right-hand side of each page. First, how many times during the past 4 weeks did the topic come up for discussion? Please give us a number such as "0," "5," or "10," not a word such as "none," "a few," or "many." Guess if you are unsure, but don't leave any blanks. Second, how hot or angry, on the average, were the discussions? If the discussions were typically very angry, circle *5*. If the discussions were typically calm, circle *1*. If the discussions were inbetween calm and angry, circle *2*, *3*, or *4* depending upon your opinion. Again, guess if you are unsure, but don't leave blank any items you circled *yes* on the left-hand side of the page. Any questions?

Check the ICs very carefully for omitted items on the right-hand side. Two common errors are failing to provide ratings for an item endorsed *yes* or writing in words such as "a few" or "often" instead of numerical frequencies.

Scoring Instructions

Three scores are obtained for each person's IC:

1. *Quantity of issues*. Sum the number of issues marked *yes*.

2. *Intensity of issues*. For the issues marked *yes*, sum the intensity ratings and divide by the number of issues marked *yes* to obtain a mean intensity.

3. *Weighted frequency-by-intensity score*. First, multiply each frequency by its associated intensity rating. Then sum these cross products, sum the frequencies, and divide the sum of the products by the sum of the frequencies.

Means for clinic and nonclinic samples may be found in Chapter 5, Table 5-2.

Issues Checklist

Below is a list of things that sometimes get talked about at home. Circle *YES* for the topics that you and your parents/son or daughter have talked about at all during the last 4 weeks. Circle *NO* for those that have not come up.

Now go back over the list. For those topics that you circled *YES*, answer these 2 questions . . .

Go down this column for all 3 pages. Then come back to this page and answer the questions on the right.

How many times during the last 4 weeks has it come up? (Give a number)

How hot are the discussions for each topic?

Topic	How many times?	Calm	A little angry		Angry
1. Telephone calls yes no		1	2	3	4	5
2. Time for going to bed yes no		1	2	3	4	5
3. Cleaning up bedroom yes no		1	2	3	4	5

Topic			How many times?	Calm	A little angry			Angry
4. Doing homework	yes	no		1	2	3	4	5
5. Putting away clothes	yes	no		1	2	3	4	5
6. Using the television	yes	no		1	2	3	4	5
7. Cleanliness (washing, showers, brushing teeth)	yes	no		1	2	3	4	5
8. Which clothes to wear	yes	no		1	2	3	4	5
9. How neat clothing looks	yes	no		1	2	3	4	5
10. Making too much noise at home	yes	no		1	2	3	4	5
11. Table manners	yes	no		1	2	3	4	5
12. Fighting with brothers and sisters	yes	no		1	2	3	4	5
13. Cursing	yes	no		1	2	3	4	5
14. How money is spent	yes	no		1	2	3	4	5
15. Picking books or movies	yes	no		1	2	3	4	5
16. Allowance	yes	no		1	2	3	4	5
17. Going places without parents (shopping, movies, etc.)	yes	no		1	2	3	4	5
18. Playing stereo or radio too loudly	yes	no		1	2	3	4	5
19. Turning off lights in house	yes	no		1	2	3	4	5
20. Drugs	yes	no		1	2	3	4	5
21. Taking care of records, games, bikes, pets and other things	yes	no		1	2	3	4	5

(continued)

Topic			How many times?	Calm		A little angry		Angry
22. Drinking beer or other liquor	yes	no		1	2	3	4	5
23. Buying records, games, toys, and things	yes	no		1	2	3	4	5
24. Going on dates	yes	no		1	2	3	4	5
25. Who should be friends	yes	no		1	2	3	4	5
26. Selecting new clothes	yes	no		1	2	3	4	5
27. Sex	yes	no		1	2	3	4	5
28. Coming home on time	yes	no		1	2	3	4	5
29. Getting to school on time	yes	no		1	2	3	4	5
30. Getting low grades in school	yes	no		1	2	3	4	5
31. Getting in trouble at school	yes	no		1	2	3	4	5
32. Lying	yes	no		1	2	3	4	5
33. Helping out around the house	yes	no		1	2	3	4	5
34. Talking back to parents	yes	no		1	2	3	4	5
35. Getting up in the morning	yes	no		1	2	3	4	5
36. Bothering parents when they want to be left alone	yes	no		1	2	3	4	5
37. Bothering teenager when he/she wants to be left alone	yes	no		1	2	3	4	5
38. Putting feet on furniture	yes	no		1	2	3	4	5
39. Messing up the house	yes	no		1	2	3	4	5
40. What time to have meals	yes	no		1	2	3	4	5

Topic	How many times?	Calm		A little angry		Angry
41. How to spend free time yes no		1	2	3	4	5
42. Smoking yes no		1	2	3	4	5
43. Earning money away from the house yes no		1	2	3	4	5
44. What teenager eats yes no		1	2	3	4	5

Now go back to the first page and follow the directions on the right-hand side of the pages.

Note. The IC is reproduced with the permission of Dr. Ronald J. Prinz.

CONFLICT BEHAVIOR QUESTIONNAIRE

The CBQ is introduced to the family by going over the instructions written on the questionnaire and asking if family members have any questions about the form. Although the CBQ was originally labeled "The Interaction Behavior Questionnaire" on the form given to families to disguise its purpose, this practice has created sufficient confusion among investigators using the instrument that we now label the questionnaire with its proper name.

Scoring Instructions: Long Version CBQs

Two scores are obtained for each family member.
Parent version:
1. Parent's report of adolescent's behavior (53 items):
   a. Add one point for each of the following items answered *true:* 1, 5, 17, 19, 22, 23, 25, 26, 28, 29, 31, 32, 35, 37, 38, 41, 43, 44, 46, 47, 49, 50, 52, 53, 55, 56, 58, 59, 61, 62, 64, 65, 67, 68, 69, 70, 71, 72, 73, 74, 75.
   b. Add one point for each of the following answered *false:* 2, 4, 7, 8, 10, 11, 13, 14, 16, 20, 34, 40
2. Parent's report of dyadic behavior (22 items):
   a. Add one point for each *true:* 9, 15, 21, 27, 36, 39, 42, 48, 51, 54, 57, 60, 66.
   b. Add one point for each *false:* 3, 6, 12, 18, 24, 30, 33, 45, 63

Adolescent version:
1. Adolescent's report of parent's behavior (51 items):
   a. Add one point for each of the following items answered *true:* 1, 2, 4, 5, 7, 8, 11, 14, 17, 19, 20, 22, 28, 31, 32, 34, 35, 37, 38, 40, 41, 43, 44, 50, 55, 56, 58, 59, 61, 62, 64, 65, 67, 68, 72, 73.

   b. Add one point for each of the following items answered *false:* 10, 13, 16, 23, 25, 26, 29, 46, 47, 49, 52, 53, 69, 70, 71.
2. Adolescent's report of dyadic behavior (22 items):
   a. Add one point for each *true:* 9, 15, 21, 27, 36, 39, 42, 48, 51, 54, 57, 60, 66.
   b. Add one point for each *false:* 3, 6, 12, 18, 24, 30, 33, 45, 63.

   We have found it convenient to construct transparent plastic overlays for scoring the CBQ. Alternatively, researchers can have families respond on standard multiple-choice, machine-scorable sheets to be read by an optical scanner.
   Normative CBQ data may be found in Chapter 5. In addition, Tables A-1 and A-2 allow raw scores to be converted to standardized *t* scores. Table A-1 presents conversions based on distressed family data, while Table A-2 is based on data from nondistressed families.

TABLE A-1 *t* Scores for Conflict Behavior Questionnaire, Based upon
Pooled Data for Distressed Families

				Converted *t* values				
Raw score	M on A	F on A	A on M	A on F	M on D	F on D	A on M-D	A on F-D
0	21	25	33	35	29	29	30	30
1	22	27	34	35	31	31	32	32
2	23	28	35	36	33	34	34	34
3	25	29	36	37	35	36	36	37
4	26	30	37	38	36	39	38	39
5	27	31	37	39	40	41	40	41
6	28	32	38	40	42	43	42	43
7	29	33	39	41	44	46	44	45
8	30	35	40	42	46	48	47	47
9	32	36	41	43	49	50	49	49
10	33	37	42	44	51	53	51	51
11	34	38	43	45	53	55	53	54
12	35	39	44	45	55	58	55	56
13	36	40	44	46	58	60	57	58
14	37	41	45	47	60	62	59	60
15	38	43	46	48	62	65	61	62
16	39	44	47	49	64	67	63	64
17	40	45	48	50	66	70	65	66
18	41	46	49	51	69	72	67	69
19	43	47	50	52	71	74	69	71
20	44	48	51	53	73	77	71	73

(*continued*)

TABLE A-1 (*continued*)

Converted *t* values

Raw score	M on A	F on A	A on M	A on F	M on D	F on D	A on M-D	A on F-D
21	45	50	51	54	75	79	73	75
22	46	51	52	55	78	81	75	77
23	47	52	53	55				
24	48	53	54	56				
25	49	54	55	57				
26	50	55	56	58				
27	52	56	57	59				
28	53	58	57	60				
29	54	59	58	61				
30	55	60	59	62				
31	56	61	60	63				
32	57	62	61	64				
33	58	63	62	65				
34	59	64	63	65				
35	61	66	64	66				
36	62	67	64	67				
37	63	68	65	68				
38	64	69	66	69				
39	65	70	67	70				
40	66	71	68	71				
41	67	73	69	72				
42	68	74	70	73				
43	70	75	71	74				
44	71	76	71	75				
45	72	77	72	75				
46	73	78	73	76				
47	74	79	74	77				
48	75	81	75	78				
49	76	82	76	79				
50	77	83	77	80				
51	79	84	77	81				
52	80	85	78	82				
53	81	86	79	83				

Note. M on A = mother's appraisal of adolescent; F on A = father's appraisal of adolescent; A on M = adolescent's appraisal of mother; A on F = adolescent's appraisal of father; M on D = mother's appraisal of dyad; F on D = father's appraisal of dyad; A on M-D = adolescent's appraisal of dyad with mother; A on F-D = adolescent's appraisal of dyad with father. Values are based on analyses of data from distressed families described in Table 5-2.

TABLE A-2 *t* Scores for Conflict Behavior Questionnaire, Based upon Pooled
Data for Nondistressed Families

	Converted *t* scores							
Raw score	M on A	F on A	A on M	A on F	M on D	F on D	A on M-D	A on F-D
0	36	34	41	38	39	34	33	33
1	38	36	42	40	43	39	40	37
2	39	37	43	42	48	45	41	41
3	41	39	45	44	53	51	46	45
4	43	40	46	46	58	56	50	49
5	45	41	48	48	62	62	54	53
6	46	43	49	50	67	67	59	58
7	48	44	50	52	72	73	63	62
8	50	46	52	54	77	78	67	66
9	52	47	53	56	81	84	72	70
10	54	48	54	58	86	89	76	74
11	55	50	56	59	91	95	80	78
12	57	51	57	61	96	101	85	83
13	59	53	58	63	100	106	89	87
14	61	54	60	65	105	112	93	91
15	62	55	61	67	110	117	98	95
16	64	57	63	69	115	123	102	99
17	66	58	64	71	120	128	107	103
18	68	60	65	73	124	134	111	108
19	69	61	67	75	129	139	115	111
20	71	63	68	77	134	145	120	115
21	73	64	69	79	139	151	124	120
22	75	65	71	81	143	156	128	124
23	76	67	72	83				
24	78	68	74	84				
25	80	70	75	86				
26	82	71	76	88				
27	83	72	78	90				
28	85	74	79	92				
29	87	75	80	94				
30	89	77	82	96				
31	90	78	83	98				
32	92	79	85	100				
33	94	81	86	102				
34	96	82	87	104				
35	97	84	89	106				
36	99	85	90	108				

(*continued*)

TABLE A-2 (*continued*)

				Converted *t* scores				
Raw score	M on A	F on A	A on M	A on F	M on D	F on D	A on M-D	A on F-D
37	101	86	91	109				
38	103	88	93	111				
39	104	89	94	113				
40	106	91	95	115				
41	108	92	97	117				
42	110	94	98	119				
43	111	95	100	121				
44	113	96	101	123				
45	115	98	102	125				
46	117	99	104	127				
47	118	101	105	129				
48	120	102	106	131				
49	122	103	108	133				
50	124	105	109	134				
51	125	106	111	136				
52	127	108	112	138				
53	129	109	113	140				

Note. M on A = mother's appraisal of adolescent; F on A = father's appraisal of adolescent; A on M = adolescent's appraisal of mother; A on F = adolescent's appraisal of father; M on D = mother's appraisal of dyad; F on D = father's appraisal of dyad; A on M-D = adolescent's appraisal of dyad with mother; A on F-D = adolescent's appraisal of dyad with father. Values are based on data from nondistressed families described in Table 5-2.

Short Forms

Users of the CBQ may wish to employ a short form for rapid screening purposes. Two short forms are available. The first is a 44-item version developed by Dr. Ronald J. Prinz, based on the data from mothers and adolescents reported in the Prinz et al. (1979) investigation. This version retains two scales for each respondent: report on the other and report on the dyad. Items that correlated highest with summary scores for each full-scale score were retained; the scales from the 44-item version correlate .98 or higher with their full-scale counterparts. Items marked with the superscript [a] on the sample CBQs that follow are included in the CBQ-44.

A shorter form of the CBQ, the CBQ-20, was developed by Robin via extensive item analyses of the long-version CBQ using the pooled data from 205 families summarized in Chapter 5. Measures of internal consistency (item-total correlations) and discriminant validity (phi coefficients) were computed for each item, and the items were rank ordered on these two variables. The 20 items for parents and adolescents with the highest item-total correlations and the highest phi coefficients were included in the short form. This form yields a single score, which correlates .96 or more with the sum of the two scales for the long form. Items marked with the superscript *b* on the sample CBQs that follow are included in the CBQ-20.

Scoring Instructions: CBQ-44

To score the CBQ-44, use the directions for the long form but score only those items included in the CBQ-44. Multiply the adolescent-report-of-parent score by 1.821 to get a long-form equivalent score. Multiply the adolescent-report-of-dyad score by 1.375, parent-report-of-teen by 1.893, and parent-report-of-dyad by 1.375. Since the CBQ-44 was developed based on teens and mothers only, scores involving the father should be interpreted cautiously.

Scoring Instructions: CBQ-20

Only one score is obtained for each CBQ:
1. Parent version:
    a. Add one point for each *true:* 15, 21, 26, 41, 42, 43, 47, 51, 55, 60, 61, 62, 66, 68.
    b. Add one point for each *false:* 2, 4, 10, 14, 16, 33.
2. Adolescent version:
    a. Add one point for each *true:* 2, 15, 19, 21, 34, 36, 38, 42, 50, 51, 55, 59.
    b. Add one point for each *false:* 3, 13, 18, 23, 25, 46, 70, 71.

Normative data for the CBQ-20 may be found in Table A-3.

TABLE A-3 Means and Standard Deviations for CBQ-20

Score	Distressed mean *(SD)*	Nondistressed mean *(SD)*	*t*	r_{pb}
Mother on adolescent	12.4 (5.0)	2.4 (2.8)	15.3*	.73
Father on adolescent	10.5 (5.0)	3.2 (3.0)	5.2*	.51
Adolescent on mother	8.4 (6.0)	2.0 (3.1)	8.2*	.50
Adolescent on father	7.6 (5.4)	1.6 (1.6)	4.1*	.42

Note. r_{pb} represents point-biserial correlation of score with distressed–nondistressed status. *t* represents value of *t*-test for differences between distressed and nondistressed families.
*$p<.001$

Conflict Behavior Questionnaire: Parent Version

You are the child's _____ mother _____ father (check one). You are filling this questionnaire out regarding your _____ son _____ daughter (check one) who is _____ years old. Think back over the last 2 weeks at home. The statements below have to do with you and your child. Read the statement, and then decide if you believe the statement is true. If it is true, then circle *true,* and if you believe the statement is not true, circle *false*. You must circle either *true* or *false*, but never both for the same item. Please answer all items. Answer for yourself, without talking it over with your spouse. Your answers will not be shown to your child.

true	false	1.	My child sulks after an argument.
true	false	2.	My child is easy to get along with. [a,b]
true	false	3.	My child and I sometimes end our arguments calmly.
true	false	4.	My child is receptive to criticism. [a,b]
true	false	5.	My child curses at me. [a]
true	false	6.	We joke around often. [a]
true	false	7.	My child, for the most part, accepts punishment.
true	false	8.	My child enjoys being with me. [a]
true	false	9.	At least once a week, we get angry with each other.
true	false	10.	My child is well behaved in our discussions. [a,b]
true	false	11.	My child lets me know when s/he is pleased with something I have done.
true	false	12.	We do a lot of things together. [a]
true	false	13.	My child almost never complains.
true	false	14.	For the most part, my child likes to talk to me. [b]
true	false	15.	We almost never seem to agree. [a,b]
true	false	16.	My child usually listens to what I tell him/her. [a,b]
true	false	17.	My child never talks when I discuss things with him/her.
true	false	18.	I enjoy the talks we have. [a]
true	false	19.	Often when I talk to my child, s/he laughs at me.
true	false	20.	My child will approach me when something is on his/her mind. [a]
true	false	21.	At least three times a week, we get angry at each other. [a,b]
true	false	22.	My child screams a lot. [a]
true	false	23.	Several hours after an argument, my child is still mad at me. [a]
true	false	24.	After an argument which turns out badly, one or both of us apologizes. [a]
true	false	25.	My child doesn't pay attention when I have discussions with him/her. [a]
true	false	26.	My child says that I have no consideration of his/her feelings. [a,b]
true	false	27.	We argue at the dinner table at least half the time we eat together. [a]
true	false	28.	My child embarrasses me in front of my friends.
true	false	29.	My child does not usually abide by decisions that the two of us reach.
true	false	30.	We listen to each other, even when we argue.
true	false	31.	When we discuss things, my child gets restless.
true	false	32.	My child usually starts our arguments.
true	false	33.	My child and I compromise during arguments. [a,b]
true	false	34.	I enjoy spending time with my child.
true	false	35.	My child mistreats me in front of his/her friends.
true	false	36.	At least once a day we get angry at each other. [a]
true	false	37.	My child leaves the house after an argument.

true	false	38.	My child runs to his/her room after an argument.
true	false	39.	We argue until one of us is too tired to go on.
true	false	40.	My child often seeks me out.[a]
true	false	41.	My child often doesn't do what I ask.[a,b]
true	false	42.	The talks we have are frustrating.[a,b]
true	false	43.	My child often seems angry at me.[a,b]
true	false	44.	My child often cries when I question him/her.[a]
true	false	45.	We have enjoyable talks at least once a week.
true	false	46.	When angry, my child becomes aggressive.
true	false	47.	My child acts impatient when I talk.[a,b]
true	false	48.	My child and I speak to each other only when we have to.[a]
true	false	49.	My child often criticizes me.
true	false	50.	My child says I don't love him/her.[a]
true	false	51.	In general, I don't think we get along very well.[a,b]
true	false	52.	My child holds a grudge.
true	false	53.	My child contradicts everything I say.[a]
true	false	54.	We argue at the dinner table almost every time we eat.[a]
true	false	55.	My child almost never understands my side of an argument.[a,b]
true	false	56.	My child lies to me often.[a]
true	false	57.	We never have fun together.[a]
true	false	58.	During a heated discussion, my child tries to hit me.[a]
true	false	59.	My child slams the door after an argument.
true	false	60.	My child and I have big arguments about little things.[a,b]
true	false	61.	My child is defensive when I talk to him/her.[a,b]
true	false	62.	My child thinks my opinions don't count.[b]
true	false	63.	We have enjoyable talks at least once a day.[a]
true	false	64.	My child does things to purposely annoy me.
true	false	65.	My child provokes me into an argument at least twice a week.[a]
true	false	66.	We argue a lot about rules.[b]
true	false	67.	My child rarely follows through with his/her end of the bargain, after we have reached an agreement.[a]
true	false	68.	My child tells me s/he thinks I am unfair.[a,b]
true	false	69.	My child compares me to other parents.
true	false	70.	My child talks under his/her breath during a discussion.
true	false	71.	My child blows up for no reason.[a]
true	false	72.	My child often isolates himself/herself in his/her room after an argument with me.
true	false	73.	If I speak calmly, my child doesn't do what I ask.[a]
true	false	74.	My child doesn't look at me when I try to talk to him/her.[a]
true	false	75.	When my child is upset about something, s/he clams up.

Note. The CBQ is reproduced with the permission of Dr. Ronald J. Prinz.
[a]Items included in the 44-item revised version
[b]Items included in the 20-item revised version.

Conflict Behavior Questionnaire: Adolescent Version for Mother

Think back over the last 2 weeks at home. The statements below have to do with you and your mother. Read the statement, and then decide if you believe the statement is true. If it is true, then circle *true*, and if you believe the statement is not true, circle *false*. You must circle either true or false, but never both for the same item. Please answer all items. Your answers will not be shown to your parents.

true	false	1.	Even when I apologize, my mother doesn't say she is sorry.
true	false	2.	My mom doesn't understand me.[b]
true	false	3.	My mom and I sometimes end our arguments calmly.[b]
true	false	4.	If I am right, my mother doesn't admit it.[a]
true	false	5.	My mom never asks me questions about things I like to talk about.
true	false	6.	We joke around often.[a]
true	false	7.	When I come up with my own ideas, she tells me I am disrespectful.
true	false	8.	I feel like I'm always wrong in an argument with my mom.
true	false	9.	At least once a week, we get angry at each other.
true	false	10.	My mom answers me when I say something.
true	false	11.	My mom picks on me.[a]
true	false	12.	We do a lot of things together.[a]
true	false	13.	My mom understand me.[a,b]
true	false	14.	My mom expects too much of us.
true	false	15.	We almost never seem to agree.[a,b]
true	false	16.	My mom stays calm during a discussion.
true	false	17.	Several hours after an argument, my mom is still mad at me.[a]
true	false	18.	I enjoy the talks we have.[a,b]
true	false	19.	When I state my own opinion, she gets upset.[b]
true	false	20.	My mom brings up a lot of my faults when we argue.[a]
true	false	21.	At least three times a week, we get angry at each other.[a,b]
true	false	22.	She says I am lazy when we argue.
true	false	23.	My mother listens when I need someone to talk to.[b]
true	false	24.	After an argument which turns out badly, one or both of us apologizes.[a]
true	false	25.	My mom is a good friend to me.[b]
true	false	26.	My mom likes my friends.[a]
true	false	27.	We argue at the dinner table at least half the time we eat together.[a]
true	false	28.	When we talk, she compares me to other kids.
true	false	29.	When we argue, my mom makes suggestions that I like.
true	false	30.	We listen to each other, even when we argue.
true	false	31.	My mom can't take jokes.
true	false	32.	My mom slaps me when she gets angry.[a]
true	false	33.	My mom and I compromise during arguments.[a]
true	false	34.	She says I have no consideration for her.[a,b]
true	false	35.	During discussions, my mom doesn't listen to my side of the story.
true	false	36.	At least once a day we get angry at each other.[a,b]

true	false	37.	She says bad things to other people about me.[a]
true	false	38.	My mother is bossy when we talk.[a,b]
true	false	39.	We argue until one of us is too tired to go on.
true	false	40.	When I try to tell her something, she doesn't let me finish.[a]
true	false	41.	My mom nags me a lot.
true	false	42.	The talks we have are frustrating.[a,b]
true	false	43.	She makes me feel that the argument is all my fault.[a]
true	false	44.	If I disagree with her, she slaps me.
true	false	45.	We have enjoyable talks at least once a week.
true	false	46.	My mom understands my point of view, even when she doesn't agree with me.[a,b]
true	false	47.	My mother can help me feel better when I am upset.
true	false	48.	My mom and I speak to each other only when we have to.[a]
true	false	49.	My mom can tell when I have something on my mind.[a]
true	false	50.	My mom seems to be always complaining about me.[b]
true	false	51.	In general, I don't think we get along very well.[a,b]
true	false	52.	My mother is interested in the things I do.[a]
true	false	53.	When my mother punishes me, she is usually being fair.[a]
true	false	54.	We argue at the dinner table almost every time we eat.[a]
true	false	55.	My mom screams a lot.[a,b]
true	false	56.	My mother never apologizes first.[a]
true	false	57.	We never have fun together.[a]
true	false	58.	My mother rarely listens to me during an argument.[a]
true	false	59.	My mom puts me down.[a,b]
true	false	60.	My mom and I have big arguments about little things.[a]
true	false	61.	She thinks my opinions are childish.[a]
true	false	62.	When I am arguing with my mother, she doesn't give me the chance to state my views.[a]
true	false	63.	We have enjoyable talks at least once a day.[a]
true	false	64.	My mom nags me about a little thing, and we end up in an argument.[a]
true	false	65.	She says I am stupid when we argue.[a]
true	false	66.	We argue a lot about rules.
true	false	67.	My mother does all the talking.
true	false	68.	My mom embarrasses me in front of my friends.
true	false	69.	Even when she doesn't let me do something I want to do, she still listens to me.[a]
true	false	70.	If I run into problems, my mom helps me out.[a,b]
true	false	71.	I enjoy spending time with my mother.[b]
true	false	72.	My mom gets angry at me whenever we have a discussion.[a]
true	false	73.	It seems like whenever I try to talk to my mother, she has something else to do.[a]

Note. To create the ACBQ-Father version, change the words "mother" to "father", "mom" to "dad", and "she" to "he" in the items. The CBQ is reproduced with permission of Dr. Ronald J. Prinz.
[a]Items included in the 44-item revised version.
[b]Items included in the 20-item version.

APPENDIX B

Interaction Behavior Code

The Interaction Behavior Code (IBC) is designed to assess global impressions of parent–adolescent problem-solving communication behavior (Prinz, 1977; Prinz & Kent, 1978). Below is a list of coding categories, incorporated into a rating form. Several coders (at least three or four) listen to an audiotaped discussion of a family attempting to resolve an issue about which they disagree. Coders are usually instructed to listen to the entire discussion twice before completing the ratings. Then the coders rate items 1–22 *no* or *yes* (scored 0 or 1), depending upon their evaluations of the presence or absence of the behaviors during the entire interaction. Items 23–32 are scored *no* (0 points), *a little* (.5 point), or *a lot* (1 point). Ratings are completed separately for each family member, and summary scores are computed for positive and negative mother, father, and adolescent behavior by summing across the following items for each rater, dividing by the number of items, then averaging across all of the raters. Thus, the *mean* of the raters' scores serves as the dependent measure.

1. *Negative behavior.* Add one point for each marked *yes*: 1, 2, 3, 4, 5, 6, 7, 8, 10, 11, 13, 14, 15, 16, 17, 18, 21. Add .5 point for each of the following marked *a little,* and one point for each marked *a lot:* 23, 24, 27, 28, 29, 30, 31, 32. Divide total by 25.
2. *Positive behavior.* Add one point for each marked *yes*: 9, 12, 19, 20, 22. Add .5 point for each of the following marked *a little,* and one point for each marked *a lot:* 25, 26. Divide total by 7.

Ratings are also completed for the dyad or triad on items 33–36. Each of these items provides a separate score. Again, the mean of the raters' scores is used for analysis.

Since the scores to be analyzed are mean scores of several raters, reliability of the mean score is computed. The Spearman-Brown formula provides an estimate for the multiple observation case based upon reliability for the single-observation case. The average interrater correlation for all possible pairs of raters is computed for the single-observation case. The Spearman-Brown formula is

$$\text{Reliability of } n \text{ raters} = \frac{n\,(x_r)}{1 + (n - 1)\,(x_r)}$$

where n refers to the number of raters and x_r refers to the average pairwise correlation, computed across all possible pairs of raters.

CATEGORY DEFINITIONS AND RATING FORM

Coder: _____

Tape: _____

Item	Mother		Son		Valence	
	No	Yes	No	Yes		
1.					—	*negative exaggeration*—putting excessive emphasis on the other person's negative qualities; overgeneralizing (look for key words "always" and "never"). Do not rate overgeneralizations said in joking fashion.
2.					—	*yelling*—raising the volume of one's voice in an angry manner.
3.					—	*ridicule, make fun of*—to tease, mock, or belittle the other aimed at hurting the other person. Intent = put down. Said in acid or sarcastic tone.
4.					—	*using big words*.
5.					—	*repeating one's opinion with insistence*—excessively and repeatedly stating the same opinion.
6.					—	*threatening*—an expression of intention to do harm or to levy negative consequences. Exclude statements in which a negative consequence is stated as a possible response to a behavior and is considered *by both parties* as a possible solution to a problem.
7.					—	*namecalling*—applying a name to the other person which connotes something negative. Must be a noun.
8.					—	*interrupting with criticism*—to break in with questions or remarks of a critical nature while the other is speaking.

Item	Mother		Son		Val-ence	
	No	Yes	No	Yes		
9.					+	*stating the other's opinion*—an effort to express the other person's views in a non-condemnatory fashion, e.g., by para-phrasing without losing the original intent (this is a positive behavior).
10.					−	*giving short unhelpful responses*—answering questions or statements with utterances that have no benefits to the dis-cussion, e.g., "Uh huh," "I don't know."
11.					−	*asking accusative questions*—asking a question which implies some wrongdoing.
12.					+	*making suggestions*—offering solutions and possible ideas (without demanding) of things that can be done differently in the future.
13.					−	*making demands*—clear-cut commands; requests which require action.
14.					−	*arguing over small points (quibbling)*—disputing minute, trivial or discussion-irrelevant aspects.
15.					−	*talking very little*—minimal participation throughout the discussion.
16.					−	*talking very much*—monopolizing the discussion.
17.					−	*disregarding the other person's points*—lack of acknowledgment of other's state-ments; speaking as though the other per-son did not say anything.
18.					−	*mind reading*—stating or attributing be-liefs to the other person.

(*continued*)

Item	Mother		Son		Val-ence	
	No	Yes	No	Yes		
19.					+	*joking (good natured)*—adding some levity to the conversation, possibly resulting in laughter, without making fun or ridiculing.
20.					+	*praising, complimenting*—expressing approval of the other person; to commend, say something positive about the other.
21.					−	*quick, negative judgment of other's suggestions*—to negate, reject, or criticize the other person's suggestions without verbal or temporal signs of taking the suggestion under consideration.
22.					+	*asking what other would like*—attempting to find out what the other person wants, expects, or prefers.

Item	Mother			Son			Val-ence	
	No	Little	Yes	No	Little	Yes		
23.							−	*abrupt changes of subject*—a sudden change of topic which leaves the original topic unresolved and does not follow from what the other person said.
24.							−	*anger*—to be annoyed, disgusted, or enraged with the other person.
25.							+	*compromise*—modifying original intentions or preferences, willingness to do so.
26.							+	*willingness to listen*—paying attention to what the other has to say; showing interest with questions and acknowledgments.
27.							−	*demanding*—making repeated demands and using tone of voice which suggests that the speaker expects compliance.

Item	Mother			Son			Val-ence	
	No	Little	Yes	No	Little	Yes		
28.							−	*sarcasm*—making sarcastic or derisive remarks about the other; implying criticism or dislike in an acid tone.
29.							−	*acquiescence*—overly accepting or agreeing.
30.							−	*silence, ignoring other*—refusing to participate, avoiding questions, not talking (for longer than a couple of seconds).
31.							−	*personal attack*—to speak of the other person accusingly; to make a verbal judgment about the other person which includes a negative trait, e.g., "You are lazy."
32.							−	*criticism*—finding fault with the other person's actions, statements or beliefs.

The following items are rated for the dyad on the scales indicated:

33. *outcome*—degree of resolution of the problems being discussed.

1	2	3	4	5
clear resolution	close to resolution	dyad unsure	far from resolution	no resolution

34. *putting each other down*—degree of belittlement and criticism, taking into account both members.

1	2	3	4
none	a little	moderate	a lot

35. *friendliness*—saying nice things to each other, keeping the discussion pleasant for both members.

1	2	3	4
none	a little	moderate	a lot

36. How effective were the two at solving problems that came up?

1	2	3	4
very effective	somewhat effective	fair	very ineffective

Note. The IBC is reproduced with the permission of Dr. Ronald J. Prinz.

Problem-Solving Exercise

SESSION ONE HOMEWORK

Name _____ Date _____

The purpose of this worksheet is to give you practice with the steps of problem solving. Write out the answers as best you can. Bring the sheet to your therapist at your next session; the therapist will go over it with you.

I. Defining the problem

A good definition of the problem tells what the other person is *doing* or *saying* that *bothers* you and *why* this bothers you. The definition is short, neutral, and does not blame the other person. Below are several definitions. Read each one. Then say whether it is good or bad. If it is bad, write down a better definition.

A. MOTHER: My problem is that I don't like to see your room dirty; all the clothes are on the bed and the dust is 2 inches thick. I'm upset when my friends come to visit and see the room looking that way.

1. Is this a good definition of a room cleaning problem?

_____ Yes _____ No

2. If you said no, write a better definition:

_____

_____

_____

B. DAUGHTER: I hate you, Mom. You just are a real pain. I'm missing out on all the fun because you make me come home by 9 p.m. on weekends.

1. Is this a good definition of a coming-home-on-time problem?

_____ Yes _____ No

2. If you said no, write a better definition:

_____

_____

_____

C. FATHER: Son, the real problem with you is that you don't respect your elders. Kids just don't know the meaning of respect today. When I was your age, I would never talk to my father the way you talk to me.

1. Is this a good definition of a talking-back problem?

_____ Yes _____ No

2. If you said no, write a better definition:

_____

_____

_____

D. SON: I get angry when you bug me 10 times a day about taking out the trash and feeding the dogs. I'm old enough to do these things without being reminded.

1. Is this a good definition for a chores problem?

_____ Yes _____ No

2. If you said no, write a better definition:

_____

_____

_____

E. Below, a mother and daughter define their problem about playing the stereo too loud. Notice how each accuses and blames the other; this is a poor way to define the problem. Read their definitions. Then write a better definition for each person.

MOTHER: You are ruining your ears with that loud stereo. You just don't have good taste in music. How can you stand all that loud noise? I can't and what's more, I won't stand for it.

DAUGHTER: Don't talk to me about taste in music. You sit around all day listening to 1940 junk music. No one listens to that stuff anymore. And get off my back about the loud stereo. I'll play it as loud as I like so I can enjoy my music.

Better definitions:

Mother: _____

_____

_____

_____

Daughter: _____

_____

_____

_____

II. Listing solutions

A. List as many ideas as you can.

B. Be creative and free.

C. Anything goes.

D. Don't say whether ideas are good or bad now. That comes later.

Make believe you are trying to solve a telephone problem. A mother is upset because her son talks on the phone 2 hours a night and runs up bills. The son says his friends live too far away to visit on weekdays; he calls them instead. Make a list of 10 ideas to solve this problem. Put down anything you can think of. Try to be creative.

List of solutions:

1. _____

2. _____

3. _____

4. _____

5. _____

6. _____

7. _____

8. _____

9. _____

10. _____

E. If you run out of ideas, here are some hints:
   1. Is a trade-off possible?
   2. Can they change anything around the house to help?
   3. Is a change of place or time possible?
   4. What about other ways to talk to friends?

III. Picking the best idea—decision making
   A. When you decide upon the best idea, you should state the good and bad points of each idea on your list. Then, rate each idea "+" or "−." Ask yourself about each idea:
      1. Will this idea solve my problem?
      2. Will this idea solve the other person's problem?
      3. Will this idea really work?
      4. Can I live with it?
   B. Consider the telephone problem we discussed above. Make believe one idea was "buy a second telephone."
      1. An adolescent might evaluate this as follows:
         "Well, this idea meets my need to talk to my friends, and my mother might get off my back for talking on her phone too much. I'll give it a '+'."

2. A parent might evaluate it as follows:

> "It is true that this would get my adolescent off my phone, but it would not solve the problem of high bills—we would have to pay for two phones. Now, if my adolescent wants to get a job to pay for the new phone, that's different. As is, I rate this idea '−'."

C. Now, write out evaluations for the first two ideas on your list for the telephone problem on the last page. For each idea write out an evaluation from the parent's side and a second evaluation from the adolescent's side.

Idea #1.

Parent's evaluation: _____

_____

_____

_____

Adolescent's evaluation: _____

_____

_____

_____

Idea #2.

Parent's evaluation: _____

_____

_____

Adolescent's evaluation: _____

_____

_____

_____

References

Adams, K. M. (1987). *Revision and validation of the parent–adolescent interaction coding system: An observational coding system for parent–adolescent conflict.* Unpublished doctoral dissertation, Wayne State University, Detroit, MI.

Alexander, J. F. (1973). Defensive and supportive communications in normal and deviant families. *Journal of Consulting and Clinical Psychology, 40,* 223–231.

Alexander, J. F., & Barton, C. (1976). Behavioral systems therapy for families. In D. H. L. Olson (Ed.), *Treating relationships* (pp. 167–168). Lake Mills, IA: Graphic Publishing Co., Inc.

Alexander, J. F., Barton, C., Schiavo, R. S., & Parsons, B. V. (1976). Systems-behavioral intervention with families of delinquents: Therapist characteristics, family behavior, and outcome. *Journal of Consulting and Clinical Psychology, 44,* 656–664.

Alexander, J. F., & Parsons, B. V. (1973). Short term behavioral intervention with delinquent families: Impact on family process and recidivism. *Journal of Abnormal Psychology, 81,* 219–225.

Alexander, J. F., & Parsons, B. V. (1982). *Functional family therapy.* Monterey, CA: Brooks/Cole.

Anderson, C. M., & Stewart, S. (1983). *Mastering resistance: A practical guide to family therapy.* New York: Guilford Press.

Aponte, H. J., & VanDeusen, J. M. (1981). Structural family therapy. In A. S. Gurman & D. P. Kniskern (Eds.), *Handbook of family therapy* (pp. 310–360). New York: Brunner/Mazel.

Azar, S. T., Robinson, D. R., Hekimian, E., & Twentyman, C. T. (1984). Unrealistic expectations and problem-solving ability in maltreating mothers. *Journal of Consulting and Clinical Psychology, 52,* 687–691.

Baer, D. M., Wolf, M. M., & Risley, T. R. (1968). Some current dimensions of applied behavior analysis. *Journal of Applied Behavior Analysis, 1,* 91–97.

Barkley, R. A. (1981). *Hyperactive children: A handbook for diagnosis and treatment.* New York: Guilford Press.

Barkley, R. A. (1987). *ADDH adolescents: Family conflicts, follow-up, and therapy.* Grant proposal submitted to the National Institute of Mental Health.

Barnes, H. L., & Olson, D. H. (1985). Parent–adolescent communication and the circumplex model. *Child Development, 56,* 438–447.

Barton, C., & Alexander, J. F. (1979, September). *The effects of competitive and cooperative set on normal and delinquent families.* Paper presented at the meeting of the American Psychological Association, New York.

Barton, C., & Alexander, J. F. (1981). Functional family therapy. In A. S. Gurman & D. P. Kniskern (Eds.), *Handbook of family therapy* (pp. 403–443). New York: Brunner/Mazel.

Barton, C., Alexander, J. F., Waldron, H., Turner, C. W., & Warburton, J. (1985). Generalizing treatment effects of functional family therapy: Three replications. *American Journal of Family Therapy, 13,* 16–26.

Bauer, W. D., & Twentyman, C. T. (1985). Abusing, neglectful, and comparison mothers' responses to child-related and non-child-related stressors. *Journal of Consulting and Clinical Psychology, 53,* 335–343.

Beck, A. T. (1967). *Depression: Clinical, experimental, and theoretical aspects.* New York: Hoeber.

Beck, A. T. (1976) *Cognitive therapy and the emotional disorders*. New York: International Universities Press.

Beck, A. T., & Emery, G. (1985). *Anxiety disorders and phobias*. New York: Basic Books.

Beck, A. T., Rush, A. J., Shaw, B. F., & Emery, G. (1979). *Cognitive therapy of depression*. New York: Guilford Press.

Bedrosian, R. C. (1981). The application of cognitive therapy techniques with adolescents. In G. Emery, S. D. Hollon, & R. C. Bedrosian (Eds.), *New directions in cognitive therapy: A casebook* (pp. 68–83). New York: Guilford Press.

Berg, I., & Fielding, D. (1979). An interview with a child to assess psychiatric disturbance: A note on its reliability and validity. *Journal of Abnormal Child Psychology, 7,* 83–89.

Bernal, G., & Flores-Ortiz, Y. (1982). Latino families in therapy: Engagement and evaluation. *Journal of Marital and Family Therapy, 8,* 357–365.

Besalel, V. A., & Azrin, N. H. (1981). The reduction of parent–youth problems by reciprocity counseling. *Behaviour Research and Therapy, 19,* 297–301.

Bienvenu, M. J. (1969). Measurement of parent–adolescent communication. *Family Coordinator, 17,* 117–121.

Blechman, E. A. (1974). The family contract game: A tool to teach interpersonal problem-solving. *Family Coordinator, 23,* 269–281.

Blechman, E. A. (1977). Objectives and procedures believed necessary for the success of a contractual approach to family intervention. *Behavior Therapy, 8,* 275–277.

Blechman, E. A. (1981). Marital therapy and child management training. In A. S. Gurman (Ed.), *Questions and answers in the practice of family therapy* (Vol. 1) (pp. 105–107). New York: Brunner/Mazel.

Blechman, E. A., & Olson, D. H. L. (1976). The family contract game: Description and effectiveness. In D. H. L. Olson (Ed.), *Treating relationships* (pp. 133–150). Lake Mills, IA: Graphic Publishing.

Bodin, A. M. (1981). The interactional view: Family therapy approaches of the mental research institute. In A. S. Gurman & D. P. Kniskern (Eds.), *Handbook of family therapy* (pp. 267–309). New York: Brunner/Mazel.

Brown, R. T., Borden, K. A., & Clingerman, M. A. (1985). Pharmacotherapy in ADD adolescents with special attention to multimodality treatments. *Psychopharmacology Bulletin, 21,* 192–211.

Carter, E. A., & McGoldrick, M. (Eds.) (1980). *The family life cycle: A framework for family therapy*. New York: Gardner Press.

Chamberlain, P., Patterson, G., Reid, J., Kavanagh, K., & Forgatch, M. (1984). Observation of client resistance. *Behavior Therapy, 15,* 144–155.

Christensen, A. (1979). Naturalistic observation of families: A system for random audio recordings in the home. *Behavior Therapy, 10,* 418–422.

Christensen, A., Sullaway, M., & King, C. E. (1983). Systematic error in behavioral reports of dyadic interaction: Egocentric bias and content effects. *Behavioral Assessment, 5,* 129–140.

Ciminero, A. R., Calhoun, K. S., & Adams, H. E. (Eds.) (1986). *Handbook of behavioral assessment* (2nd ed.). New York: Wiley.

Cone, J. D. (1979). Confounded comparisons in triple response mode assessment research. *Behavioral Assessment, 1,* 85–95.

Cone, J. D., & Foster, S. L. (1982). Direct observation in clinical psychology. In P. C. Kendall & J. N. Butcher (Eds.), *Handbook of research methods in clinical psychology* (pp. 311–354). New York: Wiley.

Conger, J. J. (1977). *Adolescence and youth: Psychological development in a changing world*. New York: Harper.

Cromwell, R. E., Olson, D. H. L., & Fournier, D. G. (1976). Tools and techniques for diagnosis and evaluation in marital and family therapy. *Family Process, 15,* 1–49.

DeRubeis, R. J., & Beck, A. T. (1988). Cognitive therapy. In K. S. Dobson (Ed.), *Handbook of cognitive–behavioral therapies* (pp. 273–306). New York: Guilford Press.

Dobson, K. S. (Ed.). (1988). *Handbook of cognitive–behavioral therapies*. New York: Guilford Press.

Doherty, W. J. (1981). Cognitive processes in intimate conflict. 1. Extending attribution theory. *American Journal of Family Therapy, 9,* 3–13.

Dryden, W., & Ellis, A. (1988). Rational–emotive therapy. In K. S. Dobson (Ed.), *Handbook of cognitive–behavioral therapies* (pp. 214–272). New York: Guilford Press.

D'Zurilla, T. J. (1988). Problem-solving therapies. In K. S. Dobson (Ed.), *Handbook of cognitive behavioral therapies* (pp. 85–135). New York: Guilford Press.

D'Zurilla, T. J., & Goldfried, M. R. (1971). Problem solving and behavior modification. *Journal of Abnormal Psychology, 78,* 197–226.

Edelbrock, C., & Costello, A. J. (1984). Structured psychiatric interviews for children and adolescents. In G. Goldstein & M. Hersen (Eds.), *Handbook of psychological assessment* (pp. 276–290). New York: Pergamon.

Edelbrock, C., Costello, A. J., Dulcan, M. K., Kalas, R., & Conover, N. C. (1985). Age differences in the reliability of the psychiatric interview of the child. *Child Development, 56,* 265–275.

Elder, G. H. (1962). Structural variations in the childrearing experience. *Sociometry, 25,* 241–262.

Ellis, A., & Grieger, R. (1977) *Handbook of rational–emotive therapy*. New York: Springer.

Emery, R. B. (1982). Interparental conflict and the children of discord and divorce. *Psychological Bulletin, 92,* 310–330.

Enyart, P. (1984). *Behavioral correlates of self-reported parent–adolescent relationship satisfaction.* Unpublished doctoral dissertation, West Virginia University, Morgantown, WV.

Epstein, N. (1982). Cognitive therapy with couples. *American Journal of Family Therapy, 10,* 5–16.

Epstein, N. B., Baldwin, L. M., & Bishop, D. S. (1983). The McMaster Family Assessment Device. *Journal of Marriage and the Family, 9,* 171–180.

Felton, J. L., & Nelson, R. O. (1984). Inter-assessor agreement on hypothesized controlling variables and treatment proposals. *Behavioral Assessment, 6,* 199–208.

Ferreira, A. J., Winter, W. D., & Poindexter, E. J. (1966). Some interactional variables in normal and abnormal families. *Family Process, 5,* 60–75.

Ferster, C., & Skinner, B. F. (1957). *Schedules of reinforcement*. New York: Appleton Century Crofts.

Filsinger, E. E. (Ed.) (1983). *Marriage and family therapy: A sourcebook for family therapy.* Beverly Hills: Sage.

Fogg, R. (1972). *Some effects of teaching adolescents some creative, peaceful approaches to international conflict.* Unpublished doctoral dissertation, Harvard University, Cambridge.

Foster, S. L. (1978). *Family conflict management: Skill training and generalization procedures.* Unpublished doctoral dissertation, SUNY, Stony Brook.

Foster, S. L., & Cone, J. D. (1986). Design and use of direct observation procedures. In A. Ciminero, K. S. Calhoun, & H. E. Adams (Eds.), *Handbook of behavioral assessment* (2nd ed.) (pp. 253–324). New York: Wiley.

Foster, S. L., & Hoier, T. S. (1982). Behavioral and systems family therapies: A comparison of theoretical assumptions. *American Journal of Family Therapy, 10,* 13–23.

Foster, S. L., Prinz, R. J., & O'Leary, K. D. (1983). Impact of problem-solving communication training and generalization procedures on family conflict. *Child and Family Behavior Therapy, 5,* 1–23.

Foster, S. L., & Robin, A. L. (1988). Family conflict and communication in adolescence. In E. J. Mash & L. G. Terdal (Eds.), *Behavioral assessment of childhood disorders* (2nd ed.) (pp. 717–775). New York: Guilford Press.

Foster, S. L., & Steinfeld, B. I. (1980). *Family conflict resolution: Patterns, correlates, and change.* Paper presented at the American Psychological Association, Montreal.

Gilbert, R., Christensen, A., & Margolin, G. (1984). Patterns of alliances in nondistressed and multiproblem families. *Family Process, 23,* 75–87.

Ginsberg, B. G. (1971). *Parent–adolescent relationship development: A therapeutic and preventive mental health program*. Unpublished doctoral dissertation, Pennsylvania State University, University Park.

Goldfried, M. R. (1979). Anxiety reduction through cognitive–behavioral intervention. In P. C. Kendall and S. D. Hollon (Eds.), *Cognitive–behavioral interventions: Theory, research, and procedures* (pp. 117–152). New York: Academic Press.

Goldfried, M. R. (1982). On the history of therapeutic integration. *Behavior Therapy, 13*, 572–593.

Goldfried, M. R., & Davison, G. C. (1976). *Clinical behavior therapy*. New York: Holt, Rinehart, & Winston.

Goldfried, M. R., Decenteceo, E. T., & Weinberg, L. (1974). Systematic rational restructuring as a self-control technique. *Behavior Therapy, 5*, 247–254.

Goldfried, M. R., & D'Zurilla, T. J. (1969). A behavioral-analytic model for assessing competence. In C. D. Spielberger (Ed.), *Current topics in clinical and community psychology* (Vol. 1) (pp. 151–196). New York: Academic Press.

Goldfried, M. R., & Goldfried, A. P. (1980). Cognitive change methods. In F. H. Kanfer & A. P. Goldstein (Eds.), *Helping people change* (2nd ed.) (pp. 97–130). New York: Pergamon Press.

Goldfried, M. R., & Kent, R. (1972). Traditional versus behavioral personality assessment: A comparison of methodological and theoretical assumptions. *Psychological Bulletin, 77*, 409–420.

Goldstein, A. P., & Myers, C. R. (1986). Relationship enhancement methods. In F. H. Kanfer & A. P. Goldstein (Eds.), *Helping people change* (3rd ed.) (pp. 19–65). New York: Pergamon Press.

Gordon, S. B., & Davidson, N. (1981). Behvioral parent training. In A. S. Gurman & D. P. Kniskern (Eds.), *Handbook of family therapy* (pp. 517–555). New York: Brunner/Mazel.

Gordon, T. (1970). *Parent effectiveness training*. New York: Wyden.

Gottman, J. M. (1979). *Marital interaction: Experimental investigations*. New York: Academic Press.

Gottman, J. M., & Levenson, R. W. (1985). A valid procedure for obtaining self-report of affect in marital interaction. *Journal of Consulting and Clinical Psychology, 53*, 151–160.

Gottman, J. M., Notarius, C., Gonso, J., & Markman, H. (1976). *A couple's guide to communication*. Champaign, IL: Research Press.

Gottman, J. M., Notarius, C., Markman, H., Bank, S., Yoppi, B., & Rubin, M. E. (1976). Behavior exchange theory and marital decision making. *Journal of Personality and Social Psychology, 34*, 14–23.

Grando, R. M. (1972). *The Parent–Adolescent Relationship Development Program: Relationships among pretraining variables, role performance, and improvement*. Unpublished doctoral dissertation, Pennsylvania State University, University Park.

Grando, R. M., & Ginsberg, B. G. (1976). Communication in the father–son relationship: The Parent Adolescent Relationship Development Program (PARD). *Family Coordinator, 4*, 465–473.

Greenson, R. R. (1967). *The technique and practice of psychoanalysis*. New York: International Universities Press, 1967.

Grotevant, H. D., & Cooper, C. R. (1983). *Adolescent development in the family*. San Francisco: Jossey-Bass.

Guerney, B. G., Jr. (1977). *Relationship enhancement*. San Francisco: Jossey-Bass.

Guerney, B. G., Jr., Coufal, J., & Vogelsong, E. L. (1981). Relationship enhancement versus a traditional approach to therapeutic/preventative/enrichment parent–adolescent programs. *Journal of Consulting and Clinical Psychology, 49*, 927–939.

Gurman, A. S. (Ed.). (1981). *Questions and answers in the practice of family therapy* (Vol. 1). New York: Brunner/Mazel.

Gurman, A. S. (Ed.). (1982). *Questions and answers in the practice of family therapy* (Vol. 2). New York: Brunner/Mazel.

Gurman, A. S., & Kniskern, D. P. (1978). Research on marital and family therapy: Progress, perspective, and prospect. In S. L. Garfield & A. E. Bergin (Eds.), *Handbook of psychotherapy and behavior change* (2nd ed.) (pp. 817–902). New York: Wiley.

Gurman, A. S., & Kniskern, D. P. (Eds.) (1981). *Handbook of family therapy*. New York: Brunner/Mazel.

Haley, J. (1976). *Problem-solving therapy*. San Francisco: Jossey-Bass.

Haley, J. (1980). *Leaving home: The therapy of disturbed young people*. New York: McGraw-Hill.

Hartmann, D. P. (1977). Considerations in the choice of interobserver reliability estimates. *Journal of Applied Behavior Analysis, 10,* 103–116.

Hartmann, D. P., & Wood, D. D. (1982). Observational methods. In A. S. Bellack, M. Hersen, & A. E. Kazdin (Eds.), *International handbook of behavior modification and therapy* (pp. 109–138). New York: Plenum.

Hay, W. M., Hay, L. R., Angle, H. V., & Nelson, R. O. (1979). The reliability of problem identification in the behavioral interview. *Behavioral Assessment, 1,* 107–118.

Haynes, S. N. (1978). *Principles of behavioral assessment*. New York: Gardner Press.

Haynes, S. N., & Jensen, B. J. (1979). The interview as a behavioral assessment device. *Behavioral Assessment, 1,* 97–106.

Haynes, S. N., Jensen, B. J., Wise, E., & Sherman, D. (1981). The marital intake interview: A multimethod validity assessment. *Journal of Consulting and Clinical Psychology, 49,* 379–387.

Henggeler, S. W., Borduin, C. M., Rodnick, J. D., & Tavormina, J. D. (1979). Importance of task content for family interaction research. *Developmental Psychology, 15,* 660–661.

Herjanic, B., & Campbell, W. (1977). Differentiating psychiatrically disturbed children on the basis of a structured interview. *Journal of Abnormal Child Psychology, 5,* 127–134.

Herjanic, B., Herjanic, M., Brown, F., & Wheatt, T. (1975). Are children reliable reporters? *Journal of Abnormal Child Psychology, 3,* 41–48.

Herjanic, B., & Reich, W. (1982). Development of a structured psychiatric interview for children: Agreement between child and parent on individual symptoms. *Journal of Abnormal Child Psychology, 10,* 307–324.

Herrnstein, R. J. (1970). On the law of effect. *Journal of the Experimental Analysis of Behavior, 13,* 243–266.

Herrnstein, R. J. (1979). Derivatives of matching. *Psychological Review, 86,* 486–495.

Hersen, M., & Barlow, D. H. (1976). *Single case experimental designs: Strategies for studying behavior change*. New York: Pergamon Press.

Hetherington, E. M., Stouwie, R. J., & Ridberg, E. H. (1971). Patterns of family interaction and child-rearing: Attitudes related to three dimensions of juvenile delinquency. *Journal of Abnormal Psychology, 78,* 160–176.

Hodges, K., Kline, J., Stern, L., Cytryn, L., & McKnew, D. (1982). The development of a child assessment interview for research and clinical use. *Journal of Abnormal Child Psychology, 10,* 173–189.

Hollon, S. D., & Beck, A. T. (1979). Cognitive therapy of depression. In P. C. Kendall & S. D. Hollon (Eds.), *Cognitive–behavioral interventions: Theory, research, and procedures* (pp. 153–203). New York: Academic Press.

Inhelder, B., & Piaget, J. (1958). *The growth of logical thinking from childhood to adolescence*. New York: Basic Books.

Jacobson, N. S., Follette, W. C., & Revensdorf, D. (1984). Psychotherapy outcome research: Methods for reporting variability and evaluating clinical significance. *Behavior Therapy, 15,* 336–352.

Jacobson, N. S., Follette, W. C., Revensdorf, D., Baucom, D. H., Hahlweg, K., & Margolin, G. (1984). Variability in outcome and clinical significance of behavioral marital therapy: A reanalysis of outcome data. *Journal of Consulting and Clinical Psychology, 53,* 497–504.

Jacobson, N.S., & Margolin, G. (1979). *Marital therapy*. New York: Brunner/Mazel.

Kazdin, A. E. (1977). Assessing the clinical or applied importance of behavior change through social validation. *Behavior Modification, 1,* 427–451.

Kazdin, A. E. (1982). *Single-case research designs: Methods for clinical and applied settings.* New York: Oxford University Press.

Kelsey-Smith, M., & Beavers, W. R. (1981). Family assessment: Centripetal and centrifugal family systems. *American Journal of Family Therapy, 9,* 3–12.

Kendall, P. C. (1982). Integration: Behavior therapy and other schools of thought. *Behavior Therapy, 13,* 559–571.

Kendall, P. C., & Hollon, S. D. (Eds.). (1981). *Assessment strategies for cognitive behavioral interventions.* New York: Academic Press.

Kent, R. N. (1976). A methodological critique of "Interventions for boys with conduct problems." *Journal of Consulting and Clinical Psychology, 44,* 297–302.

Kent, R. N., & O'Leary, K. D. (1976). A controlled evaluation of behavior modification with conduct problem children. *Journal of Consulting and Clinical Psychology, 44,* 586–596.

Kent, R. N., & O'Leary, K. D. (1977). Treatment of conduct problem children: BA and/or PhD therapists. *Behavior Therapy, 8,* 653–658.

Klein, N. C., Alexander, J. F., & Parsons, B. V. (1977). Impact of family systems intervention on recidivism and sibling delinquency: A model of primary prevention and program evaluation. *Journal of Consulting and Clinical Psychology, 45,* 759–768.

Koepke, T. (1986). *Construct validation of the Parent Adolescent Relationship Inventory: A multidimensional measure of parent–adolescent interaction.* Unpublished doctoral dissertation, Wayne State University, Detroit, MI.

Lazarus, A. A., & Fay, A. (1982). Resistance or rationalization? A cognitive–behavioral perspective. In P. L. Wachtel (Ed.), *Resistance: Psychodynamic and behavioral approaches* (pp. 115–132). New York: Plenum.

Levenson, R. W., & Gottman, J. M. (1983). Marital interaction: Physiological linkage and affective exchange. *Journal of Personality and Social Psychology, 45,* 587–597.

Linehan, M. M. (1979). Structured cognitive–behavioral treatment of assertion problems. In P. C. Kendall & S. D. Hollon (Eds.), *Cognitive–behavioral interventions: Theory, research, and procedures* (pp. 205–240). New York: Academic Press.

Lloyd, M. E. (1983). Selecting systems to measure client outcome in human service agencies. *Behavioral Assessment, 5,* 55–70.

Locke, H. J., & Wallace, K. M. (1959). Short-term marital adjustment and prediction tests: Their reliability and validity. *Journal of Marriage and Family Living, 21,* 251–255.

Loeber, R., Weissman, W., & Reid, J. B. (1983). Family interactions of assaultive adolescents, stealers, and nondelinquents. *Journal of Abnormal Child Psychology, 11,* 1–14.

Madanes, C. (1981). *Strategic family therapy.* San Francisco: Jossey-Bass.

Margolin, G. (1981). Behavior exchange in happy and unhappy marriages: A family cycle perspective. *Behavior Therapy, 12,* 329–343.

Margolin, G. (1982). Ethical and legal considerations in family and marital therapy. *American Psychologist, 37,* 788–801.

Martin, B. (1977). Brief family intervention: Effectiveness and importance of including the father. *Journal of Consulting and Clinical Psychology, 45,* 1002–1010.

Mash, E. J., & Terdal, L. G. (1988). *Behavioral assessment of childhood disorders* (2nd ed.). New York: Guilford Press.

McDowell, J. J. (1982). The importance of Herrnstein's mathematical statement of the law of effect for behavior therapy. *American Psychologist, 37,* 771–779.

McNemar, Q. (1969). *Psychological statistics* (4th ed.). New York: Wiley.

Meichenbaum, D. (1977). *Cognitive behavior modification.* New York: Plenum.

Meichenbaum, D., & Gilmore, J. B. (1982). Resistance from a cognitive–behavioral perspective. In P. L. Wachtel (Ed.), *Resistance: Psychodynamic and behavioral approaches* (pp. 133–156). New York: Plenum.

Miller, I. W., Epstein, N. B., Bishop, D. S., & Keitner, G. I. (1984, November). *The Family*

Assessment Device: Reliability and validity. Paper presented at the Association for Advancement of Behavior Therapy, Philadelphia.

Minuchin, S. (1974). *Families and family therapy.* Cambridge: Harvard University Press.

Minuchin, S., & Fishman, H. C. (1981). *Family therapy techniques.* Cambridge: Harvard University Press.

Minuchin, S., Rosman, B., & Baker, L. (1978). *Psychosomatic families.* Cambridge: Harvard University Press.

Mischel, W. (1968). *Personality and assessment.* New York: Wiley.

Mittl, V. F., & Robin, A. L. (1987). Acceptability of alternative interventions for parent–adolescent conflict. *Behavioral Assessment, 9,* 417–428.

Montemayor, R. (1983). Parents and adolescents in conflict: All families some of the time and some families most of the time. *Journal of Early Adolescence, 5,* 23–30.

Montemayor, R. (1986). Family variation in parent–adolescent storm and stress. *Journal of Adolescent Research, 1,* 15–31.

Moos, R. H., & Moos, B. S. (1981). *Family environment scale manual.* Palo Alto, CA: Consulting Psychologists Press.

Navran, L. (1967). Communication and adjustment in marriage. *Family Process, 6,* 173–184.

Nayar, M. (1982). *An analysis of the discriminant validity of self-report and behavioral measures of parent–adolescent conflict with mother–father–adolescent triads.* Unpublished master's thesis, Wayne State University, Detroit, MI.

Nayar, M. (1985). *Cognitive factors in the treatment of parent–adolescent conflict.* Unpublished doctoral dissertation, Wayne State University, Detroit, MI.

Nelson, R. O., & Haynes, S. C. (1979). Some current dimensions of behavioral assessment. *Behavioral Assessment, 1,* 1–16.

Novaco, R. W. (1975). *Anger control: The development and evaluation of an experimental treatment.* Lexington, MA: D. C. Heath.

O'Leary, K. D., Fincham, F., & Turkewitz, H. (1983). Assessment of positive feelings toward spouse. *Journal of Consulting and Clinical Psychology, 51,* 949–951.

O'Leary, K. D., & Turkewitz, H. (1978). Methodological errors in marital and child treatment. *Journal of Consulting and Clinical Psychology, 46,* 747–758.

Olson, D. H. (1977). Insiders' and outsiders' views of relationships: Research studies. In G. Levinger & H. Rausch (Eds.), *Close relationships* (pp. 115–135). Amherst: University of Massachusetts Press.

Olson, D. H., McCubbin, H. I., Barnes, H. L., Larsen, A. S., Muxen, M. J., & Wilson, M. A. (1983). *Families: What makes them work.* Beverly Hills: Sage.

Olson, D. H., Portner, J., & Bell, R. (1982). *Faces II: Family Adaptability and Cohesion Scales.* St. Paul: Family Social Science, University of Minnesota.

Olson, D. H., & Ryder, R. G. (1970). Inventory of marital conflicts (IMC): An experimental interaction procedure. *Journal of Marriage and the Family, 32,* 443–448.

Olson, D. H., Sprenkle, D. H., & Russell, C. S. (1979). Circumplex model of marital and family systems: 1. Cohesion and adaptability dimensions, family types, and clinical applications. *Family Process, 18,* 3–27.

Oltmanns, T. F., Broderick, J. E., & O'Leary, K. D. (1977). Marital adjustment and the efficacy of behavior therapy with children. *Journal of Consulting and Clinical Psychology, 45,* 724–729.

Osborn, A. F. (1963). *Applied imagination.* New York: Scribners.

Papp, P. (1980). The Greek Chorus and other techniques of paradoxical therapy. *Family Process, 19,* 45–57.

Parsons, B. V., & Alexander, J. F. (1973). Short-term family intervention: A therapy outcome study. *Journal of Consulting and Clinical Psychology, 41,* 195–201.

Patterson, G. R. (1976). The aggressive child: Victim and architect of a coercive system. In E. J. Mash, L. A. Hamerlynck, & L. C. Handy (Eds.), *Behavior modification and families* (pp. 267–316). New York: Brunner/Mazel.

Patterson, G. R. (1979). A performance theory for coercive family interaction. In R. Cairns (Ed.),

Social interaction: Methods, analysis, and illustrations (pp. 119–162). Hillsdale, NJ: Lawrence Erlbaum.

Patterson, G. R. (1982). *Coercive family process*. Eugene, OR: Castalia Press.

Patterson, G. R., & Bank, L. (1986). Bootstrapping your way in the nomological thicket. *Behavioral Assessment, 8,* 49–73.

Patterson, G. R., & Reid, J. B. (1970). Reciprocity and coercion: Two facets of social systems. In C. Neuringer and J. L. Michael (Eds.), *Behavior modification in clinical psychology* (pp. 133–177). New York: Appleton Century Crofts.

Perosa, L., Hansen, J., & Perosa, S. (1981). Development of the Structural Family Interaction Scale. *Family Therapy, 8,* 77–80.

Piaget, G. W. (1972). Training patients to communicate. In A. A. Lazarus (Ed.), *Clinical behavior therapy* (pp. 155–173). New York: Brunner/Mazel.

Porter, B., & O'Leary, K. D. (1980). Types of marital discord and child behavior problems. *Journal of Abnormal Child Psychology, 8,* 287–295.

Prinz, R. J. (1977). *The assessment of parent–adolescent relations: Discriminating distressed and non-distressed dyads.* Unpublished doctoral dissertation, SUNY, Stony Brook.

Prinz, R. J., Foster, S. L., Kent, R. N., & O'Leary, K. D. (1979). Multivariate assessment of conflict in distressed and nondistressed mother–adolescent dyads. *Journal of Applied Behavior Analysis, 12,* 691–700.

Prinz, R. J., & Kent, R. N. (1978). Recording parent–adolescent interactions without the use of frequency or interval-by-interval coding. *Behavior Therapy, 9,* 602–604.

Prinz, R. J., Rosenblum, R. S., & O'Leary, K. D. (1978). Affective communication differences between distressed and nondistressed mother–adolescent dyads. *Journal of Abnormal Child Psychology, 6,* 373–383.

Rayha, L. (1982). *A social learning analysis of reciprocity, problem-solving communication skills, and marital discord in distressed and nondistressed families.* Unpublished master's thesis, Wayne State University, Detroit, MI.

Reid, J. B. (Ed.). (1978). *A social learning approach to family intervention: Vol. 2. Observation in home settings.* Eugene, OR: Castalia Press.

Riskin, J., & Faunce, E. E. (1970a). Family interaction scales: 1. Theoretical framework and method. *Archives of General Psychiatry, 22,* 504–512.

Riskin, J., & Faunce, E. E. (1970b). Family interaction scales: 2. Data analysis and findings. *Archives of General Psychiatry, 22,* 513–526.

Robin, A. L. (1975). *Communication training: A problem-solving approach to parent–adolescent conflict.* Unpublished doctoral dissertation, SUNY, Stony Brook.

Robin, A. L. (1979). Problem-solving communication training: A behavioral approach to the treatment of parent–adolescent conflict: *American Journal of Family Therapy, 7,* 69–82.

Robin, A. L. (1980). Parent–adolescent conflict: A skill training approach. In D. P. Rathjen and J. P. Foreyt (Eds.), *Social competence interventions for children and adults* (pp. 147–211). New York: Pergamon Press.

Robin, A. L. (1981). A controlled evaluation of problem-solving communication training with parent–adolescent conflict. *Behavior Therapy, 12,* 593–609.

Robin, A. L. (1985). *Annual program report for 1985: Parent–child stress.* Report to the William T. Grant Foundation. Detroit, MI: Author.

Robin, A. L., & Canter, W. (1984). A comparison of the Marital Interaction Coding System and community ratings for assessing mother–adolescent problem-solving. *Behavioral Assessment, 6,* 303–314.

Robin, A. L., & Foster, S. L. (1984). Problem-solving communication training: A behavioral–family systems approach to parent–adolescent conflict. In P. Karoly & J. J. Steffen (Eds.), *Adolescent behavior disorders: Foundations and contemporary concerns* (pp. 195–240). Lexington, MA: D. C. Heath.

Robin, A. L., & Fox, M. (1979). *Parent–adolescent interaction system coding manual.* Unpublished manuscript, University of Maryland, College Park.

Robin, A. L., Kent, R. N., O'Leary, K. D., Foster, S. L., & Prinz, R. J. (1977). An approach to teaching parents and adolescents problem-solving communication skills: A preliminary report. *Behavior Therapy, 8,* 639–643.

Robin, A. L., & Koepke, T. (1985). *Molecular versus molar observational coding systems for assessing mother–adolescent problem-solving communication behavior.* Manuscript submitted for publication.

Robin, A. L., Koepke, T., & Hull, B. (1988). *Comparison of the Family Beliefs Inventory and the Parent–Adolescent Relationship Questionnaire.* Manuscript in preparation.

Robin, A. L., Koepke, T., & Moye, A. (1986). *Multidimensional assessment of parent–adolescent relations.* Unpublished manuscript.

Robin, A. L., Kraus, D., Koepke, T., & Robin, R. A. (1987). *Growing up hyperactive in single versus two-parent families.* Paper presented at the American Psychological Association Conference, New York, NY.

Robin, A. L., Nayar, M., & Rayha, L. (1984, August). *Quantity and quality of parent–adolescent interaction: A behavioral analysis.* Paper presented at the American Psychological Association Convention, Toronto, Ontario, Canada.

Robin, A. L., & Siegel, P. (1988). *Behavioral family systems therapy for anorexia nervoxa.* Unpublished manuscript.

Robin, A. L., & Weiss, J. G. (1980). Criterion-related validity of behavioral and self-report measures of problem-solving communication skills in distressed and non-distressed parent–adolescent dyads. *Behavioral Assessment, 2,* 339–352.

Robinson, E. A., & Jacobson, N. S. (1987). Social learning theory and family psychopathology: A Kantian model in behaviorism. In T. Jacob (Ed.), *Family interaction and psychopathology: Theories, methods, and findings* (pp. 117–162). New York: Plenum.

Rosen, A., & Proctor, E. K. (1981). Distinctions between treatment outcomes and their implications for treatment evaluation. *Journal of Consulting and Clinical Psychology, 49,* 418–425.

Ross, D. M., & Ross, S. A. (1982). *Hyperactivity: Current issues, research, and theory* (2nd ed.). New York: Wiley.

Russell, C. S. (1980). A methodological study of family cohesion and adaptibility. *Journal of Marital and Family Therapy, 6,* 459–470.

Rutter, M., & Graham, P. (1968). The reliability and validity of the psychiatric assessment of the child: 1. Interview with the child. *British Journal of Psychiatry, 114,* 563–579.

Safer, D. J., & Krager, J. M. (1985). Prevalence of medication treatment for hyperactive adolescents. *Psychopharmacology Bulletin, 21,* 212–215.

Schubiner, H., & Robin, A. (in press). Screening adolescents for depression and parent-teen conflict in an ambulatory medical setting: a preliminary investigation. *Pediatrics, 85.*

Snyder, D. K. (1979). Multidimensional assessment of marital satisfaction. *Journal of Marriage and the Family, 6,* 813–823.

Snyder, D. K. (1981). *Marital Satisfaction Inventory manual.* Los Angeles: Western Psychological Services.

Spanier, G. B. (1976). Measuring dyadic adjustment: New scales for assessing the quality of marriage and similar dyads. *Journal of Marriage and the Family, 38,* 15–28.

Spivack, G., Platt, J. J., & Shure, M. B. (1976). *The problem solving approach to adjustment.* San Francisco: Jossey-Bass.

Stanton, M. D. (1981). Strategic approaches to family therapy. In A. S. Gurman and D. P. Kniskern (Eds.), *Handbook of family therapy* (pp. 361–402). New York: Brunner/Mazel.

Steinberg, L. D. (1981). Transformations in family relations at puberty. *Developmental Psychology, 17,* 833–840.

Steinberg, L. D., & Hill, J. (1978). Patterns of family interaction as a function of age, onset of puberty, and formal thinking. *Developmental Psychology, 14,* 683–684.

Steinfeld, B. I., Foster, S. L., Prinz, R. J., Robin, A. L., & Weiss, J. G. (1980). *Issues of conflict for mothers and adolescents: A descriptive and developmental analysis.* Unpublished manuscript available from S. L. Foster, Department of Psychology, West Virginia University,

Morgantown, WV.

Steinglass, P. (1987). A systems view of family interaction and psychopathology. In T. Jacob (Ed.), *Family interaction and psychopathology: Theories, methods, and findings* (pp. 25–66). New York: Plenum.

Stern, S. (1984). *A group cognitive–behavioral approach to the management and resolution of parent–adolescent conflict.* Unpublished doctoral dissertation, University of Chicago.

Stokes, T. F., & Baer, D. M. (1977). An implicit technology of generalization. *Journal of Applied Behavior Analysis, 10,* 349–367.

Straus, M. A. (1979). Measuring intrafamily conflict and violence: The Conflict Tactics (CT) Scales. *Journal of Marriage and the Family, 41,* 75–88.

Strayhorn, J. M. (1977). *Talking it out.* Champaign, IL: Research Press.

Stuart, R. B. (1980). *Helping couples change: A social learning approach to marital therapy.* New York: Guilford Press.

Stuart, R. B., Jayaratne, S., & Tripodi, T. (1976). Changing adolescent deviant behaviour through reprogramming the behaviour of parents and teachers: An experimental evaluation. *Canadian Journal of Behavioural Science, 8,* 132–144.

Stuart, R. B., & Tripodi, T. (1973). Experimental evaluation of three time-constrained behavioral treatments for predelinquents and delinquents. In R. D. Ruben, J. P. Brady, & J. D. Henderson (Eds.), *Advances in behavior therapy* (Vol. 4, pp. 1–12). New York: Academic Press.

Stuart, R. B., Tripodi, T., Jayaratne, S., & Camburn, D. (1976). An experiment in social engineering in serving the families of predelinquents. *Journal of Abnormal Child Psychology, 4,* 243–261.

Szapocznik, J., Kurtines, W. M., Foote, F. H., Perez-Vidal, A., & Hervis, O. (1983). Conjoint versus one-person therapy: Some evidence for the effectiveness of conducting family therapy through one person. *Journal of Consulting and Clinical Psychology, 51,* 889–899.

Twentyman, C. T., Rorhbeck, C. A., & Amish, P. L. (1984). A cognitive–behavioral model of child abuse. In S. Saunders (Ed.), *Violent individuals and families: A practitioner's handbook* (pp. 86–111). Springfield, IL: Charles C. Thomas.

Valins, S., & Nisbett, R. (1976). Attribution processes in the development and treatment of emotional disorders. In J. Spence, R. Carson, & J. Thibaut (Eds.), *Behavioral approaches to therapy* (pp. 261–274). Morristown, NJ: General Learning Press.

Varley, C. K. (1985). A review of studies of drug treatment efficacy for attention deficit disorder with hyperactivity in adolescents. *Psychopharmacology Bulletin, 21,* 216–221.

Vincent-Roehling, P., & Robin, A. L. (1986). Development and validation of the Family Beliefs Inventory: A measure of unrealistic beliefs among parents and adolescents. *Journal of Consulting and Clinical Psychology, 54,* 693–697.

Vogelsong, E. L. (1975). *Preventative–therapeutic programs for mothers and adolescent daughters: A follow-up of relationship enhancement versus discussion and booster versus no-booster methods.* Unpublished doctoral dissertation, Pennsylvania State University, University Park.

Wachtel, P. (1982). What can dynamic therapies contribute to behavior therapy? *Behavior Therapy, 13,* 594–609.

Weathers, L., & Liberman, R. P. (1975). Contingency contracting with families of delinquent adolescents. *Behavior Therapy, 6,* 356–366.

Weeks, G. R., & L'Abate, L. (1982). *Paradoxical psychotherapy: Theory and technique.* New York: Brunner/Mazel.

Weiss, G., & Hechtman, L. T. (1986). *Hyperactive children grown up.* New York: Guilford Press.

Weiss, R. L. (1981). Resistance in behavioral marriage therapy. In A. S. Gurman (Ed.), *Questions and answers in the practice of family therapy* (Vol. 1) (pp. 155–159). New York: Brunner/Mazel.

Weiss, R. L., Hops, H., & Patterson, G. R. (1973). A framework for conceptualizing marital conflict, a technology for altering it, and some data for evaluating it. In L. A. Hamerlynck, L. C. Handy, & E. J. Mash (Eds.), *Behavior change: Methodology, concepts, and practice* (pp.

309–342). Champaign, IL: Research Press.

Weiss, R. L., & Margolin, G. (1986). Marital conflict and accord. In A. R. Ciminero, K. S. Calhoun, & H. E. Adams (Eds.), *Handbook of behavioral assessment* (2nd ed.) (pp. 561–600). New York: Wiley.

Weissman, M. M., Orvaschel, H., & Padian, N. (1980). Children's symptom and social functioning self-report scales. *Journal of Nervous and Mental Disease, 168,* 736–740.

Williams, A. M. (1979). The quantity and quality of marital interaction related to marital satisfaction: A behavioral analysis. *Journal of Applied Behavior Analysis, 12,* 665–678.

Wills, T. A., Weiss, R. L., & Patterson, G. R. (1974). A behavioral analysis of the determinants of marital satisfaction. *Journal of Consulting and Clinical Psychology, 42,* 802–811.

Witkin, S. L. (1981). Resistance to role-playing in marital group therapy. In A. Gurman (Ed.), *Questions and answers in the practice of family therapy* (Vol. 1) (pp. 168–172). New York: Brunner/Mazel.

Wolf, M. M. (1978). Social validation: The case for subjective measurement, or how applied behavior analysis is finding its heart. *Journal of Applied Behavior Analysis, 11,* 203–214.

Yarrow, M. R., Campbell, J. D., & Burton, R. V. (1970). Recollections of childhood: A study of the retrospective method. *Monographs of the Society for Research in Child Development, 35* (Serial No. 138).

Youniss, J., & Smollar, J. (1985). *Adolescent relations with mothers, fathers, and friends.* Chicago: The University of Chicago Press.

Zuckerman, E., & Jacob, T. (1979). Task effects in family interaction. *Family Process, 18,* 47–53.

Index